PHARMACY
TERMINOLOGY

PHARMACY TERMINOLOGY

Jahangir Moini, MD, MPH, CPhT

Professor and Former Director, Allied
Health Sciences

Pharmacy Technician Program
Everest University
Melbourne, Florida

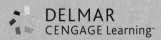

DELMAR
CENGAGE Learning™

Australia • Brazil • Japan • Korea • Mexico • Singapore • Spain • United Kingdom • United States

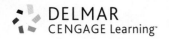

DELMAR
CENGAGE Learning

Pharmacy Terminology
Jahangir Moini, MD, MPH, CPhT

Vice President, Career and Professional Editorial: Dave Garza

Director of Learning Solutions: Matthew Kane

Acquisitions Editor: Tari Broderick

Managing Editor: Marah Bellegarde

Senior Product Manager: Darcy M. Scelsi

Editorial Assistant: Ian J. Lewis

Vice President, Career and Professional Marketing: Jennifer McAvey

Marketing Manager: Kristin McNary

Marketing Coordinator: Erica Ropitzky

Production Director: Carolyn Miller

Content Project Manager: Anne Sherman

Senior Art Director: Jack Pendleton

For product information and technology assistance, contact us at
Cengage Learning Customer & Sales Support, 1-800-354-9706

For permission to use material from this text or product, submit all requests online at **www.cengage.com/permissions**. Further permissions questions can be e-mailed to **permissionrequest@cengage.com**

Library of Congress Control Number: 2009930899

ISBN-13: 978-1-4283-1787-1

ISBN-10: 1-4283-1787-2

Delmar
5 Maxwell Drive
Clifton Park, NY 12065-2919
USA

Cengage Learning is a leading provider of customized learning solutions with office locations around the globe, including Singapore, the United Kingdom, Australia, Mexico, Brazil, and Japan. Locate your local office at: **international.cengage.com/region**

Cengage Learning products are represented in Canada by Nelson Education, Ltd.

To learn more about Delmar, visit **www.cengage.com/delmar**

Purchase any of our products at your local college store or at our preferred online store **www.ichapters.com**

Notice to the Reader

Publisher does not warrant or guarantee any of the products described herein or perform any independent analysis in connection with any of the product information contained herein. Publisher does not assume, and expressly disclaims, any obligation to obtain and include information other than that provided to it by the manufacturer. The reader is expressly warned to consider and adopt all safety precautions that might be indicated by the activities described herein and to avoid all potential hazards. By following the instructions contained herein, the reader willingly assumes all risks in connection with such instructions. The publisher makes no representations or warranties of any kind, including but not limited to, the warranties of fitness for particular purpose or merchantability, nor are any such representations implied with respect to the material set forth herein, and the publisher takes no responsibility with respect to such material. The publisher shall not be liable for any special, consequential, or exemplary damages resulting, in whole or part, from the readers' use of, or reliance upon, this material.

Printed in the United States of America
1 2 3 4 5 6 7 12 11 10 09

Dedication

*This book is dedicated to
my wife Hengameh, and daughters
Mahkameh and Morvarid.*

Contents

Section II Terminology of the Body Systems

Section III Terminology of Special Populations

Section IV Terminology Related to the Pharmacy Profession

Section V   Mathematics Review

Preface

This first-edition textbook is designed as a thorough introduction to pharmacy and medical terminology. The importance of understanding and remembering the terms used in the daily practices of pharmacy and medicine cannot be overstated. Everyone whose work influences the health of patients must be fluent in the terminology that their jobs will require them to know. This text will ensure that the terminology skills of students are of the highest level, ensuring the highest-quality patient care when they enter the workforce.

ORGANIZATION

This book is organized so that general terminology for each chapter is discussed first, followed by pathological conditions related to the subject matter. Abbreviations are covered thoroughly, as are medications used for specific disorders, and related drug terminology. The book is divided into 5 sections and 30 chapters. Part 1 is an introduction to terminology, Part 2 discusses terminology of the body systems, and Part 3 covers terminology of special populations. Part 4 deals with terminology related to the pharmacy profession, and Part 5 is a mathematics review. Additionally, there is a glossary and an index at the end of the book.

FEATURES

Each chapter of this textbook contains an outline of key topics, objectives that students must be able to meet upon completion of their reading, bolded key terms, many figures and tables, and review questions in several formats (multiple choice, fill in the blank, true/false, labeling, definitions, abbreviations, matching, and spelling).

Acknowledgments

The author would like to acknowledge the following individuals for their time and efforts in aiding him with their contributions to this book.

Darcy Scelsi
Senior Product Manager
Academic and Professional Group
Delmar Cengage Learning

Greg Vadimsky, Pharmacy Technician
Melbourne, Florida

The author also would like to thank all of the reviewers and the entire production team for their contributions to this book. It would not have been possible without their long hours of work and patience.

REVIEWERS

John Colaizzi, PhD, RPh
Rutgers, The State University of New Jersey
Piscataway, New Jersey

David Elder, RPh
Skagit Valley College
Mount Vernon, Washington

Stephanie Gardner, PharmD, EdD
University of Arkansas for Medical Sciences
Little Rock, Arkansas

William J. Havins, BUS, CPhT
Central New Mexico Community College
Albuquerque, New Mexico

Paul Lee, CPhT
CVS
Mechanicsville, Virginia

Lia Mays, CPhT
Everest College
Arlington, Texas

Michelle McCranie, CPhT, AAS
Ogeechee Technical Institute
Statesboro, Georgia

Michelle Miller, PharmD, RPh
Kirkwood Community College
Cedar Rapids, Iowa

James Mizner, RPh, MBA
Applied Career Training
Arlington, Virginia

Rebekah Schneider, PharmD
Shenandoah University
Winchester, Virginia

Steven Clark Stoner, PharmD, BCPP
UMCK School of Pharmacy
Kansas City, Missouri

Sandy Tschritter, CPhT, BA
Spokane Community College
Spokane, Washington

Lorraine Zentz, CPhT, PhD
Gatlin Education Services
Fort Worth, Texas

About the Author

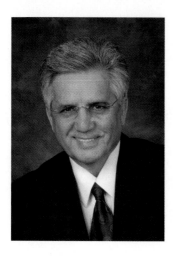

Dr. Moini was assistant professor at Tehran University School of Medicine for 9 years teaching medical and allied health students. The author is a professor and former director (for 15 years) of allied health programs at Everest University. Dr. Moini established, for the first time, the associate degree program for pharmacy technicians in 2000 at EU's Melbourne campus. For 5 years, he was the director of the pharmacy technician program. He also established several other new allied health programs for EU. As a physician and instructor for the past 35 years, he believes that pharmacy technicians should be skillful in various types of pharmacy settings and have confidence in their duties and responsibilities in order to prevent medication errors.

Dr. Moini is actively involved in teaching and helping students to prepare for service in various health professions, including the roles of pharmacy technicians, medical assistants, and nurses. He worked with the Brevard County Health Department as an epidemiologist and health educator consultant for 18 years, offering continuing education courses and keeping nurses up-to-date on the latest developments related to pharmacology, medications errors, immunizations, and other important topics. He has been an internationally published author of various allied health books since 1999.

How to Use StudyWARE™ to Accompany Pharmacy Terminology

The StudyWARE™ software helps you learn terms and concepts in *Pharmacy Terminology*. As you study each chapter in the text, be sure to explore the activities in the corresponding chapter in the software. Use StudyWARE as your own private tutor to help you learn the material in your *Pharmacy Terminology* textbook.

Getting started is easy. Visit the Online Companion website for the product at www.delmarlearning.com/companions. Look for and click on the title of the book. Click on StudyWARE and click on the link to launch the program. When you launch the program, enter your first and last name so the software can store your quiz results. Then choose a chapter from the menu to take a quiz or explore one of the activities.

MENUS

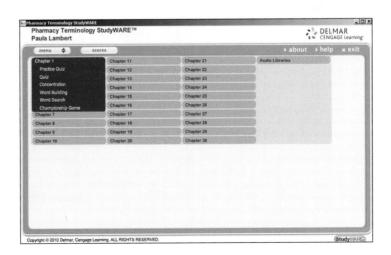

You can access the menus from wherever you are in the program. The menus include quizzes and other activities.

QUIZZES

Quizzes include multiple-choice, fill-in-the-blank, matching, and word-building questions. You can take the quizzes in both practice mode and quiz mode. Use practice mode to improve your mastery of the material. You have multiple tries to get the answers correct. Instant feedback tells you whether you're right or wrong and helps you learn quickly by explaining why an answer was correct or incorrect. Use quiz mode when you are ready to test yourself and keep a record of your scores. In quiz mode, you have one try to get the answers right, but you can take each quiz as many times as you want.

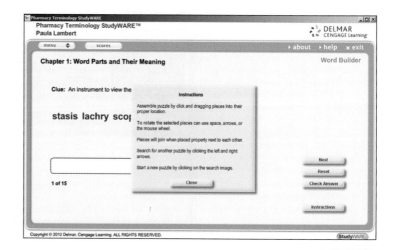

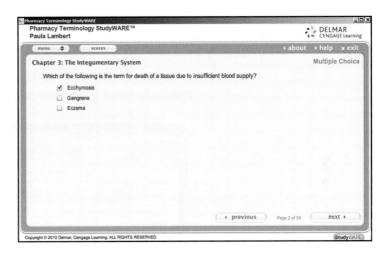

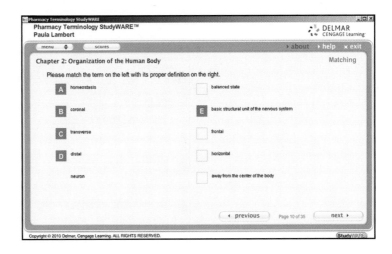

SCORES

You can view your last scores for each quiz and print your results to hand in to your instructor.

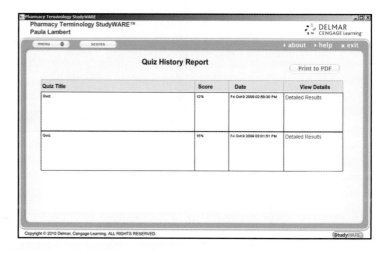

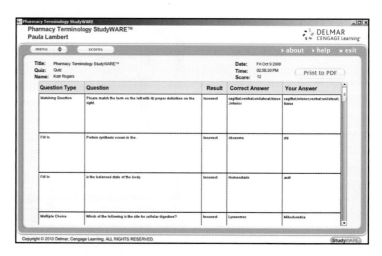

ACTIVITIES

Activities include image-labeling, concentration, word-search puzzles, and a championship game. Have fun while increasing your knowledge!

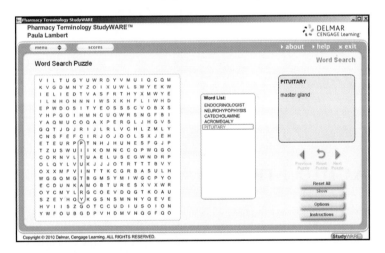

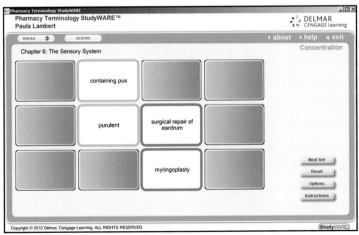

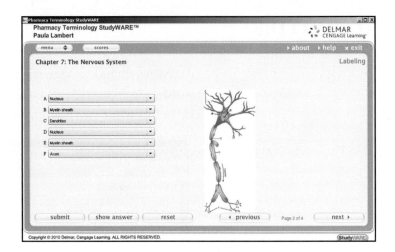

AUDIO LIBRARY

The StudyWARE Audio Library is a reference that includes audio pronunciations and definitions for medical terms and drugs found in the text. Use the audio library to practice pronunciation and review definitions for medical terms and drugs. You can browse terms by chapter or search by keyword. Listen to pronunciations of the terms you select or listen to an entire list of terms.

INTRODUCTION TO TERMINOLOGY

1 Word Parts and Their Meanings

OBJECTIVES

Upon completion of this chapter, the reader should be able to:

1. Describe the origin of medical language.
2. Explain the importance of knowing medical terminology for the pharmacy profession.
3. Define the terms *word root, suffix, prefix*, and *combining form*.
4. Define a prefix and state the rule for using prefixes in words.
5. Define a suffix and state the rule for using suffixes in words.

OVERVIEW

Medical terminology is the language of medicine and is used in all areas of the health care industry. Learning medical terminology is very similar to learning a foreign language. Many medical terms are derived from Greek and Latin prefixes, roots, and suffixes (these are called *word parts*). Most of the terms related to diagnosis and surgery have Greek origins, and most anatomic terms come from Latin. Many new terms are derived from the universal language, which is English.

The pharmacy technician will need to effectively communicate with the pharmacist and a variety of other health care professionals using the medical language. Memorizing word parts and rules will aid in understanding medical terminology. By learning to analyze word parts, it is possible to determine the meaning of medical words. The ability to understand and define the parts of the medical term will make understanding the whole word easier, therefore enhancing the ability to communicate precisely with other health care professionals.

WORD PARTS

Most terms have three components: the word root, prefix, and suffix. The ability to use these common roots, prefixes, and suffixes is known as *word building*, an essential skill needed by pharmacy staff members. The ability to define and identify these components of words will aid the technician in understanding the meanings of medical and pharmacological terminology and abbreviations.

Word Roots

The **word root** is the core of a word. It is also called the *stem* or the *base* of a word, and usually has a Greek or Latin origin. All medical words have at least one word root; some have multiple roots that are joined by a vowel called a combining vowel (use of this will be discussed later). The word *root* most commonly identifies the body part involved; some word roots also indicate color. Table 1-1 shows common word roots.

TABLE 1-1   Common General Word Roots

Root	Meaning	Example
aden/o	gland	**aden**oid
adip/o	fat	**adip**ose
aer/o	air	**aer**osol
alb	white	**alb**umin
ambul/o	walk	**ambul**atory
andr/o	male	**andro**gen
angi/o	vessel	**angio**gram
arthr	joint	**arthr**itis
bucc	cheek	**bucc**al
canc	crab	**canc**er
carcin/o	cancer	**carcin**ogen
cardi	heart	**cardi**ology
cereb	brain	**cereb**rum
chem/o	chemistry	**chem**otherapy
chol	bile	**chol**angiogram
cyan	blue	**cyan**osis
cyst/o	urinary bladder	**cyst**oscopy
cyt	cell	**cyt**ology
dactyl	finger	syn**dactyl**ism

(continues)

TABLE 1-1 Common General Word Roots (*continued*)

Root	Meaning	Example
dermat/o	skin	**dermat**ology
encephal/o	brain	electro**encephal**ogram
erythr/o	red	**erythr**ocyte
gastr	stomach	**gastr**ic acid
gluco	sugar	**gluco**se
hema	blood	**hema**toma
hepat/o	liver	**hepat**oma
hydro	water	**hydro**cephalus
lachry	tear	**lachry**mal fluid
lact/o	milk	**lact**ose
lapar/o	abdomen	**lapar**oscope
laryng	larynx (voice box)	**laryng**itis
leuk/o	white	**leuk**emia
lingua	tongue	sub**lingua**l
mast, mamm	breast	**mast**ectomy, **mamm**ogram
melan/o	black	**melan**oma
meter	measure	thermo**meter**
my	muscle	**my**algia
nas	nose	**nas**al
necr/o	dead	**necr**osis
nephr/o	kidney	**nephr**osis
ocul	eye	**ocul**ar
odont	tooth	orth**odont**ist
onc/o	tumor	**onc**ology
ophthalm/o	eye	**ophthalm**oscope
optic	eye	**optic**ian
oste/o	bone	**oste**oarthritis
ot	ear	**ot**algia
path/o	disease	**path**ology
phleb/o	vein	**phleb**otomy
proct/o	rectum	**proct**ologist
psych/o	mind	**psych**ology
ren	kidney	**ren**al
rhin/o	nose	**rhin**ovirus
spir/o	breathing	**spir**ometer

thromb/o	blood clot	**thromb**olysis
tox, toxo	poisonous	**tox**ic, **toxo**plasmosis
ur/o	urine	**ur**ology
uter/o	uterus	intra**uter**ine
vas/o	blood vessel	**vas**oconstriction
xanth/o	yellow	**xanth**in

Prefixes

A short word part added to the beginning of a word root that modifies the meaning of the word root is a **prefix**. Prefixes tend to indicate numbers, measurements, position, placement, and color. Not all medical words require a prefix. Look at the example to see how a prefix alters the meaning of a word root. Table 1-2 shows general prefixes.

EXAMPLE

Word root – *cardi* (heart)

Prefixes – *brady-* (slow) or *tachy-* (fast)

   Bradycardia: a slow heartbeat

   Tachycardia: a fast heartbeat

Word root – *pne* (breathing)

Prefixes – *brady-, tachy-, dys-* (difficult)

   Bradypnea: slow breathing

   Tachypnea: rapid breathing

   Dyspnea: difficult breathing

TABLE 1-2 General Prefixes

Prefix	Meaning	Example
a-	without, not, no	**a**phasia (without speech)
ab-	away from	**ab**duct (to move away from the body's midline)
ad-	toward	**ad**duct (to move toward the body's midline)
ante-	before, forward	**ante**partum (before birth)
anti-	against	**anti**biotic (against life)
auto-	self	**auto**graft (a graft from one's own body)
bio-	life	**bio**logy (study of life)
brady-	slow	**brady**cardia (slow heartbeat)

(continues)

TABLE 1-2   General Prefixes (*continued*)

Prefix	Meaning	Example
circum-	around	**circum**cision (circular incision to remove the foreskin of the penis)
con-	together	**con**genital (relating to a condition present at birth)
contra-	against	**contra**indication (a factor that indicates something should not be done, or should not be given)
dys-	painful, difficult	**dys**uria (painful urination)
ecto-	out, outside	**ecto**pic (congenitally displaced, or out of place)
endo-	within, inner	**endo**scope (instrument to view within)
epi-	upon, above	**epi**dermic (upon or over the skin)
eu-	good, normal	**eu**phoria (a feeling of well-being)
ex-, exo-	out, away from	**ex**cision (the act of cutting out)
extra-	outside	**extra**cellular (outside the cells)
hyper-	over, above	**hyper**glycemia (high blood glucose)
hypo-	below, deficient, under	**hypo**tension (low blood pressure)
infra-	below, under, beneath	**infra**costal (below the ribs)
inter-	between, among	**inter**vertebral (between the vertebrae)
intra-	within, inside	**intra**dermal (inside the skin)
macro-	large	**macro**cephalic (having a large head)
mal-	bad, poor	**mal**aise (a feeling of sickness)
micro-	small	**micro**cephalic (having a small head)
multi-	many	**multi**lobular (having many lobules)
neo-	new	**neo**natal (relating to a newborn infant)
pan-	all	**pan**carditis (heart structure inflammation)
para-	near, beside, abnormal, alongside	**para**thyroid (near the thyroid gland)
per-	through	**per**cutaneous (through the skin)
peri-	around	**peri**cardial (around the heart)
poly-	many, excessive	**poly**cystic (composed of many cysts)
post-	after	**post**partum (after birth)
pre-	before, in front of	**pre**mature (occurring before the expected time)
retro-	behind, backward	**retro**version (turning backward)
sub-	below, under	**sub**lingual (below the tongue)
super-	above, excess	**super**numerary (above the normal number)
supra-	above	**supra**renal (above the kidneys)
tachy-	fast, rapid	**tachy**pnea (rapid breathing)
trans-	across, through	**trans**hepatic (across the liver)
ultra-	beyond, excess	**ultra**sound (high-frequency sound waves)

Prefixes Used to Indicate Numbers

Prefixes with meanings such as "one," "two," "three," "many," and "half" are sometimes combined with roots or suffixes to define numbers. Table 1-3 shows general numerical prefixes.

TABLE 1-3   Number Prefixes

Prefix	Meaning	Example (Definition)
bi-	two	**bi**lateral (two sides)
hemi-	half	**hemi**plegia (paralysis of one side of the body)
mono-	one	**mono**plegia (paralysis of one extremity)
multi-	many	**multi**gravida (a woman who has been pregnant more than once)
nulli-	none	**nulli**gravida (a woman who has not been pregnant)
poly-	many	**poly**uria (large amounts of urine)
quad-	four	**quad**riplegia (paralysis of all four extremities)
semi-	partial, half	**semi**conscious (partially conscious)
tri-	three	**tri**ceps (a muscle with three "heads")
uni-	one	**uni**lateral (one side)

Prefixes Used to Indicate Measurements

Prefixes that express measurements include those that signify "excessive," "many," or "much." They often refer to multiple amounts or to conditions that are greater than or less than normal. Table 1-4 shows prefixes that relate to measurements.

TABLE 1-4   Prefixes Related to Measurements

Prefix	Meaning	Example
hyper-	excessive	**hyper**tension (an excessive or above-normal level of blood pressure)
hyp-	under, below, beneath, less than normal	**hyp**oxemia (lower-than-normal blood oxygen level)
hypo-	under, below, beneath, less than normal	**hypo**glycemia (lower-than-normal blood sugar)
multi-	many	**multi**para (to bear many children)
poly-	many, much	**poly**uria (the excretion of large amounts of [much] urine) **poly**arthritis (inflammation of many joints)

Prefixes Indicating Position and Placement

Prefixes that pertain to position or placement are often combined with roots or suffixes. These prefixes may signify positions or placements such as "above," "below," and "toward." Table 1-5 shows prefixes that signify position or placement.

TABLE 1-5 Prefixes for Position and Placement

Prefix	Meaning	Example
ab-	from, or away from	**ab**duct (to move away from the body's midline)
ad-	toward, or increase	**ad**duct (to move toward the body's midline)
ambi-	both	**ambi**dextrous (able to use both hands equally well)
cata-	down	**cata**bolism (breaking down into smaller parts)
circum-	around	**circum**oral (around the mouth)
de-	down, or from	**de**scend (coming down from)
ecto-	outside	**ecto**pic (outside of a normal location)
endo-	within	**endo**cervical (relating to the cervix's inner lining)
epi-	upon, or over	**epi**gastric (upon the stomach)
ex-	out, away from, or outside	**ex**tract (removal of a tooth away from the oral cavity)
extra-	outside, or beyond	**extra**hepatic (outside of the liver)
hyper-	above, beyond, excessive	**hyper**tension (excessive blood pressure)
hypo-	under, below, beneath, or less than normal	**hypo**glossal (under the tongue)
inter-	between	**inter**costal (between the ribs)
intra-	within	**intra**venous (within a vein)
meso-	middle	**meso**derm (the middle of the three skin layers)
para-	near, beside, beyond, or two "like" parts	**para**cervical (near or beside the cervix)
peri-	around	**peri**anal (around the anus)
pre-	in front	**pre**cordial (the section of the "chest wall" in front of the heart)
pro-	before, or preceding	**pro**gravid (preceding pregnancy)
retro-	behind	**retro**flexion (an abnormal organ position, such as when it is tilted backward)
sub-	under, or below	**sub**lingual (under the tongue)
supra-	above, or over	**supra**pubic (above or over the pubic area)

Prefixes Indicating Color

Prefixes that signify color may refer to reactions, growths, rashes, or body fluids. Color prefixes may be "pure," or combining forms.

TABLE 1-6 Prefixes (with Combining Forms) for Color

Prefix	Meaning	Example
chlor/o	green	**chlor**ophyll (green pigment in plants that accomplishes photosynthesis)
cirrh/o	yellow or tawny	**cirrh**osis (chronic liver degeneration with resulting yellowness of the liver and skin)
cyan/o	blue	**cyan**oderma (slightly bluish, grayish, slate-like, or dark skin discoloration)
eosin/o	red or rosy	**eosin**ophil (a bi-lobed leukocyte that stains a red or rosy color with an acid dye)
erythr/o	red	**erythr**ocyte (a mature red blood cell)
jaund/o	yellow	**jaund**ice (yellow skin discoloration)
leuk/o	white	**leuk**oplasia (white, hardened, and thick patches firmly attached to mucous membranes in the mouth, vulva, or penis)
melan/o	black	**melan**oma (darkly pigmented cancerous tumors)
poli/o	gray	**poli**omyelitis (inflammation of the spinal cord's gray matter)
purpur/o	purple	**purpur**a (blood collected beneath the skin as pinpoint hemorrhages that appear red/purple and discolor the skin)
xanth/o	yellow	**xanth**oderma (yellow skin coloration)

Suffixes

A word ending that modifies the meaning of the word root is called a **suffix**. When the word root is attached to a suffix, it may require a combining vowel, though not always. Not all words have a suffix. Most medical terms have a suffix.

- *-itis* = inflammation   **example:** arth**ritis** = inflammation of a joint

- *-logy* = study of   **example:** patho**logy** = study of diseases

- *-plasty* = surgical repair   **example:** rhino**plasty** = surgical repair of the nose

Examples of common suffixes are shown in Table 1-7.

EXAMPLE

Word root – *pharmac/o* (pharmacy)

Suffix – *-logy* (the study of)

    Pharmaco**logy**: the study of pharmacy

Word root – *path/o* (disease)

Suffix – *-logy*

    Patho**logy**: the study of disease

TABLE 1-7   General Suffixes

Suffix	Meaning	Example
-ac	pertaining to	cardi**ac** (pertaining to the heart)
-al	pertaining to	sublingu**al** (pertaining to the esophagus)
-algia	pain	neur**algia** (nerve pain)
-ary	pertaining to	pulmon**ary** (pertaining to the lungs)
-cele	hernia (bulging)	hydro**cele** (bulging, due to fluid, in the tissue surrounding the testis)
-centesis	surgical puncture to remove fluid	amnio**centesis** (surgical puncture to remove fluid from the amniotic sac)
-cyte	cell	erythro**cyte** (red blood cell)
-dipsia	thirst	poly**dipsia** (excessive, constant thirst)
-dynia	pain	cephalo**dynia** (pain in the head)
-eal	pertaining to	esophag**eal** (pertaining to the esophagus)
-ectomy	excision, surgical removal	hyster**ectomy** (surgical removal of the uterus)
-emia	blood condition	leuk**emia** (condition of abnormal white blood cells)
-genic	producing, forming	carcino**genic** (producing cancer)
-gram	record, picture	electrocardio**gram** (a record of electronic heart activity)
-graph	instrument for recording	electrocardio**graph** (the instrument that records electronic heart activity)
-graphy	process of recording	sono**graphy** (the process of recording sound)
-iasis	pathological condition	cholelith**iasis** (condition of having gallstones)
-iatry	treatment	psych**iatry** (treatment of mental conditions)
-ic	pertaining to	cephal**ic** (pertaining to the head)
-itis	inflammation	arthr**itis** (inflammation of the joints)
-lepsy	seizure	epi**lepsy** (seizure disorder)
-logist	specialist	neuro**logist** (specialist of the nerves and nervous system)
-logy	study of	bio**logy** (study of life)
-lysis	destruction, breaking down	neuro**lysis** (destruction of nervous tissue)
-lytic	reduce, destroy	hemo**lytic** (referring to destruction of red blood cells)
-malacia	softening	osteo**malacia** (bone softening)
-megaly	enlargement, enlarged	acro**megaly** (enlargement of tissues due to excessive growth hormone produced after puberty)
-meter	instrument to measure	cyto**meter** (instrument that measures or counts cells)
-metry	process of measuring	pelvi**metry** (process of measuring structures of the pelvis)
-oid	resembling, like	muc**oid** (resembling mucus)
-oma	tumor	melan**oma** (tumor resulting from melanocytes)
-opia	vision	dipl**opia** (double vision)

-osis	condition (abnormal condition)	cyan**osis** (a bluish condition of the skin and mucous membranes)
-partum	birth, labor	post**partum** (following birth)
-pathy	disease	osteo**pathy** (bone disease)
-penia	deficiency, decreased number	leukocyto**penia** (decreased amount of white blood cells)
-pepsia	digestion	dys**pepsia** (indigestion)
-pexy	surgical fixation	masto**pexy** (plastic surgery to correct "sagging" breasts)
-philia	attraction to	chromo**philia** (attraction to specific dyes in a staining process)
-phonia	sound, voice	a**phonia** (inability to speak)
-phobia	fear	aero**phobia** (fear of air, specifically drafty air)
-plasty	surgical repair	rhino**plasty** (surgical repair of the nose)
-ptosis	drooping, sagging	blepharo**ptosis** (drooping of the eyelids)
-rrhage	bursting forth of blood	hemo**rrhage** (bursting forth of blood from blood vessels)
-rrhea	flow, discharge	dia**rrhea** (flowing stool; loose bowel movements)
-sclerosis	hardening	arterio**sclerosis** (hardening of the arteries)
-scope	instrument to view	laryngo**scope** (instrument used to view the larynx)
-scopy	process of viewing	endo**scopy** (process of viewing body canals or hollow organs)
-stasis	control, stopping, stop	hemo**stasis** (stopping bleeding)
-stenosis	narrowing	tracheo**stenosis** (narrowing of the trachea)
-stomy	creation of an artificial opening	colo**stomy** (creation of an opening out of the colon)
-therapy	treatment	hydro**therapy** (treatment using water)
-tomy	incision	cranio**tomy** (incision into the cranium)
-tripsy	crushing, rubbing	litho**tripsy** (crushing of kidney stones using shock waves)
-trophy	nourishment, development	a**trophy** (lack of nourishment causing wasting away)
-tropia	turning	exo**tropia** (turning of one eye away from the other)
-uria	urine, urination	noct**uria** (nighttime urination)

Combining Forms and Vowels

A **combining form** or **combining vowel** is a letter that joins a word root with a suffix. It can also be used between two word roots. The most common combining vowel is the letter "o," and the next most common is the letter "i." The combining form also helps in pronunciation by making the word more "smooth" in sound. If a suffix begins with a vowel, a combining vowel is not required (such as in the term "arthr/itis"). If a suffix begins with a consonant, a combining vowel should be added (such as in the term "ot/o/scope."

EXAMPLE	
oste/o	**osteo**arthritis
cardi/o	**cardio**gram
hepat/o	**hepato**logy

See Table 1-8 for common combining forms.

TABLE 1-8   Common General Combining Forms

Combining Form	Meaning	Example
abdomin/o	abdomen	**abdomin**ocentesis
aden/o	gland	**aden**oma
angi/o	vessel	**angi**ogram
arteri/o	artery	**arteri**ograph
arthr/o	joint	**arthr**oscopy
ather/o	fatty	**ather**osclerosis
balan/o	glans penis	**balan**oplasty
bronch/o	bronchus	**bronch**oscope
bucc/o	cheek	**bucc**olingual
burs/i	bursa, sac	**burs**itis
carcin/o	cancer, cancerous	**carcin**ogenic
cardi/o	heart	**cardi**ologist
carp/o	wrist	**carp**al
cephal/o	head	**cephal**odynia
cerebr/o	cerebrum, brain	cerebrospinal
cheil/o	lip	**cheil**otomy
chol/e	gall, bile	**chol**elithiasis
cost/o	rib	inter**cost**al
crani/o	cranium (skull)	**crani**otomy
cyst/o	urinary bladder	**cyst**oscopy
cyt/o	cell	**cyt**ology
derm/o, dermato/o	skin	dermatologist
encephal/o	brain	hydro**encephal**itis
electr/o	electricity, electrical activity	**electro**encephalogram

enter/o	intestines	**enter**itis
esophag/o	esophagus	**esophag**eal
gastr/o	stomach	**gastr**otomy
gingiv/o	gums	**gingiv**itis
gynec/o	woman	**gynec**omastia
hem/o, hemat/o	blood	**hemat**olysis
hepat/o	liver	**hepat**oma
hist/o	tissue	**hist**ology
hydr/o	water	**hydr**ocele
hyster/o	uterus	**hyster**ectomy
kerat/o	cornea	**kerat**otomy
lacrim/o	tear duct, tears	**lacrim**al
lact/o	milk	**lact**ose
lapar/o	abdomen	**lapar**oscopy
laryng/o	larynx (voice box)	**laryng**itis
lingu/o	tongue	sub**lingu**al
lip/o	fat	**lip**oma
mast/o	breast	**mast**ectomy
men/o	menses, menstruation	**men**arche
my/o	muscle	**my**algia
myel/o	spinal cord, bone marrow	**myel**ogram
nas/o	nose	**nas**al
nat/o	birth	pre**nat**al
necr/o	death	**necr**osis
nephr/o	kidney	**nephr**otomy
neur/o	nerve	**neur**opathy

PLURAL WORDS

When the plural form of a word is used, the end of the word changes. For example, the term "nucleus" (as of a cell) is the singular form, while the term "nuclei" is the plural form, signifying more than one nucleus. Table 1-9 shows some examples of singular-to-plural suffix changes.

TABLE 1-9 Singular-to-Plural Suffix Changes

Singular Form	Plural Form
ap**ex**	ap**ices**
append**ix**	append**ices**
atri**um**	atri**a**
bacteri**um**	bacteri**a**
biops**y**	biops**ies**
cris**is**	cris**es**
fibr**oma**	fibr**omata**
gangli**on**	gangli**a**
metastas**is**	metastas**es**
nucle**us**	nucle**i**
ov**um**	ov**a**
phalan**x**	phalan**ges**
pleur**a**	pleur**ae**
sarc**oma**	sarc**omata**
sept**um**	sept**a**
thor**ax**	thor**aces**
thromb**us**	thromb**i**
vertebr**a**	vertebr**ae**

REVIEW EXERCISES

Multiple Choice

Select the best answer and write the letter of your choice to the left of each number.

1. When the prefix cyan/o is used, it means that:

   A. The object is blue.
   B. The object is oily.
   C. The object is dry.
   D. Something is poisonous.

2. The most common combining vowel is:

   A. i
   B. a
   C. o
   D. e

3. The underlined portion of the word *hypolipemia* represents which of the following word parts?

   A. suffix
   B. prefix
   C. root
   D. combining form

4. The prefix *retro-* means:

   A. below
   B. around
   C. after
   D. behind

5. The prefix *ambi-* means:

   A. under
   B. self
   C. both
   D. without

6. If a suffix begins with a vowel, the _____ will attach directly to it.

   A. hyphen
   B. prefix
   C. word root
   D. combining form

7. The basic foundation of a word is known as the:

    A. prefix
    B. word root
    C. suffix
    D. hyphen

8. A word root + a vowel is known as a:

    A. suffix
    B. word root
    C. prefix
    D. combining form

9. The combining form *ren/o* refers to the:

    A. chest
    B. kidneys
    C. abdomen
    D. urinary bladder

10. A word element that is added at the end of a word is a:

    A. hyphen
    B. suffix
    C. prefix
    D. word root

11. One prefix indicating number is:

    A. *poly-*
    B. *para-*
    C. *peri-*
    D. *purpur-*

12. In the term *polycystic, cyst-* is which word part?

    A. prefix
    B. word root
    C. suffix
    D. combining form

13. In the term *dysuria, dys-* is which word part?

    A. prefix
    B. word root
    C. suffix
    D. combining form

14. In the term *cardiopulmonary, -ary* is which word part?

    A. prefix
    B. word root
    C. suffix
    D. combining form

15. The term *cardiology* means
    A. pertaining to the heart
    B. inflammation of the heart
    C. study of the heart
    D. one who specializes in heart diseases

Fill in the Blank

Complete each statement with the most appropriate answer.

1. The basic foundation of a word is known as the
   _____.

2. The word element that is attached directly to the beginning
   of a word is known as a _____.

3. The component part of a word that is usually an *o* (or
   sometimes an *i*) is called the _____.

4. A word ending is called a _____.

5. A word root and a vowel are known as a _____.

6. A woman who is pregnant for the *first* time is termed a
   _____-*gravida*.

7. The medical term that means "being *without* pain," or refers
   to an agent that is given to relieve pain, is ___-*algesic*.

8. A person who is paralyzed on *one-half* (one side) of the
   body is known to have _____-*plegia*.

9. A tooth having *two cups* or points is known as a ___-*cuspid*
   tooth.

10. The excretion of large amounts of urine (*much* urine) is
    known as _____-*uria*.

True / False

Identify each of the following statements as true or false by
placing a "T" or "F" on the line beside each number.

_____ 1. The plural of *nucleus* is "nuclea."

_____ 2. The suffix meaning "surgical repair" is -*plasty*.

_____ 3. The word root *dactyl* means "finger."

_____ 4. The combining form *bucc/o* means "tongue."

_____ 5. The suffix that means "pain" is -*algia*.

_____ 6. The plural of *atrium* is "atria."

_____ **7.** The correct spelling of the plural form of *appendix* is "appendixes."

_____ **8.** The suffix that means "flow" or "discharge" is *-rrhea*.

_____ **9.** The plural of *septum* is "septae."

_____ **10.** The prefix that means "bad, difficult, painful" is *dys-*.

Definitions

Define the following roots and give one example of each.

	Meaning	Example
1. andro	_____	_____
2. dermat	_____	_____
3. hydro	_____	_____
4. angio	_____	_____
5. ambulo	_____	_____
6. hema	_____	_____
7. cyt	_____	_____
8. arthr	_____	_____
9. alb	_____	_____
10. lacto	_____	_____

Organization of the Human Body

OBJECTIVES

Upon completion of this chapter, the reader should be able to:

1. Describe the structural units of the human body.

2. Describe four types of tissues.

3. List the body cavities and their contents.

4. Describe major body planes.

5. Identify regions of the body.

6. Define, pronounce, and spell the medical terms and anatomical structures related to body structure.

7. Interpret the meanings of the abbreviations presented in this chapter.

OVERVIEW

Modern medicine began long ago with observations of the normal function of the human body. Once normal body function was understood, it could be determined why and how things malfunctioned. Anyone working in health care professions, including the pharmacy technician, must have a basic understanding of normal body function in order to recognize and problem-solve disease processes and injury. A basic understanding of the organization of the body will aid in understanding normal anatomy and in communicating with other health care workers.

STRUCTURAL UNITS OF THE BODY

The human body consists of a variety of structural units: cells, tissues, organs, and various systems (Figure 2-1). Cells, the smallest units of life, form tissues. Tissues form organs. Organs make up individual body systems.

Cells

The most basic unit of structure and function in the human body is the **cell**. Cells are not visible to the human eye, but may be observed under a microscope. Although cells vary in size, shape, and specialized functions, all share certain structural characteristics. The **cell membrane** encloses the cell, the **nucleus** houses the genetic material and controls cellular activities, the **cytoplasm** fills out the cell, and the **organelles** help the cell to function (Figure 2-2).

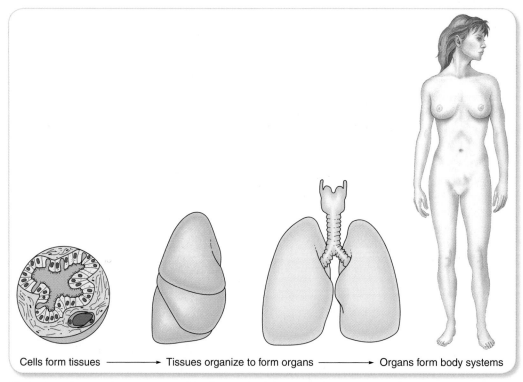

Cells form tissues ⟶ Tissues organize to form organs ⟶ Organs form body systems

Figure 2-1 Structural components of the human body.

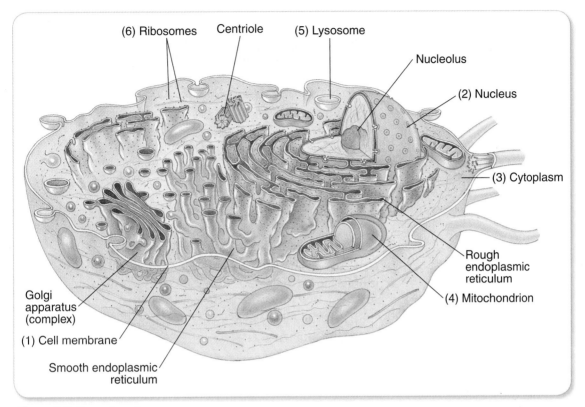

(6) Ribosomes   Centriole   (5) Lysosome

Nucleolus

(2) Nucleus

(3) Cytoplasm

Rough
endoplasmic
reticulum

(4) Mitochondrion

Golgi
apparatus
(complex)

(1) Cell membrane

Smooth endoplasmic
reticulum

Figure 2-2 Parts of a cell.

The cell membrane (also called the *plasma membrane*) is more than a simple boundary surrounding the cellular contents. It is an actively functioning part of the living material. The cell membrane regulates movement of substances in and out of the cell, and is the site of much biological activity.

The nucleus houses the genetic material, called *chromosomes* (deoxyribonucleic acid), which contains the information required for cell reproduction and protein synthesis.

The cytoplasm is the gel-like material that makes up most of a cell's volume. It contains networks of membranes as well as the organelles.

The organelles carry out specific activities. Examples of organelles include **endoplasmic reticulum, ribosomes, mitochondria, lysosomes, Golgi apparatus, cilia, flagellum,** and **centrioles** (Table 2-1). Individual cells perform specific functions, such as energy production, absorption, excretion, hormone secretion, and reproduction.

TABLE 2-1   Function of Organelles

Organelle	Function
endoplasmic reticulum	provides passages through which transport of substances occurs in cytoplasm
ribosomes	sites for protein synthesis
mitochondria	sites of cellular respiration and energy production
lysosomes	site for cellular digestion
Golgi apparatus	manufactures carbohydrates and packages secretions for discharge from cell
cilia and flagella	aid in cell movement or particle movement away from cells
centrioles	cell division

Tissues

Cells are organized into groups and layers called **tissues**. Each type of tissue is composed of similar cells specialized to carry out a particular function. The tissues of the human body are of four major types: epithelial, connective, muscle, and nervous.

1. The **epithelial tissues**, or **epithelium**, form protective coverings and function in secretion and absorption. They are the covering for and lining of body structures. For example, the top layer of skin and the lining of the uterus both consist of epithelial tissues.

2. The **connective tissues** support soft body parts and bind structures together. They serve as frameworks, fill spaces, store fat, produce blood cells, protect against infections, and help repair tissue damage. Examples of connective tissues are blood, bones, tendons, and adipose.

3. The **muscle tissues** produce body movements. They are able to contract and relax. The three types of muscle tissue are skeletal muscle, smooth muscle, and cardiac muscle. **Skeletal muscles** attach to bones and are controlled by conscious effort. For this reason, they are often called *voluntary* muscle tissue. **Smooth muscle** is the tissue that comprises the walls of hollow internal organs, such as the stomach, intestine, urinary bladder, uterus, and blood vessels. Unlike skeletal muscle, smooth muscle usually cannot be stimulated to contract by conscious effort. Thus, its action is *involuntary*. Smooth muscle is also called **visceral muscle**. **Cardiac muscle** is found only in the heart and, like smooth muscle, it is controlled involuntarily. This tissue makes up the bulk of the heart and pumps blood through the heart chambers and into blood vessels.

4. **Nerve tissues** are found in the brain, spinal cord, and peripheral nerves. The basic cells are called **neurons,** or nerve cells. Because neurons communicate with each other and with muscle and gland cells, they can coordinate, regulate, and integrate many body functions.

Organs

Groups of different tissues that interact form **organs**. They are complex structures with specialized functions. Examples of organs are the kidneys, lungs, brain, heart, testes, and pancreas.

Body Systems

Groups of organs that function closely together comprise **body systems**. The human organism consists of several body systems. Each system includes a set of interrelated organs that work together by allowing each system to provide specialized functions that contribute to **homeostasis** (a balanced state). The organ systems include:

- skeletal
- muscular
- integumentary
- lymphatic
- nervous
- endocrine
- cardiovascular
- male and female reproductive
- digestive
- respiratory
- urinary

BODY CAVITIES

The human body can be divided into two major cavities: the **ventral cavity** and the **dorsal cavity**. The ventral cavity includes the **thoracic cavity** and the **abdominopelvic cavity**. The organs within these last two cavities are called *viscera*. The dorsal cavity includes the **cranial cavity** and the **vertebral canal** (Figure 2-3).

The thoracic cavity contains the heart, great blood vessels, lungs, trachea, and esophagus. The thoracic cavity is separated from the lower abdominopelvic cavity by a broad, thin muscle called the *diaphragm*. This cavity includes an upper abdominal portion and a lower pelvic portion.

The **abdominal cavity** includes the stomach, liver, spleen, gallbladder, kidneys, and most of the small and large intestines. The **pelvic cavity** contains the terminal portion of the large intestine, the urinary bladder, and the internal reproductive organs.

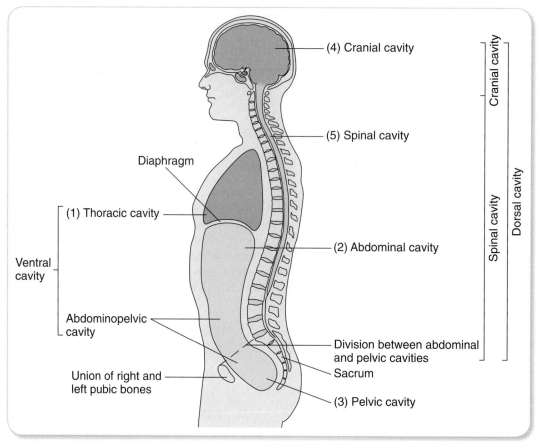

Figure 2-3 Body cavities.

The cranial cavity contains the brain and the vertebral canal, or spinal cavity, which contains the spinal cord, and is part of the dorsal cavity.

BODY PLANES

Observing the relative locations and organization of internal body parts requires cutting or sectioning the body along various planes (Figure 2-4). The following terms describe such planes and sections:

1. **Sagittal** – refers to a length-wise plane that divides the body into right and left portions. If a sagittal plane passes along the midline, the body is divided into equal parts; this is called *midsagittal*. A sagittal section lateral to the midline is called *parasagittal*.

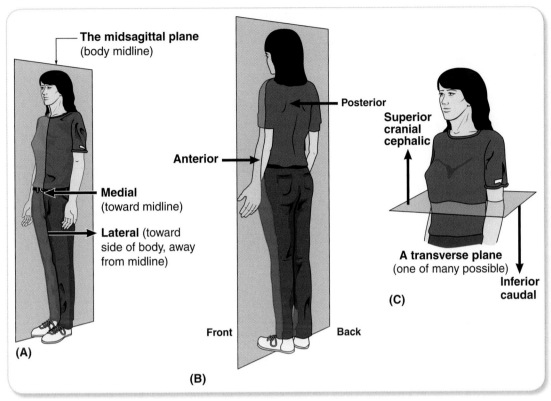

Figure 2-4 Body planes.

2. **Coronal** (or *frontal*) – refers to a plane that divides the body into anterior and posterior portions.

3. **Transverse** (or *horizontal*) – refers to a plane that divides the body into superior and inferior portions.

The terms of relative position describe the location of one body part with respect to another. Examples of these terms are **anterior**, **posterior**, **superior**, and **inferior**.

BODY REGIONS

A number of terms designate body regions. The abdominal area, for example, is subdivided into the following nine regions (Figure 2-5).

1. **Epigastric region** – refers to the upper middle portion.

2. **Left and right hypochondriac regions** – lie on each side of the epigastric region.

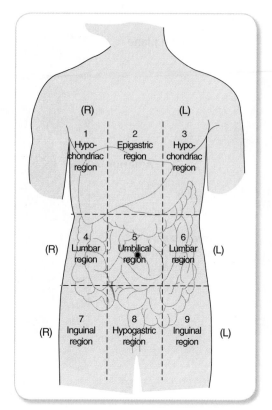

Figure 2-5 Abdominal regions.

3. **Umbilical region** – refers to the middle portion.
4. **Left and right lumbar regions** – lie on each side of the umbilical region.
5. **Hypogastric region** – refers to the lower middle portion.
6. **Left and right iliac regions** (left and right inguinal regions) – lie on each side of the hypogastric region.

The abdominal area is also often subdivided into four quadrants (Figure 2-6). These imaginary divisions are useful to describe the location of abdominopelvic pain, or in determining the location of abdominal organs.

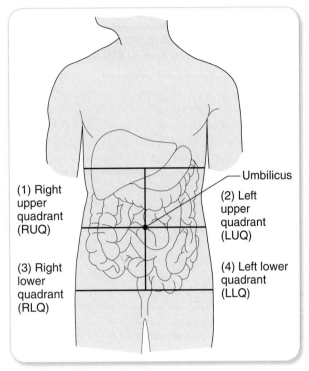

Figure 2-6 Abdominal quadrants.

GENERAL TERMINOLOGY RELATED TO THE BODY

The following are common terms that relate to the body in health and disease.

TABLE 2-2   General Anatomical Terminology

Term	Pronunciation	Definition
abdominal	ab-DAH-mih-nul	pertaining to the part of the body between the chest and pelvis
anatomy	uh-NAH-toh-mee	the study of the structures of the body
anterior	an-TEE-ree-or	the front surface of the body; or "situated in front"
bilateral	by-LAH-teh-rul	having two sides
caudal	KAW-dul	pertaining to or nearer to the tail
cell	sell	the smallest unit of life that can live independently of a larger creature

(continues)

TABLE 2-2 General Anatomical Terminology (*continued*)

Term	Pronunciation	Definition
cell membrane	SELL MEM-brayn	a semi-permeable membrane that encloses a cell's cytoplasm; also called *plasma membrane*
centrioles	SEN-tree-olz	rod-shaped bodies (usually numbering two) near the nucleus; they help separate the chromosomes during cell division
cephalic	seh-FAH-lik	pertaining to or nearer to the head
chromosome	KRO-moh-zoam	a thread-like body in a cell's nucleus that contains genetic information
cilia	SIH-lee-uh	short, hair-like projections from a cell that move fluids around the cell
coronal	koh-ROH-nul	a vertical plane dividing the body into anterior and posterior portions
cranial	KRAY-nee-ul	pertaining to the cranium (the portion of the skull that contains the brain)
cytology	sy-TAW-loh-jee	the study of the cell
cytoplasm	SY-toh-plah-zum	a colloidal suspension that fills the cell from the nuclear membrane to the plasma membrane; it consists of cytosol and organelles
cytosol	SY-toh-sol	the fluid portion of the cytoplasm; it surrounds the organelles
distal	DIS-tul	situated away from the center of the body
dorsal	DOR-sul	pertaining to the back; or "situated behind"
endoplasmic reticulum	en-doh-PLAZ-mik reh-TIH-kyoo-lum	a network of membranes within the cytoplasm
epigastric region	eh-pih-GAS-trik REE-jun	the abdominal region above the stomach
flagellum	flah-JEH-lum	a long, whip-like extension from a cell that provides movement for the cell
frontal	FRUN-tul	a vertical plane dividing the body into anterior and posterior portions
gene	jeen	a fundamental physical and functional unit of heredity
Golgi apparatus	GOL-jee ah-puh-RAH-tus	layers of membranes that make compounds containing proteins, sorting and preparing these compounds for transport to other parts of the cell or out of the cell
histology	his-TAW-loh-jee	the study of the function of tissues
homeostasis	ho-mee-oh-STAY-sis	a steady state; a condition of internal stability and constancy

hypochondriac region	hy-poh-KON-dree-ak REE-jun	the upper, lateral portion of the abdomen, just below the ribs, on each side of the body
hypogastric region	hy-poh-GAS-trik REE-jun	the abdominal region below the stomach
iliac region	IH-lee-ak REE-jun	the lower, lateral portion of the abdomen, between the abdomen and thigh, on each side of the body
inferior	in-FEE-ree-or	situated below
lateral	LAH-teh-rul	a part of the body that is farther from the middle or center of the body
lysosomes	LY-soh-sohmz	small sacs of digestive enzymes; they digest substances within the cell
medial	MEE-dee-ul	pertaining to the middle; or near the middle of the body
mitochondria	my-toh-KON-dree-uh	large organelles with folded membranes inside; they convert energy from nutrients into ATP
neuron	NOO-ron	the basic structural element of the nervous system
nucleus	NOO-klee-us	the cell's control center; it directs all cell activities based on the information contained in its chromosomes
organ	OR-gun	a part of the body with a specific function or a component of a body system
organelles	or-gah-NELZ	specialized structures in the cytoplasm of a cell
pathology	pah-THAW-loh-jee	the study of the nature and causes of disease and its relation to changes in structure and function
pelvic cavity	PEL-vik CAH-vih-tee	the area of the body below the abdomen between the pelvis and pelvic girdle
physiology	fih-zee-AW-loh-jee	the study of the functions of the structures of the body
posterior	pos-TEE-ree-or	the back surface of the body; or "situated behind"
proximal	PROK-sih-mul	situated nearest the center of the body
ribosomes	RY-boh-zohmz	small, free bodies in the cytoplasm or attached to the endoplasmic reticulum; they are composed of ribonucleic acid and protein, and manufacture proteins
sagittal	SAH-jih-tul	a vertical plane through the body dividing it into right and left portions
skeletal muscle	SKEH-leh-tul MUH-sul	the type of muscle that provides skeletal movement
smooth muscle	SMOOTH MUH-sul	the type of muscle that forms the supporting tissue of blood vessels and hollow organs
superficial	soo-per-FIH-shul	on the surface, or shallow
superior	soo-PEE-ree-or	situated above
tissue	TIH-shoo	a group of cells that act together for a specific purpose

(continues)

TABLE 2-2   General Anatomical Terminology (*continued*)

transverse	tranz-VERS	a horizontal plane dividing the body into upper and lower portions
umbilical region	um-BIH-lih-kul REE-jun	pertaining to the umbilicus, or the center of the abdomen
unilateral	yoo-nih-LAH-teh-rul	pertaining to one side of the body
ventral	VEN-trul	pertaining to the belly, or situated nearer to the surface of the belly
vesicles	VEH-sih-kulz	small membrane-bound sacs in the cytoplasm; they store materials and move materials into or out of the cell in bulk amounts
visceral	VIH-seh-rul	pertaining to body organs enclosed within a cavity, especially the abdominal organs
voluntary muscle	VAW-lun-teh-ree MUH-sul	the type of muscle that may be controlled by conscious effort

ABBREVIATIONS

The following abbreviations relate to the organization of the body.

TABLE 2-3   General Anatomical Abbreviations

Abbreviation	Meaning
abd	abdomen, abdominal
AP	anteroposterior
cyt	cytology, cytoplasm
D	dorsal
DNA	deoxyribonucleic acid
ER	endoplasmic reticulum
HIS	histology
LAT, lat	lateral
LLQ	left lower quadrant
LUQ	left upper quadrant
P	posterior
PA	posteroanterior
RLQ	right lower quadrant
RNA	ribonucleic acid
RUQ	right upper quadrant
umb	umbilical
V, vent	ventral

REVIEW EXERCISES

Multiple Choice

Select the best answer and write the letter of your choice to the left of each number.

1. The small, free bodies in the cytoplasm that may be attached to the endoplasmic reticulum are called:

    A. ribosomes
    B. mitochondria
    C. genes
    D. cilia

2. A group of cells that act together for a specific task is referred to as a(n):

    A. organ
    B. cytosol
    C. tissue
    D. organelle

3. Which of the following medical terms means "the study of the tissues"?

    A. physiology
    B. cytology
    C. pathology
    D. histology

4. A vertical plane dividing the body into anterior and posterior portions is called:

    A. transverse
    B. sagittal
    C. vertical
    D. frontal

5. A component of body systems with a specific function is referred to as a(n):

    A. tissue
    B. organ
    C. organelle
    D. mitochondria

6. Which of the following encloses the cell?

    A. nucleus
    B. cytoplasm
    C. organelle
    D. cell membrane

7. Which of the following consists of cytosol and organelles?

   A. cytoplasm
   B. lysosome
   C. ribosome
   D. vesicle

8. The abdominal region above the stomach is known as the:

   A. hypochondriac region
   B. iliac region
   C. epigastric region
   D. hypogastric region

9. Which of the following medical terms is used for a condition of internal stability and constancy of the body?

   A. physiology
   B. anabolism
   C. anaphylaxis
   D. homeostasis

10. The medical term "coronal" is synonymous with:

    A. sagittal
    B. transverse
    C. horizontal
    D. frontal

11. Which of the following terms pertains to the "tail"?

    A. bilateral
    B. caudal
    C. proximal
    D. medial

12. Which of the following organelles is *not* within the cytoplasm?

    A. mitochondria
    B. vesicles
    C. nucleus
    D. lysosomes

13. Which of the following types of muscle is known as "voluntary"?

    A. skeletal
    B. cardiac
    C. smooth
    D. uterus

14. Which of the following terms is the opposite of "distal"?

    A. superior
    B. lateral
    C. dorsal
    D. proximal

15. Which of the following is the basic structural element of the nervous system?

    A. nucleus
    B. neuron
    C. Golgi apparatus
    D. chromosome

Fill in the Blank

Use your knowledge of medical terminology to insert the correct term from the list below.

gene	coronal	cytoplasm
cilia	Golgi apparatus	flagellum
ventral	cephalic	neuron
superficial	hypochondriac	sagittal
organ	endoplasmic reticulum	chromosome

1. The basic structural element of the nervous system is the _____.

2. A thread-like body in a cell's nucleus that contains genetic information is called a _____.

3. A vertical plane dividing the body into anterior and posterior portions is referred to as the _____ plane.

4. The term meaning "situated nearer to the head" is _____.

5. Hair-like projections from the cell that move fluids around the cell are called _____.

6. The term meaning "situated nearer to the surface of the belly" is _____.

7. A network of membranes within the cytoplasm is the _____.

8. A colloidal suspension that fills the cell inside the plasma membrane is called _____.

9. A whip-like extension from the cell that causes movement of the cell is referred to as a _____.

10. A fundamental physical and functional unit of heredity is called a _____.

Labeling – The Abdominal Regions

Write in the terms below that correspond with each letter on the figure (left).

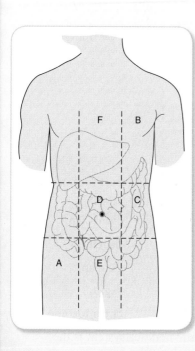

A. _____

B. _____

C. _____

D. _____

E. _____

F. _____

True / False

Identify each of the following statements as true or false by placing a "T" or "F" on the line beside each number.

_____ **1.** The connective tissues support soft body parts and bind structures together.

_____ **2.** Smooth muscles are found in the upper extremities and attach to the bones.

_____ **3.** There are only three types of tissues: epithelial, connective, and muscle.

_____ **4.** Cardiac muscle is controlled involuntarily.

_____ **5.** The thoracic cavity is separated by the stomach and liver from the lower abdominopelvic cavity.

_____ **6.** The pelvic cavity contains the terminal portion of the large intestine.

_____ **7.** The cranial cavity contains the spinal cord.

_____ **8.** The hypogastric region refers to the upper middle portion of the abdomen.

_____ **9.** The left and right hypochondriac regions lie on each side of the epigastric region.

_____**10.** "Sagittal" refers to a lengthwise plane that divides the body into right and left portions.

Definition

Define each of the following words in one sentence.

1. midsagittal: _____

2. anatomy: _____

3. inferior: _____

4. homeostasis: _____

5. histology: _____

6. iliac region: _____

7. cell: _____

8. physiology: _____

9. tissue: _____

10. neuron: _____

Abbreviations

Write the full meaning of each abbreviation.

Abbreviation	Meaning
1. ER	_____
2. DNA	_____
3. AP	_____
4. LLQ	_____
5. LAT	_____
6. vent	_____
7. P	_____
8. RNA	_____
9. RUQ	_____
10. umb	_____

Matching – Terms and Definitions

Match each term at the left with its corresponding definition by placing the correct letter on the line to the left of each number.

_____ 1. Golgi apparatus

_____ 2. nucleus

_____ 3. cell membrane

A. rod-shaped bodies near the nucleus involved with separation of the chromosomes during cell division

_____ 4. lysosome

_____ 5. ribosome

_____ 6. endoplasmic reticulum

_____ 7. cilia

_____ 8. centrioles

_____ 9. flagellum

_____ 10. mitochondria

B. a network of membranes within the cytoplasm

C. short, hair-like projections from a cell

D. a long, whip-like extension from a cell that provides movement for the cell

E. convert energy from nutrients into ATP

F. a small sac filled with digestive enzymes

G. a semi-permeable membrane that encloses a cell's cytoplasm

H. layers of membranes that make compounds containing proteins

I. are attached to the endoplasmic reticulum and manufacture proteins

J. the cell's control center

Spelling

Circle the correct spelling from each pairing of words.

1. hemeostasis   homeostasis

2. lisosome   lysosome

3. sagittal   sagital

4. hypokondriac   hypochondriac

5. flagelum   flagellum

6. visceral   viceral

7. umbilical   umbillical

8. mitochondria   mytochondria

9. nuclus   nucleus

10. chromosome   chromossome

SECTION II

TERMINOLOGY OF THE BODY SYSTEMS

CHAPTER

3

The Integumentary System

OBJECTIVES

Upon completion of this chapter, the reader should be able to:

1. Name the tissues in the different layers of the skin.
2. Identify the functions of the different skin layers.
3. Describe certain conditions affecting the superficial layers of the skin.
4. List five medications used for skin conditions.
5. Interpret the meaning of the abbreviations presented in this chapter.
6. Define, pronounce, and spell the diseases and disorders in this chapter.
7. Recognize common pharmacological agents used in treating disorders of the integumentary system.
8. Describe the common types of drugs used for integumentary system conditions.

STRUCTURE AND FUNCTION OF THE INTEGUMENTARY SYSTEM

The primary organ of the **integumentary system** is the **skin**. The skin serves several functions:

- protection for underlying tissues and organs
- regulation of body temperature
- manufacture of vitamin D, which is necessary for bone and tooth development
- site of nerve endings producing sensory receptors
- storage site for fat, glucose, water, and salts

The Skin

The skin is the heaviest body organ. It contains various accessory structures, including hair, nails, sensory receptors, and glands. The skin consists of three layers. The outer layer is called the **epidermis**. The thicker inner layer is called the **dermis**. The dermis is made of connective tissue, consisting of various types of protein fibers, epithelial tissue, smooth muscle tissue, nervous tissue, and blood. Beneath the dermis is a loose connective tissue, mostly made of **adipose** (fat) tissue, that binds the dermis to the organs beneath, forming the **subcutaneous** layer. Figure 3-1 shows the skin layers and the associated structures of the skin.

The Epidermis

The epidermis contains stratified squamous epithelium, and does not contain blood vessels. Specialized epidermal cells called **melanocytes** produce a dark pigment (**melanin**), which provides color in the skin and absorbs ultraviolent radiation from sunlight. Melanocytes lie deep within the epidermis. The deepest layer of epidermal cells, called the **stratum basale** or **stratum germinativum**, is close to the dermis and is nourished by dermal blood vessels.

As epidermal cells age, they are pushed outward from the dermis toward the skin surface. They receive less nutrients as they age, and then die. These older cells, known as **keratinocytes**, harden as part of a process called **keratinization**.

The Dermis

The dermis is largely composed of dense connective tissues made of tough collagenous fibers. Networks of these fibers give the skin

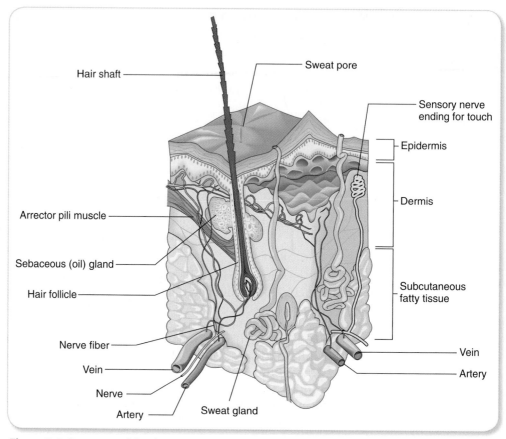

Figure 3-1 Structures of the skin.

toughness and elasticity. Dermal blood vessels supply nutrients to all skin cells. These vessels also help regulate body temperature.

The Subcutaneous Layer

The subcutaneous layer consists mainly of loose connective tissue and fatty tissue. It serves to insulate and protect the deeper tissues.

The Accessory Structures

Sebaceous glands contain groups of specialized epithelial cells and are usually associated with hair follicles. They secrete an oily mixture of fatty material and cellular debris called **sebum** through small ducts into the hair follicles. Sebum helps keep the hair and skin soft, pliable, and waterproof.

Sweat glands, or *sudoriferous* glands, are exocrine glands that are widespread throughout the skin. Each gland consists of a tiny tube that originates as a ball-shaped coil in the deeper dermis.

Hair covers the majority of the surface area of the body. The color and texture of the hair are dependent upon the melanin cells surrounding the hair shaft and the shape of the hair follicle.

Nails are protective coverings for the tips of the fingers and toes.

GENERAL TERMINOLOGY RELATED TO THE INTEGUMENTARY SYSTEM

The following are common terms that are related to the integumentary system.

Word	Pronunciation	Definition
albino	al-BYE-noh	an individual with albinism (deficiency or absence of pigment in hair, skin, and eyes due to abnormal melanin production)
amputation	am-pew-TAY-shun	severing of a limb, part of a limb, breast, or another body part
cerumen	seh-ROO-men	the soft, brownish-yellow waxy secretion from the ceruminous glands of the external auditory meatus
collagen	KOL-ah-jen	the main protein in bone, cartilage, and connective tissue; provides support and strength for these structures
corium	KOH-ree-um	the layer of skin just under the epidermis, also known as the *dermis*
debridement	deh-BRIDE-ment	surgical removal of dead or contaminated tissue from a wound
dermis	DER-mis	the lowest layer of skin; positioned above the subcutaneous fat (adipose) layer
diaphoresis	dye-ah-foh-REE-sis	the secretion of sweat
epidermis	ep-ih-DER-mis	the outermost layer of the skin
keratin	KAIR-ah-tin	the tough protein that forms most skin structures, including hair and nails
keratolytic	KAIR-ah-toh-LIT-ic	an agent used to break down or loosen the horny (hardened) layer of the skin
mast cell	MAST cell	a large connective tissue cell containing biochemicals, including histamine; may be related to allergic reactions and are involved in secondary inflammation from injuries and infections
melanin	MEL-an-in	dark-brown or black pigments occurring in the skin, hair, and retina
melanocytes	MEL-an-oh-sights or mel-AN-oh-sights	pigment-producing cells in the epidermis's basal layer that result in epidermal pigmentation
sebaceous gland	see-BAY-shus	an oil gland located in the dermis that usually opens into the hair follicles
sebum	SEE-bum	the oily secretions of the sebaceous glands
sudoriferous gland	soo-door-IF-er-us	a sweat gland
ultraviolet light	ul-trah-VYE-oh-let	artificial sunlight used to treat some skin lesions

PATHOLOGICAL CONDITIONS OF THE INTEGUMENTARY SYSTEM

Following are the disorders and conditions of the integumentary system:

Abscess – a localized infection that causes a pocket of pus

Acne vulgaris – a common inflammatory disorder seen on the face, chest, and upper back that affects adolescents during puberty

Alopecia – hair loss anywhere on the body, or the condition of "baldness"

Blister – a fluid-filled, thin-walled structure under or within the epidermis

Burn – disruption or destruction of tissue that has been exposed to fire, a toxin, or excessive energy (heat); may be minor and quickly healed (such as sunburn) or may be extensive and fatal (such as chemical or thermal burns)

Carbuncle – a deep-seated abscess that forms inside a hair follicle

Cellulitis – a subcutaneous tissue infection that is usually painful and may spread rapidly over a large skin area

Cyanosis – a bluish discoloration of the skin

Dermatitis – inflammation of the skin, which may be acute or chronic, contact (in response to an irritant or allergen), or seborrheic (related to areas where oil glands are most prevalent)

Ecchymosis – blood that has pooled inside the skin; usually a large, irregular, and purplish patch of skin that may result from trauma or a bleeding condition

Eczema – a chronic condition of the skin with inflammation, scaling, discharge of serous fluid, and (usually) itching that may be caused by allergies, toxins, or other causes

Erythema – skin inflammation and reddening

Fissure – a split, groove, or gap that may be either part of normal anatomy or the result of disease or injury; for example, an anal fissure is a painful crack in the lining of the anus

Fistula – an abnormal passageway from an abscess, cavity, or hollow organ to another structure, or to the skin surface

Furuncle – a localized pus-producing infection originating deep in a hair follicle; also known as a *boil*

Gangrene – death of tissue due to insufficient supply of blood; it may be caused by bacteria or an infection that invades dead tissue

Herpes zoster – a viral infection of the nerve roots in the skin; commonly called "shingles"

Hives – circumscribed, slightly elevated lesions of the skin that are paler in the center than on the edges; also known as *wheals* or as a part of the condition known as "urticaria"

Hyperkeratosis – overgrowth of the epidermis's horny layer

Impetigo – a bacterial skin infection usually seen in children that is highly contagious; appears initially as a fluid-filled blister that, upon bursting, leaves a crusty border around the lesion

Keloid – a firm, nodular, and usually linear mass of hyperplastic, thick scar tissue in the dermis; consists of irregular bands of collagen, and usually occurs after trauma, surgery, burns, or severe skin disease

Keratosis – thickening and overgrowth of the cornified epithelium of the skin; *seborrheic keratosis* is also known as "senile warts"

Laceration – a jagged skin cut or wound

Nevus (mole) – a pigmented skin blemish that is usually benign, but may become malignant; composed of nevus cells derived from melanocytes, and may be referred to as a "birthmark" or "mole"

Papule – a small, solid, circumscribed skin elevation

Pediculosis – an infestation of lice, usually affecting hairy areas of the body, including the top of the head, eyebrows, eyelids, underarms, chest, and pubic area

Pemphigus – a serious skin condition with unknown cause characterized by large, fluid-filled blisters that rupture easily, leaving the skin raw; if untreated, this condition is usually fatal

Petechiae – tiny, pinhead-sized hemorrhagic spots in the skin

Polyp – a small, stalk-like growth that protrudes upward or outward from a mucous membrane surface, resembling a mushroom stalk

Pruritus – itching

Psoriasis – a chronic skin disorder characterized by raised, reddish patches covered with white scale; most often appears on the elbows, knees, scalp, genitalia, and trunk; patches may also appear at sites of trauma

Purpura – hemorrhaging into the skin

Pustule – a small elevation of the skin filled with pus; a small abscess

Scleroderma – an immune system disorder that causes the skin to become tight, tough, and hyperpigmented; may progress to the kidneys, lungs, heart, and digestive tract

Systemic lupus erythematosus – a chronic, inflammatory disease affecting many body systems that is an example of a collagen disease; primary cause has not been determined, but viral infection or immune system dysfunction is suggested

Tinea – a fungal infection of skin or related structures, also known as "ringworm;" most commonly treated with topical antifungal medications, but in some cases, oral therapy may be required

Tinea pedis – a fungal infection of the foot, also known as "athlete's foot"

Ulcer – an erosive or penetrating lesion on a skin or mucosal surface, usually involving inflammation

Wart (verruca) – a defined skin elevation with a rough surface, usually appearing on the hands, face, neck, and knees, and caused by a localized virus; genital warts are contagious

Xanthosis – a yellow discoloration of the skin caused by tissue destruction, often from cancer; may also be caused by ingestion of foods with yellow pigments, such as carrots and squash (this type of xanthosis is usually harmless)

Xeroderma – a dermatologic condition characterized by rough, dry skin

ABBREVIATIONS RELATED TO THE INTEGUMENTARY SYSTEM

The following are common abbreviations related to the integumentary system.

Abbreviation	Meaning
BSA	body surface area
Bx, bx	biopsy
derm.	dermatology
DLE	discoid lupus erythematosus
FS	frozen section
FTSG	full-thickness skin graft

I&D	incision and drainage
LE	lupus erythematosus
PPD	purified protein derivative
PSS	progressive systemic scleroderma
SLE	systemic lupus erythematosus
SPF	sun protection factor
TENS	transcutaneous electrical nerve stimulation
ung.	ointment
UV	ultraviolet (light)
UVA	ultraviolet A
UVB	ultraviolet B
XP, XDP	xeroderma pigmentosum

MEDICATIONS USED TO TREAT INTEGUMENTARY SYSTEM DISORDERS

The following are common medications used for integumentary system disorders.

Generic Name	Trade Name	Drug Class	Use
benzocaine	Anbesol®, Orajel®	anesthetic	to relieve pain
dibucaine	Nupercainal®		
lidocaine	Lidoderm®		
clotrimazole	Lotrimin®	antifungal	to slow or stop fungi growth
ketoconazole	Nizoral®		
tolnaftate	Absorbine®, Desenex®		
diphenhydramine	Allerdryl®, Benadryl®	antihistamine	to slow, stop, or prevent allergic reactions
fexofenadine	Allegra®		
loratadine	Claritin®		
bacitracin	Neosporin®	antibacterial	to slow or stop bacterial growth
benzoyl peroxide	Clearasil®		
neomycin	Myciguent®		
doxepin	Zonalon®	antipruritic	to relieve itching
hydrocortisone	Bactine®, Caldecort®		
betamethasone	Diprosone®, Betnovate®	anti-inflammatory (corticosteroid)	to reduce inflammation
triamcinolone	Aristocort®, Triamolone®		

DRUG TERMINOLOGY

The following are common types of drugs used for the integumentary system:

Word	Pronunciation	Definition
alpha hydroxy acid	AL-fa hye-DROK-see	agent added to cosmetics to improve skin appearance
anesthetic	an-es-THET-ik	agent that relieves pain by blocking nerve sensations
antibacterial	an-tye-bak-TEER-ee-all	agent that kills or slows the growth of bacteria
antibiotic	an-tye-bye-OT-ik	agent that kills or slows the growth of microorganisms
antifungal	an-tye-FUN-gall	agent that kills or slows the growth of fungi
antihistamine	an-tye-HISS-tah-meen	agent that controls allergic reactions by blocking the effectiveness of histamines in the body
anti-inflammatory	an-tye-in-FLAH-mah-tor-ee	agent that relieves the symptoms of inflammations
antipruritic	an-tye-proo-RIT-ik	agent that controls itching
antiseptic	an-tye-SEP-tik	agent that, like an antibiotic, kills or slows the growth of microorganisms
astringent	as-TRIN-jent	agent that removes excess oils and impurities from the skin's surface
corticosteroid	kor-tih-ko-STAIR-oid	agent with anti-inflammatory properties
emollient	eh-MOH-lee-ent	agent that smoothes or softens skin
parasiticide	pah-rah-SIT-ih-side	agent that kills or slows the growth of parasites

REVIEW EXERCISES

Multiple Choice

Select the best answer and write the letter of your choice to the left of each number.

1. Which of the following vitamins may be produced by the skin?

   A. vitamin C
   B. vitamin A
   C. vitamin D
   D. vitamin E

2. Which of the following structures is not contained in the dermis?

   A. receptors
   B. capillaries
   C. follicles
   D. nails

3. Which of the following is a congenital lesion of the skin that is commonly called a "birthmark"?

   A. melanoma
   B. nevus
   C. papule
   D. vesicle

4. Which of the following is the medical term for "shingles"?

   A. impetigo
   B. pediculosis
   C. erysipelas
   D. herpes zoster

5. An ointment, cream, or spray prescribed to relieve itching is called a(n):

   A. keratolytic
   B. antibacterial
   C. antipruritic
   D. antipyretic

6. Which of the following is referred to as "subcutaneous fat"?

   A. dermis
   B. hypodermis
   C. epidermis
   D. adipose tissue

7. Raised, irregular, lumpy, or shiny scars caused by excess collagen fiber produced during wound healing are known as:

   A. keloids
   B. macrophages
   C. abrasions
   D. edemas

8. Partial or complete hair loss, either naturally or from medication, is known as:

   A. sebum
   B. dandruff
   C. alopecia
   D. albinism

9. A small elevation of the skin that contains pus is referred to as a(n):

   A. furuncle
   B. pustule
   C. sebum
   D. impetigo

10. An inflammatory skin disease, often with a serous discharge, is referred to as:

    A. dermatitis
    B. decubitus ulcer
    C. pediculosis
    D. eczema

11. Which of the following is produced by sebaceous glands?

    A. melanin
    B. oil
    C. sweat
    D. hair

12. Which of the following is a superficial skin infection characterized by pustules and caused by bacteria?

    A. impetigo
    B. scabies
    C. shingles
    D. gangrene

13. A yellowing discoloration of the skin caused by destruction of tissue is called:

    A. warts
    B. tinea

C. xanthosis
D. cyanosis

14. Which of the following conditions is characterized by bleeding into the skin?

   A. purpura
   B. pustule
   C. papule
   D. polyp

15. A common inflammatory disorder seen on the face, chest, and upper back in adolescents during puberty is known as:

   A. dermatitis
   B. eczema
   C. hyperkeratosis
   D. acne vulgaris

Fill in the Blank

Use your knowledge of medical terminology to insert the correct term from the list below.

amputation	fistula	sebum
abscess	gangrene	ulcer
carbuncle	keratin	hives
diaphoresis	mast cells	furuncle
ecchymosis	melanocyte	erythema

1. _____ contain a wide variety of biochemicals, including histamine.

2. The secretion of sweat is referred to as _____.

3. A pocket of pus that is caused by a localized infection is called a(n) _____.

4. _____ is due to insufficient blood supply, which may be caused by an infection or bacteria that may invade dead tissue.

5. An _____ is an erosive or penetrating lesion on the skin or a mucosal surface, usually with inflammation.

6. The oily secretion of the sebaceous glands is called _____.

7. _____ is a tough protein that forms the basis for most skin structures, including nails.

8. A pigment-producing cell located in the basal layer of the epidermis is referred to as a _____.

9. A _____ is a deep-seated abscess that forms in a hair follicle.

10. Reddening of the skin is referred to as _____.

Labeling

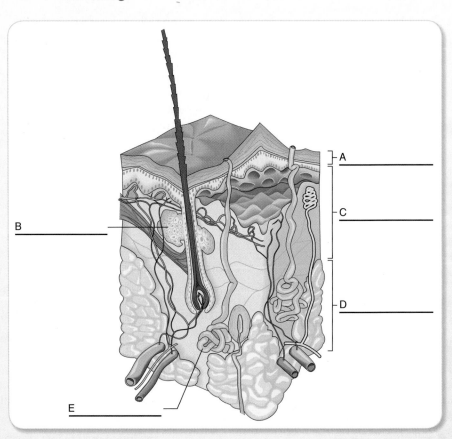

A. _____

B. _____

C. _____

D. _____

E. _____

Write in the terms below that correspond with each letter on the figure above.

A. _____

B. _____

C. _____

D. _____

E. _____

True / False

Identify each of the following statements as true or false by placing a "T" or "F" on the line beside each number.

_____ 1. Hair loss anywhere on the body is called "acne vulgaris."

_____ 2. A fluid-filled, thin-walled structure under the dermis is referred to as a "blister."

_____ 3. Erythema consists of skin inflammation and reddening.

_____ 4. A bluish discoloration of the skin is called "jaundice."

_____ 5. A small, solid, circumscribed skin elevation is referred to as a "nevus" or "mole."

_____ 6. A thick scar tissue in the dermis is known as a "keloid."

_____ 7. Herpes zoster is a viral infection of the nerve roots in the skin.

_____ 8. Impetigo is a bacterial skin infection usually seen in children that is highly contagious.

_____ 9. A jagged skin cut or wound is called a "senile wart."

_____10. Tiny, pinhead-sized hemorrhagic spots in the skin signify a condition known as "petechiae."

Definitions

Define each of the following words in one sentence.

1. pruritus: _____

2. sudoriferous gland: _____

3. keratin: _____

4. erythema: _____

5. exfoliation: _____

6. ecchymosis: _____

7. cellulitis: _____

Abbreviations

Write the full meaning of each abbreviation.

Abbreviation	Meaning
1. DLE	_____
2. Bx	_____
3. XP	_____
4. UVA	_____
5. SPF	_____
6. LE	_____
7. PPD	_____
8. I&D	_____
9. FS	_____
10. BSA	_____

Matching – Terms and Definitions

Match each term at the left with its corresponding definition by placing the correct letter on the line to the left of each number.

_____ **1.** xanthosis

_____ **2.** tinea

_____ **3.** wart

_____ **4.** pustule

_____ **5.** melanin

_____ **6.** petechiae

_____ **7.** sebum

_____ **8.** blister

_____ **9.** gangrene

_____ **10.** mast cell

A. a small elevation of the skin filled with pus

B. pinhead-sized hemorrhagic spots in the skin

C. the oily secretions of the sebaceous glands

D. a fluid-filled, thin-walled structure under the epidermis

E. contains histamine and may be related to allergic reactions

F. death of tissue due to insufficient supply of blood

G. a fungal infection of the skin

H. dark pigments occurring in the skin

I. a defined skin elevation with a rough surface that is caused by a localized virus

J. a yellow discoloration of the skin

Spelling

Circle the correct spelling from each pairing of words.

_____ 1. zeroderma   xeroderma

_____ 2. veruca   verruca

_____ 3. tinea   tenea

_____ 4. psoriasis   soriasis

_____ 5. pemfigus   pemphigus

_____ 6. nevus   nevos

_____ 7. pruritus   proritus

_____ 8. empetigo   impetigo

_____ 9. ecchymosis   eckymosis

_____ 10. melanocyte   melenosite

The Skeletal System

OBJECTIVES

Upon completion of this chapter, the reader should be able to:

1. Explain the main functions of the skeletal system.
2. Identify the bones of the human skeleton.
3. Describe common skeletal diseases.
4. Define, pronounce, and spell the diseases and disorders covered in this chapter.
5. Define common skeletal abbreviations.
6. Correctly spell and pronounce skeletal terms.
7. Recognize common pharmacological agents used in treating disorders of the skeletal system.
8. Describe the common types of drugs used for skeletal system conditions.

STRUCTURE AND FUNCTION OF THE SKELETAL SYSTEM

The **skeletal system** consists of the bony framework for the human body. Bones have many different functions:

- support body structures and provide shape for the body
- protect internal organs and tissues
- allow movement and points of attachment for muscles
- storage sites for minerals
- sites of blood cell formation

Bones

Bones differ greatly in size and shape, but are similar in their structure, how they develop, and how they function. Bones are classified as follows:

- **long bones** – long longitudinal axes, expanded ends (examples: forearm and thigh bones)
- **short bones** – cube-like, with lengths and widths nearly equal (examples: wrist bones)
- **flat bones** – plate-like, with broad surfaces (examples: ribs, scapulae, and some skull bones)
- **irregular bones** – variety of shapes, usually connected to other types of bones (examples: vertebrae and many facial bones)
- **sesamoid (round) bones** – usually small, nodular, and embedded within tendons near joints (example: kneecap and elbow bones)

Skeletal Structure of the Body

The skeleton is divided into two portions: the axial skeleton and the appendicular skeleton. There are a total of 206 bones in the body. The major bones of the skeleton are shown in Figure 4-1.

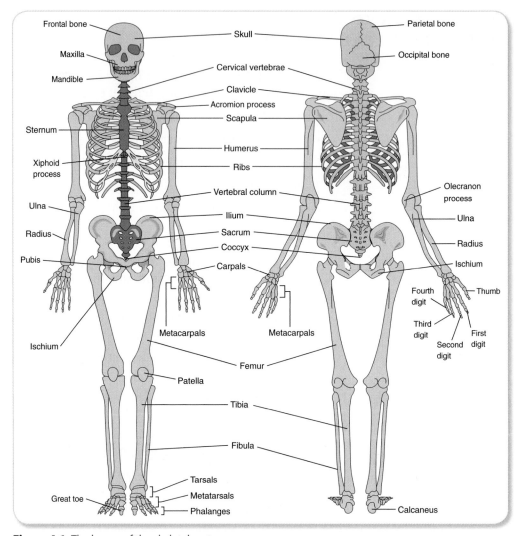

Figure 4-1 The bones of the skeletal system.

Axial skeleton	80 bones
Skull: *8 cranial bones:* frontal, parietal (2), occipital, temporal (2), sphenoid, ethmoid *14 facial bones:* maxilla (2), zygomatic (2), palatine (2), inferior nasal concha (2), mandible, lacrimal (2), nasal (2), vomer	22
Middle ear bones: malleus (2), incus (2), stapes (2)	6
Hyoid	1

Vertebral column: cervical vertebrae (7), thoracic vertebrae (12), lumbar vertebrae (5), sacrum, coccyx	26
Thoracic cage: ribs (24), sternum	25
Appendicular skeleton	**126 bones**
Pectoral girdle: scapula (2), clavicle (2)	4
Upper limbs: humerus (2), radius (2), ulna (2), carpal (16), metacarpal (10), phalanx (28)	60
Pelvic girdle: hips (2)	2
Lower limbs: femur (2), tibia (2), fibula (2), patella (2), tarsal (14), metatarsal (10), phalanx (28)	60
Entire body	**206**

Bones of the Skull

The human skull consists of 22 bones that, except for the lower jaw, are firmly interlocked along sutures (Figure 4-2). Eight of these bones make up the cranium. Fourteen bones form the facial area. The mandible (or lower jawbone) is movable.

The bones of the cranium, their pronunciations, and definitions are listed below.

ethmoid bone	ETH-moyd	lies just behind the nasal bone, in front of the *sphenoid bone*, and separates the nasal cavity from the brain
frontal bone	FRUN-tall	forms the forehead (front of the skull) and upper part of bony cavities that contain the eyeballs and nasal cavities; includes the frontal sinuses, just above where the frontal bone joins the nasal bones
occipital bone	ock-SIP-it-tall	forms the back of the head and base of the skull; contains the foramen magnum, which is a large opening through which the spinal cord passes
parietal bones	pah-REYE-eh-tall	form the sides and roof of the cranium
sphenoid bone	SFEE-noyd	located at the base of the skull in front of the temporal bones; anchors the frontal, parietal, occipital, temporal, and ethmoid bones, and forms part of the base of the eye orbits
temporal bones	TEM-por-all	two bones forming the lower sides and part of the cranium's base; contain the middle and inner ear structures and the mastoid sinuses, and are located immediately behind the external parts of the ear and project downward to form the **mastoid process**

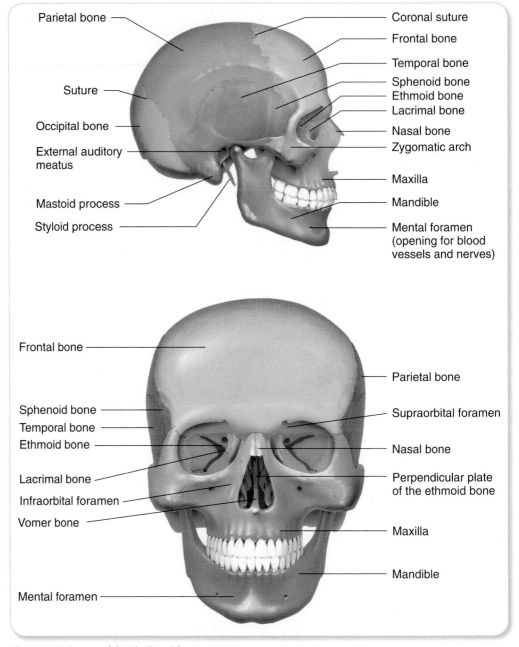

Figure 4-2 Bones of the skull and face.

The facial bones, their pronunciations, and definitions are listed below.

lacrimal bones	LACK-rim-all	two fragile bones resembling the shape of fingernails; located at the inner corner of each eye, and join the cheek bones to form the **fossa**, housing the tear (lacrimal) ducts
mandibular bone	man-DIB-yoo-lar	the lower jaw bone, also known as the **mandible**; the largest and strongest facial bone and the only movable bone of the skull; meets the temporal bone in a movable **temporomandibular joint (TMJ)** and contains tooth sockets along its upper margin
maxillary bones	MACK-sih-ler-ee	two bones also known as **maxillae**; the upper jaw bones, and also form the hard palate (the front part of the roof of the mouth)
nasal bones	NAY-zall	two oblong bones that form the "bridge" of the nose; meet at the face's midline and join the frontal bone, ethmoid bone, and the maxillae
nasal conchae	NAY-zall KONG-kee	long, curved, spongy bones that help to form the side and lower walls of the nasal cavity; connect with the maxillae, lacrimal, ethmoid, and palatine bones
palatine bones	PAL-ah-tine	bones in the palate that form the nasal cavity's rear sidewall as well as the back part of the roof of the mouth (hard palate)
vomer	VOH-mer	a thin, flat bone that forms the lower portion of the nasal septum and joins with the sphenoid, palatine, ethmoid, and maxillary bones
zygomatic bones	zeye-go-MAT-ik	the "cheek bones"; located on each side of the face, they form the high part of the cheek and the outer border of the eye orbits

Bones of the Spine

The **spine** or **vertebral column** extends from the skull to the pelvis. It forms the skeleton's vertical axis, and is made up of many bony sections called **vertebrae**, which are separated by intervertebral discs (Figure 4-3). The vertebral column supports the head and trunk, and protects the spinal cord.

cervical vertebrae	SIR-vih-kall VER-the-bray	the first segment of the vertebral column, consisting of the first 7 bones of the vertebral column, located immediately behind the skull
thoracic vertebrae	tho-RASS-ik	the next 12 vertebrae, progressing down the vertebral column; connect with the 12 pairs of ribs, and increase in size as they approach the lumbar vertebrae
lumbar vertebrae	LUM-bar	third segment consisting of the next 5 vertebrae, which are the largest parts of the movable section of the vertebral column; support the back and lower trunk of the body
sacrum	SAY-krum	fourth segment, a large, triangular bone (in adults); develops from 5 sacral bones that fuse upon reaching adulthood
coccyx	COCK-six	fifth segment (the *tailbone*) located at the very end of the vertebral column; in adults, it develops from the fusion of 4 individual coccygeal bones that exist during childhood

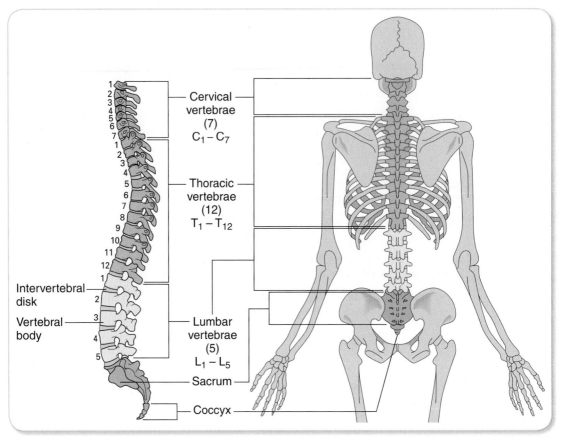

Figure 4-3 Bones of the spine.

The segments of the vertebral column, their pronunciations, and definitions are listed below. This table is listed in order from the neck to the sacrum, and not alphabetically.

Bones of the Thorax

The thoracic (chest) cavity is created by the ribs and sternum (Figure 4-4). The thoracic cage protects the organs of the thoracic cavity and the upper abdominal cavity. It is composed of 12 pairs of ribs, which are divided into **true ribs** (the first 7 ribs), **false ribs** (ribs 8 through 10), and **floating ribs** (ribs 11 and 12). The **sternum** (breastbone) is a long, flat bone in the center of the chest that is shaped slightly like a sword. It forms the midline portion of the front of the thorax.

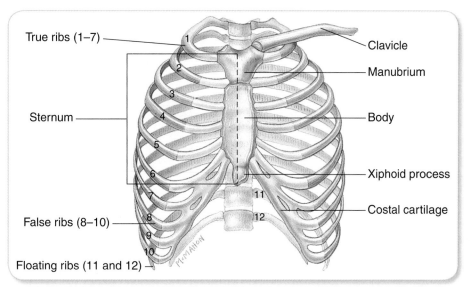

Figure 4-4 Bones of the thorax.

Bones of the Upper and Lower Extremities

The appendicular skeleton consists of the bones of the upper and lower extremities, and the bones that anchor the limbs to the axial skeleton. The bones of the upper extremities include the **scapula** (shoulder blade), which is a large, triangular bone that connects the humerus to the clavicle (Figure 4-5).

The bones of the upper limbs, their pronunciations, and definitions are listed below. These bones are listed in descending order as they are located in the body, not alphabetically.

humerus	HYOO-mer-us	the long upper arm bone, joining the scapula above and radius and ulna below
radius	RAY-dee-us	one of the two bones of the forearm, joining the humerus above and wrist bones below; on the lateral (thumb side) of the arm
ulna	UHL-nah	the second of the two bones of the forearm, joining the humerus above and wrist bones below; on the medial (little finger side) of the arm, and has a large projection at its end called the **olecranon process**, which forms the joint of the elbow
carpals	CAR-pals	the 8 wrist bones; each wrist has two rows of four bones each
metacarpals	met-ah-CAR-pals	the bones of the hand that join with the carpals (wrist bones) and the phalanges (finger bones)
phalanges	fah-LAN-jeez	the bones of the fingers; each finger has 3 of these bones except for the thumb, which has only 2 (this term also applies to the bones of the toes)

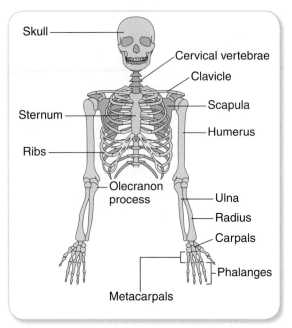

Figure 4-5 Bones of the upper extremities.

The **pelvis** is the bony structure at the base of the spine, formed by the hip bones (the ilium, ischium, and pubis), the sacrum, and the coccyx. It is shown in Figure 4-6.

The bones of the lower limbs are shown in Figure 4-7 and include those listed in the table.

The bones of the lower limbs, their pronunciations, and definitions are listed below. They are listed in descending order, not alphabetically.

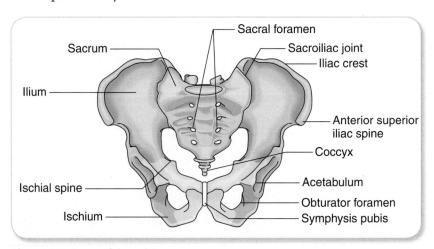

Figure 4-6 Bones of the pelvis.

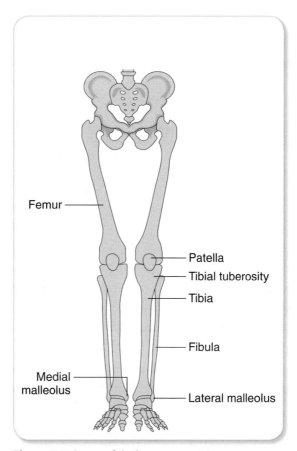

Figure 4-7 Bones of the lower extremities.

femur	FEE-mer	the thigh bone; the longest, strongest bone in the body; has a large rounded head and forms part of the hip as well as part of the knee
patella	pah-TELL-ah	the knee bone or *kneecap*; the largest sesamoid bone in the body, and covers and protects the knee joint
tibia	TIB-ee-ah	the larger and stronger of the 2 bones of the lower leg, between the ankle and knee; also called the **shin bone**
fibula	FIB-yoo-lah	the smaller and more slender of the 2 bones of the lower leg; also called the "calf bone"
tarsals	TAR-sals	the 7 bones of the ankle, the largest of which is the **calcaneous** (*heel bone*); the entire weight of the body is supported by the talus bone (found at the ankle joint)
metatarsals	met-ah-TAR-sals	the 5 long bones of the foot, which are very important for weight-bearing
phalanges	fah-LAN-jeez	the bones of the toes (this term also applies to the bones of the fingers); each toe has 3 phalangeal bones, except for the great toe, which has only 2

GENERAL TERMINOLOGY RELATED TO THE SKELETAL SYSTEM

The following vocabulary words are commonly used when discussing the skeletal system.

Word	Pronunciation	Definition
bone processes	—	projections or outgrowths of bones
cancellous bone	CAN-sell-us	spongy or "trabecular" bone; of low density and strength, but has a very high surface area
cervical vertebrae	SIR-vih-kal VER-teh-bray	vertebrae of the neck (C1 to C7); found immediately behind the skull
compact bone	—	hard, dense bone that is usually found at the periphery of skeletal structures, as distinguished from spongy bone
diaphysis	dye-AFF-ih-sis	main or middle shaft-like section of a bone
epiphyseal line	ep-ih-FIZZ-ee-all	an elevated ridge of cartilage separating the diaphysis from the epiphysis
epiphysis	eh-PIFF-ih-sis	the end of a long bone; has a bulb-like shape and provides space for muscles to be attached
false ribs	—	five lower ribs on either side of the ribcage that do not unite directly with the sternum
Fissure	FISH-er	a groove, cleft, or depression (*sulcus*) in a bone
flat bones	—	bones that are broad and thin, with curved or flat surfaces (flat bones are found in the skull, pelvis, sternum, ribcage, and scapula)
floating ribs	—	the two lower false ribs on either side of the ribcage that are not attached anteriorly; also known as "vertebral ribs"
fontanelle (or fontanel)	fon-tah-NELL	space between an infant's cranium bones; the "soft spot"
foramen	for-AY-men	hole in a bone where blood vessels or nerves pass through
Fossa	FOSS-ah	hollow or concave depression in bone
hematopoiesis	hem-ah-toh-poy-EE-sis	the formation of cellular components in the blood
long bones	—	bones that are longer rather than wider, with distinctively shaped ends, such as the femur; grow mostly by elongation of the diaphysis
lumbar vertebrae	LUM-bar VER-teh-bray	the lower back vertebrae (L1 to L5), which are the largest segments of the movable part of the vertebral column
medullary cavity	MED-u-lair-ee	the center cavity of a shaft of a long bone, containing the yellow marrow (adipose tissue)

ossification	oss-sih-fih-KAY-shun	the process of bone formation by conversion of cartilage and fibrous connective tissue
osteoblasts	OSS-tee-oh-blasts	immature bone cells, each with a single nucleus, that actively produce bone tissue
osteoclasts	OSS-tee-oh-clasts	large bone cells that absorb or digest older bone tissue
osteocytes	OSS-tee-oh-sites	star-shaped, mature bone cells, which are the most abundant type found in bone
periosteum	pair-ee-AH-stee-um	thick, white, fibrous membrane covering the surface of long bones
red bone marrow	—	soft, semi-fluid tissue found in the small spaces of cancellous bone; it is the source of blood cell production
sinus	SY-nuss	a cavity, opening, or hollow space within a bone or other body structures
thoracic vertebrae	tho-RASS-ik	the 12 chest vertebrae (T1 to T12), composing the middle section of the vertebral column
true ribs	—	the first 7 rib pairs located towards the top of the ribcage, connecting to the vertebrae in back and to the sternum in front
yellow bone marrow	—	marrow in the diaphysis of long bones composed mostly of fatty tissue
xiphoid process	ZY-foyd PRAW-ses	a small downward extension from the lower part of the sternum

PATHOLOGICAL CONDITIONS RELATED TO THE SKELETAL SYSTEM

Following are the disorders and conditions of the skeletal system.

Arthritis – an inflammation in a joint; the two most common types of arthritis are rheumatoid arthritis (which involves the immune system) and osteoarthritis

Fracture – a traumatic injury to a bone in which the continuity of the bone tissue is broken; there are various types of fractures:

- A **closed fracture** is a break with no open wound.

- A **comminuted fracture** occurs with more than two pieces. It may have significant associated soft tissue trauma.

- A **compound fracture** is when skin is broken over the fracture; also known as an *open fracture*.

- A **displaced fracture** is when one, both, or all fragments are out of normal alignment.
- A **greenstick fracture** is an incomplete break of a soft bone. It occurs primarily in children.
- An **impacted fracture** occurs with one end wedged into the opposite end, or inside the fractured fragment.
- An **oblique fracture** is at an oblique angle across the bone.
- A **pathologic fracture** occurs at the site of bone already damaged by disease.
- A **spiral fracture** is a fracture that curves around bone and may become displaced by twisting.
- A **stress fracture** is a crack in one cortex of bone.
- A **transverse fracture** occurs as a horizontal break through bone.

Gout – a metabolic disorder that causes excessive production of uric acid, depositing it in joints (often in the great toe); also known as "gouty arthritis"

Herniated disk – also called "spinal disk herniation"; occurs when an intervertebral disk is torn, allowing the soft material in its center to bulge out (Figure 4-8)

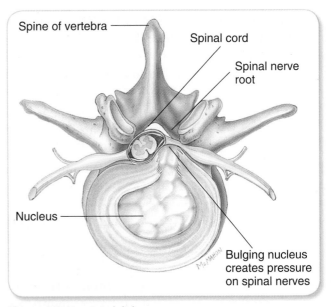

Figure 4-8 Herniated disk.

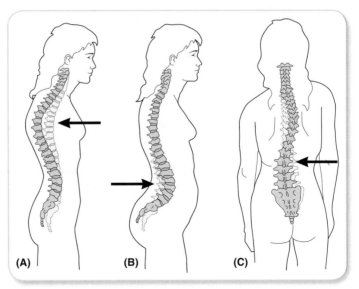

Figure 4-9 Abnormal curvature of the spine (a) kyphosis (b) lordosis (c) scoliosis.

Kyphosis – a hunched deformity of the back; common in patients with osteoporosis (Figure 4-9)

Lordosis – an inward, forward curvature known as "swayback" (Figure 4-9)

Lyme arthritis – joint inflammation caused by infection from the bite of a tick carrying *Borrelia burgdorferi*

Osteoarthritis – degenerative joint disease characterized by bone hypertrophy, and the deterioration of articular cartilage

Osteomalacia – softening of the bones due to defective bone mineralization, mostly due to deficiencies of calcium and phosphorus in the blood; results in fractures and deformities of weight-bearing bones, and is called "**rickets**" when it occurs in children

Osteomyelitis – a serious bone infection that requires aggressive antibiotic treatment, usually resulting from a bacterial infection that has spread through the blood to bone tissue

Osteoporosis – a bone disease involving loss of normal bone density that increases the risk of fracture; literally means "porous bones"

Scoliosis – a lateral (sideward) curvature either to the left or right (see Figure 4-9)

ABBREVIATIONS RELATED TO THE SKELETAL SYSTEM

The following are common abbreviations related to the skeletal system.

Abbreviation	Meaning
AP	anteroposterior
BMD	bone mineral density
CDH	congenital dislocation of the hip
C1 – C7	cervical vertebra 1 – 7
CT	computerized tomography
DIP	distal interphalangeal
fib	fibula
Fx	fracture
L1 – L5	lumbar vertebra 1 – 5
OA	osteoarthritis
PIP	proximal interphalangeal joints
RA	rheumatoid arthritis
S1 – S5	sacrum (the disc space between the last lumbar vertebra and the sacrum may be described as S1 – S5)
T1 – T12	thoracic vertebra 1 – 12
THR	total hip replacement
TKR	total knee replacement
TMJ	temporomandibular joint

MEDICATIONS USED TO TREAT SKELETAL SYSTEM DISORDERS

The following are common medications used for the skeletal system.

Drug Class	Generic Name	Pronunciation for Generic Name	Trade Name	Use
analgesic (NSAIDs are also analgesics)	acetaminophen (paracetamol)	ah-see-tah-MIN-oh-fen (pah-ra-SEE-ta-mall)	Tylenol®, Anacin-3®, etc.	to relieve pain
	aspirin	AS-pih-rin (or AS-prin)	Bayer®, Excedrin®, etc.	
anti-inflammatory (corticosteroids) (aspirin and NSAIDs also reduce inflammation)	prednisone	PRED-nih-zoan	Cortan®, Deltasone®, etc.	to reduce inflammation
nonsteroidal anti-inflammatory drugs (NSAIDs)	ibuprofen	eye-byoo-PRO-fen	Advil®, Motrin®, etc.	to reduce inflammation, but these are not steroids
	ketorolac, tromethamine	keh-TOR-oh-lak, tro-METH-ah-meen	Toradol® (IV)	
	nabutemone	nah-BYOO-teh-moan	Relafen®, Relifex®, etc.	
	naproxen	nah-PROK-sen	Naproxyn®, Aleve®, etc.	

DRUG TERMINOLOGY

The following are common types of drugs used to treat skeletal conditions.

Drug	Pronunciation	Definition
analgesic	an-al-JEE-zik	agent that relieves pain
anti-inflammatory (corticosteroid)	kor-tih-koh-STAIR-oyd	agent that reduces inflammation
muscle relaxant	MUS-sel ree-LAK-sent	agent that relieves muscle stiffness
narcotic	nar-KOT-ik	agent that relieves pain by affecting the body in ways that are similar to opium
nonsteroidal anti-inflammatory drug (NSAID)	non-stair-OY-dal	agent that reduces inflammation without the use of steroids

REVIEW EXERCISES

Multiple Choice

Select the best answer and write the letter of your choice to the left of each number.

1. A disease in which the bones become abnormally soft due to deficiencies of calcium and phosphorus in the blood is known as:

   A. osteoporosis
   B. osteomalacia
   C. osteomyelitis
   D. Ewing's sarcoma

2. Bones that are longer than they are wide, with distinctively shaped ends (such as the femur) are known as:

   A. compact bones
   B. sesamoid bones
   C. short bones
   D. long bones

3. A long, flat bone located in the center of the chest (thorax) that connects to the rib bones is known as the:

   A. sesamoid
   B. sternum
   C. vomer
   D. scapula

4. Which of the skull bones is movable?

   A. zygomatic
   B. vomer
   C. mandible
   D. maxillae

5. A disease characterized by bones becoming fragile (due to loss of bone density) is called:

   A. osteomalacia
   B. osteoporosis
   C. osteomyelitis
   D. osteochondroma

6. The medical term for an extreme outward curvature of the upper spine (commonly known as "humpback" or "hunchback") is:

   A. scoliosis
   B. lordosis

    C. kyphosis

    D. osteochondroma

7. The medical term for an inward, forward curvature of the lumbar part of the spine (commonly known as "swayback") is:

    A. osteochondroma

    B. kyphosis

    C. lordosis

    D. scoliosis

8. The medical term for an abnormal sideward (lateral) curvature of part of the spine to the left or right is:

    A. lordosis

    B. scoliosis

    C. kyphosis

    D. osteochondroma

9. An elevated ridge of cartilage separating the diaphysis from the epiphysis is known as the:

    A. epiphyseal line

    B. intervertebral disc

    C. crest

    D. cancellous bone

10. A hole in a bone through which blood vessels or nerves pass is known as a:

    A. fissure

    B. fontanel

    C. fossa

    D. foramen

11. Which of the following terms refers to the shaft of a long bone?

    A. epiphysis

    B. metaphysic

    C. diaphysis

    D. sulcus

12. The two divisions of the skeleton are appendicular and _____.

    A. cranial

    B. thoracic

    C. vertebral

    D. axial

13. Which of the following is not a function of the skeletal system?

    A. hemopoiesis
    B. protection
    C. hormone secretion
    D. body movement

Fill in the Blank

Use your knowledge of medical terminology to insert the correct term from the list below into the appropriate statement.

femur	fibula	carpal
patella	ulna	scapula
humerus	conchae	tibia
coccyx	sphenoid	diaphysis
vomer	zygomatic	osteoblast

1. The _____ is an immature bone cell.

2. The shin bone is also called the _____.

3. The longest, strongest bone in the body is the _____.

4. The largest sesamoid bone in the body is the _____.

5. The _____ joins the humerus above and wrist bones below.

6. The _____ joins the scapula above and the radius and ulna below.

7. The tailbone is also called the _____.

8. A thin, flat bone that forms the lower portion of the nasal septum is referred to as the _____.

9. The _____ is a large, triangular bone that connects the humerus to the clavicle.

10. The _____ is a long, curved, spongy bone that helps to form the side and lower walls of the nasal cavity.

Labeling the Skull

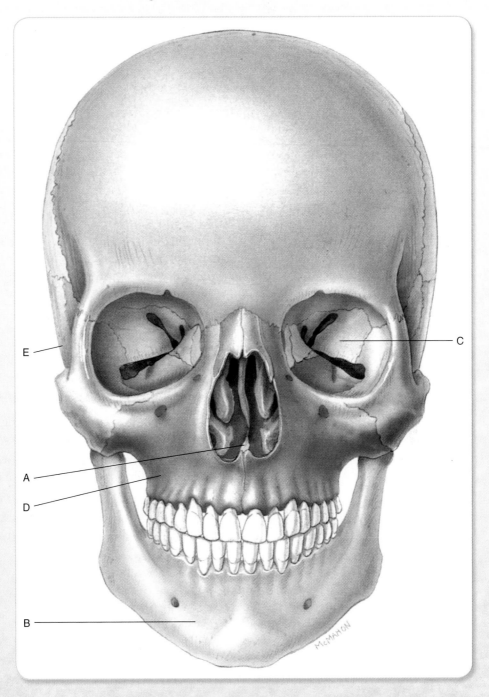

Write in the sections of the skull that correspond with each letter on the figure above.

A. _____

B. _____

C. _____

D. _____

E. _____

True / False

Identify each of the following statements as true or false by placing a "T" or "F" on the line beside each number.

_____ 1. The nasal bones form the "bridge" of the nose.

_____ 2. The two fragile nasal bones that resemble the shape of fingernails are referred to as "nasal conchae."

_____ 3. Joint inflammation as a result of the bite of a tick may cause osteomalacia.

_____ 4. An inward, forward curvature of the spine is known as "humpback."

_____ 5. The fibrous membrane covering the surface of long bones is called the *periosteum.*

_____ 6. Osteoporosis is a serious bone infection that requires aggressive antibiotic treatment.

_____ 7. Corticosteroids are used to reduce inflammation.

_____ 8. An agent that relieves pain by affecting the body in ways similar to opium is called a *narcotic.*

_____ 9. The process of bone formation by conversion of cartilage and fibrous connective tissue is referred to as *ossification.*

_____10. The two upper, false ribs on either side of the ribcage that are not attached anteriorly are known as floating ribs.

Labeling – The Anterior View of the Ribs, Shoulder, and Arm

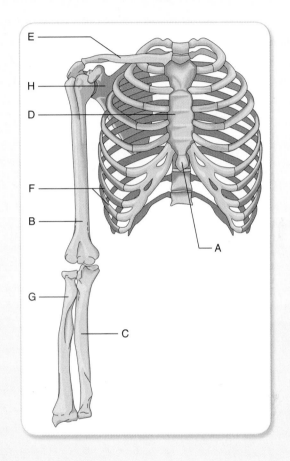

Write in the sections below that correspond with each letter on the figure above.

A. _____

B. _____

C. _____

D. _____

E. _____

F. _____

G. _____

H. _____

Definitions

Define each of the following words or phrases in one sentence.

1. long bone: _____

2. axial skeleton: _____

3. middle ear bones: _____

4. parietal bone: _____

5. nonsteroidal anti-inflammatory drug (NSAID): _____

6. false ribs: _____

7. osteoblasts: _____

8. sinus: _____

9. kyphosis: _____

10. osteomalacia: _____

Abbreviations

Write the full meaning of each abbreviation.

Abbreviation	Meaning
1. Fx	_____
2. THR	_____
3. TMJ	_____
4. L1 – L5	_____
5. T1 – T12	_____
6. CT	_____
7. ERT	_____
8. OA	_____
9. RA	_____
10. C1 – C7	_____

Matching–Terms and Definitions

Match the following terms with their definitions by placing the correct letter on the line to the left of each number.

_____ 1. bone processes

_____ 2. fissure

_____ 3. epiphysis

_____ 4. foramen

_____ 5. hematopoiesis

_____ 6. fontanelle

_____ 7. sinus

_____ 8. red bone marrow

_____ 9. yellow bone marrow

_____ 10. epiphyseal line

A. an elevated ridge of cartilage separating the diaphysis from the epiphysis

B. composed mostly of fatty tissue

C. a cavity or hollow space

D. the formation of cellular components in blood

E. space between an infant's cranial bones

F. hole in a bone where blood vessels or nerves pass through

G. the end of a long bone

H. the source of blood cell production

I. projections or outgrowths of bones

J. a groove, cleft, or depression in a bone

Spelling

Circle the correct spelling from each pairing of words.

1. osteoporosis   osteopurosis

2. artthritis   arthritis

3. osteomalasia   osteomalacia

4. scoliosis   skoliosis

5. analgasic   analgesic

6. zygumatic bone   zygomatic bone

7. sesamoid bone   sessamoid bone

8. hyoeid bone   hyoid bone

9. vertebrae   vertebrea

10. fisurre   fissure

The Muscular System and Joints

OBJECTIVES

Upon completion of this chapter, the reader should be able to:

1. Compare the location and function of skeletal, smooth, and cardiac muscle.

2. List major muscles of the trunk and upper extremities.

3. Describe the main disorders that affect muscles.

4. Identify at least 10 abbreviations common to muscles and joints.

5. List four names of major muscles of the head and neck.

6. Explain how muscles work together to produce movement.

7. Describe the major muscles of the lower extremities.

8. Recognize common pharmacological agents used in treating disorders of the muscular system.

STRUCTURE AND FUNCTION OF THE MUSCULAR SYSTEM

The primary organs of the muscular system are the muscles. There are three types of muscles—skeletal muscle, smooth muscle, and cardiac muscle. The main functions of the muscular system are:

- to allow body movement
- to provide form and shape to the body
- to maintain body temperature by generating heat

Skeletal Muscle

Skeletal muscles are also called **voluntary muscles** because they are consciously controlled. The bony framework of the skeleton provides points of attachment for the muscles. Skeletal muscles often work in pairs, using **contraction** and **relaxation** to coordinate movement. Skeletal muscle is striated, and contractions are rapid and forceful. About 40 percent of an individual's weight is attributed to muscle mass in average adults.

Smooth Muscle

Smooth muscles are also known as visceral muscles, and are found in the stomach, respiratory system, blood vessels, and intestines. Smooth muscle doesn't attach to bones. The contraction of smooth muscles (**involuntary muscles**) is unconscious and is regulated by the autonomic nervous system. Smooth muscle is not striated, and contraction is rhythmic and slow.

Cardiac Muscle

Cardiac muscle is found only in the heart, and it controls the heart's contractions. It is the only involuntary muscle that is also striated.

MUSCLES OF THE HEAD AND NECK

The important muscles of the head and neck are listed in Table 5-1 and are also shown in Figure 5-1.

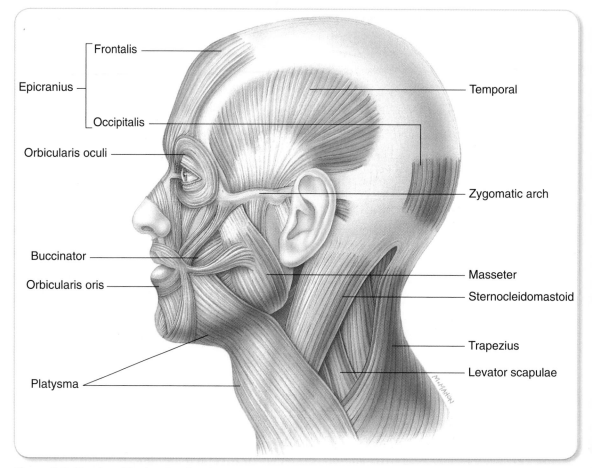

Figure 5-1 Muscles of the head and neck.

TABLE 5-1 Muscles of the Head and Neck

buccinator	BUCK-sin-ay-tor	a thin muscle located between the maxilla and mandible on each side of the face
masseter	mass-SEE-ter	used for chewing, this muscle is located at the angle of the jaw
orbicularis oculi	or-BIH-kyoo-lah-rus AW-kyoo-lie	located around the eyes
orbicularis oris	or-BIH-kyoo-lah-rus OH-ris	located around the mouth
sternomastoid	stir-no-MASS-toyd	also known as the *sternocleidomastoid*, this muscle flexes and rotates the head; it is located in the anterior portion of each side of the neck
temporalis	tem-ph-RAL-is	used for chewing, this muscle links the mandible to the temple on each side of the face

MUSCLES OF THE TRUNK AND UPPER EXTREMITIES

The **trunk** (or **torso**) is the main part of the body. Torso muscles include the **diaphragm**, as well as the muscles of the abdomen and perineum. The important muscles of the trunk and upper extremities are listed in Table 5-2 and are also shown in Figure 5-2.

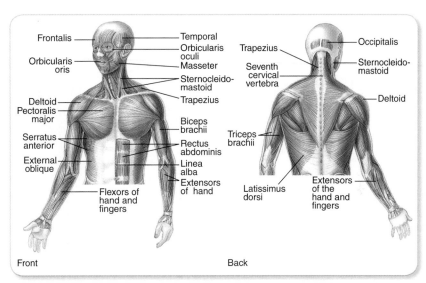

Figure 5-2 Muscles of the upper extremities.

TABLE 5-2   Muscles of the Trunk and Upper Extremities

biceps brachii	BYE-seps BRAY-kee-eye	located on the upper arm; important in the movements of the elbow and forearm
deltoid	DELL-toyd	located above and controls movements of the shoulder
diaphragm	DYE-uh-fram	also known as the "thoracic diaphragm"; extends across the bottom of the ribcage and is crucial for breathing and respiration
flexor carpi	FLEK-sor KAR-pee	a group of muscles located along the anterior surface of the forearm
latissimus dorsi	lah-TIS-ih-mus DOR-sigh	large, flat muscle of the trunk stretching from the armpit to just above the gluteus; responsible for shoulder and lumbar spine movements
pectoralis major	peck-toh-RAY-lis MAY-jor	commonly referred to as "pecs"; located at the upper front of the chest wall and controls movements of the arm
serratus anterior	seh-RAH-tus an-TEE-ree-or	a thin muscle of the chest wall extending from the ribs under the arm to the scapula
teres minor	TEH-res MY-nor	a cylindric, elongated muscle of the shoulder
trapezius	trah-PEE-zee-us	extends from the occipital bone to the lower thoracic vertebrae, and supports the upper arm and shoulder
triceps brachii	TRY-seps BRAY-kee-eye	located posteriorly in the upper arm; mostly controls movements of the elbow

MUSCLES OF THE LOWER EXTREMITIES

The important muscles of the lower extremities are listed in Table 5-3 and are also shown in Figure 5-3.

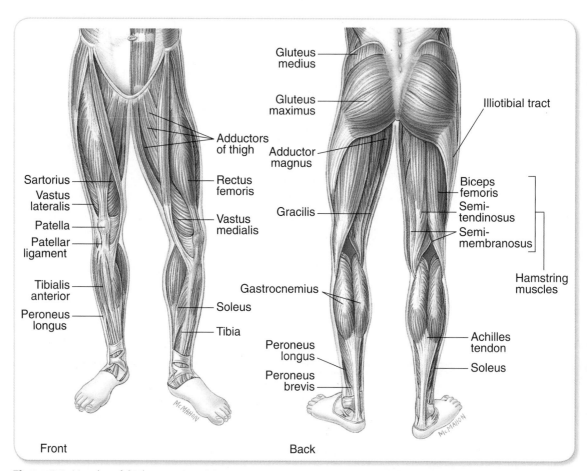

Figure 5-3 Muscles of the lower extremities.

TABLE 5-3   Muscles of the Lower Extremities

gastrocnemius	gas-trok-NEE-mee-us	located in the calf of the leg and is important for all movements of the leg
gluteus maximus	GLOO-tee-us MACKS-ih-mus	the largest of the three gluteus muscles; important in maintaining erect posture of the torso
gluteus medius	GLOO-tee-us MEE-dee-us	located on the outer surface of the pelvis; assists in movements of the thigh and hip

hamstring	HAM-string	tendons behind the knee and near the posterior part of the femur; primarily acts in movements of the knee and hip
quadriceps femoris	KWAHD-drih-seps FEM-or-iss	subdivided into four smaller muscles on the front of the thigh; together, they act in movements of the knee, hip, and leg
rectus femoris	REK-tus FEH-moh-ris	a fusiform muscle of the anterior thigh; one of the four parts of the quadriceps femoris
sartorius	sar-TOH-ree-us	the longest muscle in the body, extending from the pelvis to the calf of the leg
tibialis anterior	tib-ee-AY-lis an-TEER-ee-or	located in the shin of the leg; important for movements of the ankle and foot
vastus lateralis	VAS-tus lah-teh-RAH-lis	the largest of the four muscles of the quadriceps femoris group, situated on the lateral side of the thigh

JOINTS

The place where two or more bones come together is called a **joint**. Most joints are constructed so that movement of both bones is possible. Joints are classified by their structure or function. Types of joints include fibrous, cartilaginous, and synovial joints. Muscle contractions and the range of motion of the body's joints allows for many different types of body movements.

GENERAL TERMINOLOGY RELATED TO THE MUSCULAR SYSTEM AND JOINTS

The following terms are used in discussing the muscular system.

Term	Pronunciation	Definition
abduction	ab-DUCK-shun	movement away from the median plane of the body; the opposite of adduction
adduction	ad-DUCK-shun	movement toward the median plane of the body; the opposite of abduction
articular cartilage	ar-TIK-yoo-lar CAR-tih-laj	also known as *hyaline cartilage*; dense, white, connective tissue that covers all freely moveable joints in the body
articulation (joint)	ar-tik-yoo-LAY-shun (JOYNT)	where several bones come together; there are three types of joints: immovable, slightly moveable, and freely moveable

(continues)

Term	Pronunciation	Definition
circumduction	sir-kum-DUK-shun	movement of a limb in a circular manner; true circumduction can only occur at ball-and-socket joints (the hip and shoulder)
contraction	con-TRACK-shun	the generation of tension in a muscle that may lengthen or shorten the muscle, though shortening or reduction is usually implied
contracture	con-TRACK-cher	shortening of a muscle or tendon in response to stress
dislocation	dis-loh-KAY-shun	movement of a joint out of its normal position as a result of an injury
dorsiflexion	dor-see-FLEK-shun	an ankle movement involving the flexing of the foot towards the leg; the opposite of plantarflexion
extension	eks-TEN-shun	a movement of a joint that increases the angle between the bones of (usually) a limb; for example, straightening of the arm is produced by extending the elbow
fascia	FASH-ee-ah	soft tissue throughout the body that interpenetrates and surrounds bones, muscles, nerves, organs, vessels, and other structures
flexion	FLEK-shun	the opposite of extension; a movement of a joint that decreases the angle between the bones of (usually) a limb
insertion	in-SIR-shun	the point of attachment of a ligament or tendon onto the skeleton or another body part
involuntary muscle	in-VOL-un-tair-ree	smooth muscle that is not consciously controllable; for example, the pupil of the eye is controlled by involuntary muscle
ligaments	LIG-ah-ments	fibrous tissues that connect bones to other bones, composed of long, stringy fibers of collagen
muscle fiber	—	contractile tissue of the body that is labeled individually based on its location and function
origin	OR-ih-jin	the point at which a muscle attaches to a bone or another muscle that is less movable
plantarflexion	plan-tar-FLEK-shun	a movement that increases the angle between the foot and the leg, which occurs at the ankle; the opposite of "dorsiflexion"
pronation	proh-NAY-shun	a rotation movement, such as the turning of the palm of the hand downward or backward
rotation	roh-TAY-shun	movement in a circular motion; for example, rotating the neck and head to reduce stress on the neck muscles
skeletal muscle	SKELL-eh-tal	a type of striated muscle, usually attached to the skeleton, that voluntarily creates movement
smooth muscle	—	non-striated, involuntary muscle found in the tunica media of vessels, bladder, uterus, GI tract, respiratory tract, kidneys, and eyes
spasm	SPAH-zum	sudden, involuntary muscle contraction

striated muscle	STRY-ay-ted	skeletal or cardiac muscle that appears striped; it is formed from separate, parallel fibers
supination	soo-pin-AY-shun	rotation of a body part that turns it upward or forward, such as when the palm faces the front of the body
tendon	TEN-dun	a sinew; a tough band of fibrous tissue usually connecting muscles to bones
trunk	TRUNK	the torso; the main part of the body, extending from the neck down to the genitals, including the thorax and abdomen
voluntary muscle	VOL-un-tair-ee	muscle that may be consciously controlled, usually striated; includes skeletal muscles and those in the eyes, face, mouth, and throat

PATHOLOGICAL CONDITIONS OF THE MUSCULAR SYSTEM AND JOINTS

Muscular and joint diseases and disorders may occur at any age, and may be experienced throughout life. Some of these diseases and disorders are chronic and may require medications, treatments, or surgery to correct them.

Ankylosing spondylitis – a chronic form of arthritis affecting the vertebral column and causing spinal deformities and fusion, believed to be of genetic cause

Arthralgia – joint pain, generally without joint inflammation (the term "arthritis" is used when there is inflammation)

Arthritis – a group of damaging inflammatory joint conditions caused by trauma, infection, or aging

Asthenia – weakness

Ataxia – lack of muscle coordination

Atrophy – a decrease in the size of a tissue or organ; also, the partial or complete wasting away of a body part

Bunion (hallux valgus) – an abnormal enlargement of the joint at the base of the great toe that causes structural deformity (Figure 5-4)

Dislocation – displacement of a bone from its normal location within a joint, often caused by a sudden impact, that results in loss of joint function

Dystonia – abnormal tone in tissues

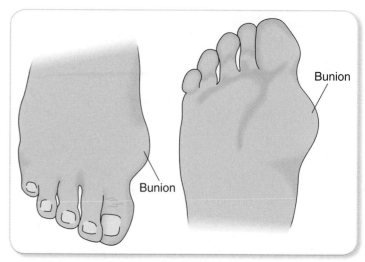

Figure 5-4 Bunion.

Ganglion cyst – a cystic tumor developing on a tendon, near a joint; a common site of ganglion cyst is the wrist (Figure 5-5)

Hypertrophy – abnormal increase, as in muscle size

Hypotonia – abnormally reduced muscle tension

Leiomyoma – a benign tumor of smooth muscle

Leiomyosarcoma – a malignant tumor of smooth muscle

Malaise – general discomfort or a feeling of uneasiness; often the first indication of disease

Muscular dystrophy – a group of genetic, hereditary muscle diseases causing progressive muscle weakness; most types of MD can affect the entire body eventually, often beginning in childhood

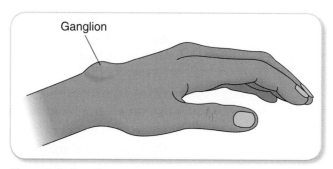

Figure 5-5 Ganglion.

Myalgia – muscle pain

Osteoarthritis – also known as "degenerative arthritis;" caused by the breakdown of cartilage in the joints; the most common form of arthritis, affecting more than 20 million people in the U.S. (Figure 5-6)

Polymyositis – a type of inflammatory muscle disease that affects many different muscles, with progressively weakening effects

Rhabdomyoma – a benign tumor in striated muscle

Rheumatoid arthritis – a chronic, systemic autoimmune disorder that attacks the joints, causing inflammation (of mainly the small joints), and can also harm the lungs and skin; it can become completely disabling (Figure 5-7)

Sciatica – inflammation of the sciatic nerve, causing a set of symptoms, including pain commonly felt on one side of the body, radiating through the lower back, buttock, leg, and foot

Sprains – injuries to ligaments caused by overstretching; if the sprain involves tearing of the ligament, immobilization and surgery may be required

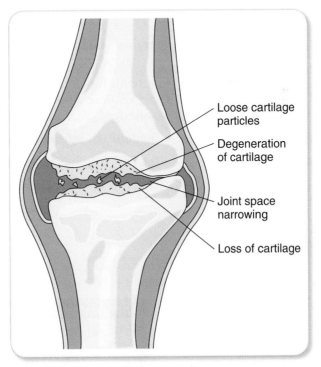

Figure 5-6 Osteoarthritis (knee joint).

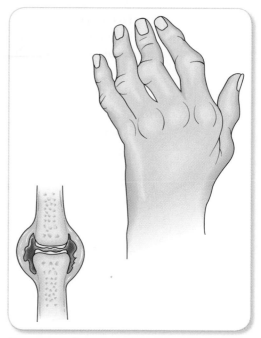

Figure 5-7 Rheumatoid arthritis.

Strains – injuries to muscles that involve muscular tearing, also known as "pulled muscles"

Systemic lupus erythematosus – also known as "SLE" or "lupus," this chronic autoimmune disease can be fatal; it attacks the tissues and cells, resulting in tissue damage and inflammation

Tendonitis – inflammation of a tendon

Tetany – painfully long muscle contraction

Tremor – abnormal, repetitive muscle contractions

ABBREVIATIONS

The following are common abbreviations related to the muscular system.

Abbreviation	Meaning
CTS	carpal tunnel syndrome
DJD	degenerative joint disease
DTR	deep tendon reflexes
EMG	electromyography

LLE	left lower extremity
LUE	left upper extremity
MCP	metacarpophalangeal (joint)
MD	muscular dystrophy
MTP	metatarsophalangeal (joint)
PIP	proximal interphalangeal (joint)
RA	rheumatoid arthritis
RF	rheumatoid factor
RLE	right lower extremity
ROM	range of motion
RUE	right upper extremity
SLE	systemic lupus erythematosus

MEDICATIONS USED TO TREAT MUSCULAR SYSTEM DISORDERS

The following medications are commonly used for muscular system disorders.

Drug Class	Generic Name	Pronunciation For Generic Name	Trade Name	Use
analgesics	acetaminophen	ah-see-toh-MIN-oh-fen	Tylenol	to relieve pain
	codeine	KOH-deen	(various)	
	hydrocodone	hi-droh-KOH-doan	Vicodin®	
	meperidine	meh-PAIR-ih-deen	Demerol®	
	morphine	MOR-feen	(various)	
	oxycodone	ok-see-KOH-doan	(various)	
anti-inflammatories	aspirin	ASS-pir-in	(various)	to counteract or suppress inflammation
	celecoxib	seh-leh-KOK-sib	Celebrex®	
	ibuprofen	eye-byoo-PRO-fen	Motrin	
	indomethacin	in-doh-METH-ah-sin	Indocin®	
	naproxen sodium	nah-PROK-sen SOH-dee-um	Anaprox®, Aleve	
corticosteroids	cortisone	KOR-tih-zoan	(various)	to alleviate or decrease inflammation
	hydrocortisone	hi-droh-KOR-tih-zoan	Cortef®, Hydrocortone®	
	prednisone	PRED-nih-zoan	(various)	
muscle relaxants	chlorzoxazone	klor-ZOK-zah-zoan	Paraflex®, Remular®	to lessen muscle tension
	cyclobenzaprine	sy-klo-BEN-zah-preen	Flexeril®	
	diazepam	dy-AZ-eh-pam	Valium®	

DRUG TERMINOLOGY

The following are common types of drugs used for muscular system conditions.

Word	Pronunciation	Definition
analgesic	an-al-JEE-zik	a medicine that relieves pain
anti-inflammatory	AN-ti-in-FLAH-mah-tor-ree	a medicine that prevents or reduces inflammation
corticosteroid	kor-tih-koh-STAIR-oyd	any of a variety of steroid hormones that prevents or relieves inflammation
muscle relaxant	MUS-sel ree-LAK-sent	a medicine that affects skeletal muscle function and decreases muscle tone

REVIEW EXERCISES

Multiple Choice

Select the best answer and write the letter of your choice to the left of each number.

1. Which of the following muscles is used for chewing?

   A. trapezius
   B. torso
   C. masseter
   D. buccinator

2. Which of the following muscles is located at the upper front of the chest wall?

   A. diaphragm
   B. deltoid
   C. trapezius
   D. pectoralis

3. A movement of a joint that increases the angle between the bones of a limb is referred to as:

   A. flexion
   B. insertion
   C. extension
   D. rotation

4. A tough band of fibrous tissue usually connecting muscles to bones is called a(n):

   A. origin
   B. ligament
   C. fascia
   D. tendon

5. A cystic tumor developing on a tendon is called:

   A. cancer
   B. ganglion cyst
   C. atrophy
   D. herniated cyst

6. A group of genetic, hereditary muscle diseases causing progressive muscle weakness is referred to as:

   A. muscular atrophy
   B. muscular hypertrophy
   C. muscular dystrophy
   D. myasthenia gravis

7. Injuries to ligaments caused by overstretching are known as:

   A. strains
   B. sprains
   C. spondylitis
   D. spondylosis

8. Which of the following are also known as *visceral muscles*?

   A. cardiac
   B. voluntary
   C. skeletal
   D. smooth

9. Which of the following muscles is crucial for breathing and respiration?

   A. pectoralis major
   B. trapezius
   C. latissimus dorsi
   D. diaphragm

10. Which of the following muscles primarily acts to move the knee and hip?

    A. hamstring
    B. quadriceps femoris
    C. tibialis anterior
    D. sternomastoid

11. An abnormal enlargement of the joint at the base of the great toe that causes structural deformity is referred to as a(n):

    A. ganglion cyst
    B. pronation
    C. bunion
    D. adduction

12. Which of the following terms means "movement that decreases the angle between the foot and the leg, which occurs at the ankle"?

    A. circumduction
    B. adduction
    C. pronation
    D. dorsiflexion

13. Which of the following medications may decrease muscle tone?

    A. muscle relaxants
    B. analgesics
    C. antibiotics
    D. antihistamines

14. The partial or complete wasting away of a body part is referred to as:

    A. hypertrophy
    B. adduction
    C. articulation
    D. atrophy

15. Which of the following muscles is important for movements of the ankle and foot?

    A. hamstring
    B. gluteus medius
    C. tibialis anterior
    D. gluteus maximus

Fill in the Blank

Use your knowledge of medical terminology to insert the correct term from the list below.

dorsiflexion	pronation	fascia
arthralgia	ataxia	ligament
origin	asthenia	tendon
sciatica	strains	adduction
supination	insertion	contraction

1. A soft tissue throughout the body that interpenetrates and surrounds muscles, organs, and other structures is known as _____.

2. Lack of muscle coordination is referred to as _____.

3. A term generally used when there is no joint inflammation that means "joint pain" is _____.

4. A movement of the ankle involving the flexing of the foot towards the leg is known as _____.

5. A rotation movement is called _____.

6. Rotation of a body part that turns it upward or forward is known as _____.

7. The point of attachment of a ligament or tendon onto the bones is called _____.

8. Injuries to muscles that involve muscular tearing are referred to as _____.

9. Movement toward the median plane of the body is called _____.

10. The point at which a muscle attaches to a bone or another muscle that is less movable is known as the _____.

Labeling – Superficial Muscles of the Body (Anterior View)

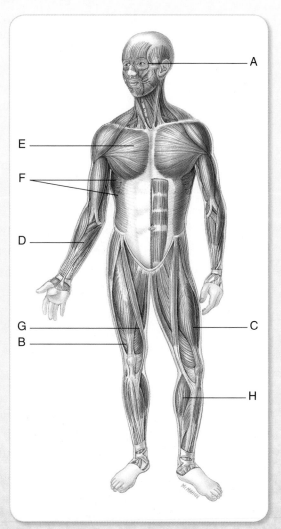

Write in the name of the muscle below that corresponds with each letter on the figure above.

A. _____

B. _____

C. _____

D. _____

E. _____

F. _____

G. _____

H. _____

True / False

Identify each of the following questions as true or false by placing a "T" or "F" beside each number.

_____ 1. Asthenia is a chronic form of arthritis affecting the vertebral column that causes spinal deformities and fusion.

_____ 2. Dislocation is the displacement of a bone from its normal location within a joint.

_____ 3. A herniated disk is also called "spinal disk herniation."

_____ 4. Rheumatoid arthritis causes inflammation of large joints.

_____ 5. Lupus is a chronic disease caused by excessive uric acid in the serum.

_____ 6. A bunion is an abnormal enlargement of the joint bone of the great toe.

_____ 7. The gluteus medius is the largest of the three gluteus muscles.

_____ 8. The deltoid muscle is located in the calf of the leg.

_____ 9. The diaphragm is the muscle that extends across the bottom of the ribcage.

_____ 10. The temporalis muscles are used for chewing.

Labeling – Superficial Muscles of the Body (Posterior View)

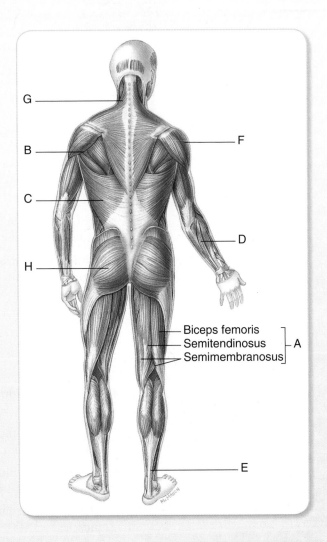

Write in the muscle name below that corresponds with each letter on the figure above.

A. _____

B. _____

C. _____

D. _____

E. _____

F. _____

G. _____

H. _____

Definitions

Define each of the following words in one sentence.

1. flexion: _____

2. contracture: _____

3. arthralgia: _____

4. trunk: _____

5. supination: _____

6. rotation: _____

7. muscle fiber: _____

8. ligament: _____

9. malaise: _____

10. striated muscle: _____

Abbreviations

Write the full meaning of each abbreviation.

Abbreviation	Meaning
1. SLE	_____
2. RA	_____
3. MD	_____
4. EMG	_____
5. RF	_____
6. DTR	_____
7. MTP	_____
8. LUE	_____
9. MCP	_____
10. RLE	_____

Matching – Terms and Definitions

Match the following terms with their definitions by placing the correct letter on the line to the left of each number.

_____ 1. triceps brachii

_____ 2. quadriceps femoris

_____ 3. sternocleidomastoid

_____ 4. buccinator

_____ 5. latissimus dorsi

_____ 6. voluntary muscle

_____ 7. ligament

_____ 8. involuntary muscle

_____ 9. tendon

_____ 10. origin

A. the point at which a muscle attaches to a bone or another muscle, and is less movable

B. a tough band of fibrous tissue

C. fibrous tissues that connect bones to other bones

D. located between the maxilla and mandible on each side of the face

E. flexes and rotates the head

F. located posteriorly in the upper arm

G. muscle that may be consciously controlled

H. flat muscle of the trunk that stretches from the armpit to just above the gluteus

I. located on the front of the thigh

J. also called "smooth muscle"

Spelling

Circle the correct spelling from each pairing of words.

1. tremar   tremor
2. dystrophy   distrophy
3. gangleon   ganglion
4. lyomyoma   leiomyoma
5. ataxia   atacia
6. sciateca   sciatica
7. asthenia   asthonia
8. supenation   supination
9. fascia   fastia
10. myaljia   myalgia

CHAPTER

6

The Sensory System

OBJECTIVES

Upon completion of this chapter, the reader should be able to:

1. Identify the major structures of the eyes.
2. Describe the functions of the eyes and ears.
3. Define, pronounce, and spell the diseases and disorders of the eyes and ears.
4. Identify the major structures of the ears.
5. Recognize common pharmacological agents used in treating disorders of the eyes and ears.
6. Describe the common types of drugs used for the eyes.
7. Interpret abbreviations used in the study of the eyes and the ears.
8. Describe the main disorders pertaining to the eyes and the ears.

Structure and Function of the Sensory System

The sensory system consists of the organs that allow sensations of touch, vision, hearing, smell, and taste. These senses receive stimuli from sensory receptors and transmit these impulses to the brain for interpretation. This chapter focuses specifically on the eye (vision) and the ear (hearing).

The Eye

The eyes are the organs of vision (or *sight*). The eye is housed in and protected by a bony socket, or **orbit**. Each eye orbit is lined with bone and contains blood vessels, connective tissue, fat, and nerves. The eyes are also protected by the **eyelids**, made up of conjunctiva, connective tissue, muscle, and very thin skin. The white portion of the eye is known as the **sclera**, an opaque structure that maintains the shape of the eyeball and also protects it. The **iris** is a muscular ring that controls the size of the **pupil**, which is the light-conducting opening at the center of the iris. The iris is most commonly known as the "colored portion" of the eye, lying between the cornea and lens. When the iris contracts or relaxes, it regulates the pupil's diameter. The transparent **cornea** covers the iris, helps focus light rays, and is continuous with the anterior portion of the sclera.

The **conjunctiva** is a thin mucous membrane that lines the eyelids and covers the anterior portion of the eye, excluding the cornea. This membrane folds back to form a narrow space between the eyeball and the eyelid. The lacrimal apparatus contains the **lacrimal gland**, located in the inner corner of each eye, which produces tears that cleanse and lubricate the conjunctival surfaces. Tears drain through the **lacrimal duct**, which is located at the inner edge (canthus) of the eye, which carries tears into the nasal cavity. The **eyelashes** are located along the edges of the eyelids, and help to prevent materials from contacting the surface of the eyeball (Figure 6-1). The **extrinsic muscles** of the eye control eye movements.

The vascular middle layer of the eye contains the **choroid coat**, which contains extensive capillaries providing a blood supply and provides nourishment for the **retina**, the inner lining of the eyeball. The retina's role in eyesight is in the focusing of an object's image, a process that bends light waves (also known as **refraction**). The choroid coat contains pigment-producing melanocytes that absorb light and help to keep the inside of the eye dark. The **ciliary body** contains a muscle that controls the shape of the **lens**, allowing for near and far vision. This process is known as **accommodation**. The lens must become more rounded in order to view closer objects. Straight *suspensory ligaments*, radiating inward from folds in the ciliary body (known as *ciliary processes*) attach to the lens and hold it in place.

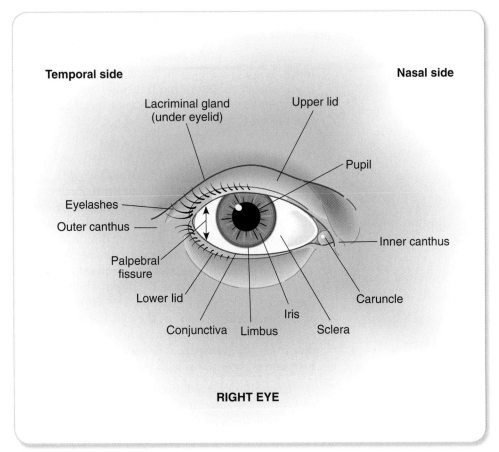

Figure 6-1 Structures of the eye.

Nerve cells in the retina called **rods** and **cones** are highly specialized for stimulation by light rays. The light-sensitive biochemical in the rods of the eye is called "visual purple," or **rhodopsin**. The majority of cones occur in the **fovea centralis**, a small depression located within the *macula lutea*, an oval, yellowish spot near the center of the retina. Impulses from the retina are transmitted through the **optic nerve**, located in the back of the eye, to the brain, where they are interpreted as vision. The section of the retina that is insensitive to light is the **optic disc**, or "blind spot," of the eye. The optic disc is the point where nerve fibers leave the eye and connect to the optic nerve. A lateral cross section of the eye is shown in Figure 6-2.

The eyeball is filled with a jelly-like substance called **vitreous humor**, which fills the posterior cavity of the eye, helps maintain the shape of the eye, and also refracts light. The **aqueous humor** is the watery fluid that fills the eye anterior to the lens, maintaining

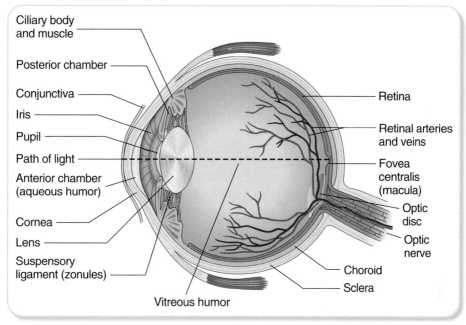

Ciliary body and muscle

Posterior chamber

Conjunctiva

Iris

Pupil

Path of light

Anterior chamber (aqueous humor)

Cornea

Lens

Suspensory ligament (zonules)

Vitreous humor

Retina

Retinal arteries and veins

Fovea centralis (macula)

Optic disc

Optic nerve

Choroid

Sclera

Figure 6-2 Cross-section of the eye.

the shape of the cornea and refracting light. This fluid is constantly produced and drained from the eye.

The Ear

The ears are the organs of hearing (sound). The ear has receptors for both hearing and **equilibrium** (balance). It may be divided into three parts: the outer, middle, and inner ear. The outer ear consists of the **pinna** (**auricle**), which is the funnel-shaped flap of cartilage that makes up the **earlobe,** and the **external auditory canal** (**meatus**). This S-shaped canal ends at the **tympanic membrane**, or **eardrum**, which transmits sound waves to the middle ear. Tiny hairs called cilia line this canal, as well as modified **ceruminous glands** (sweat glands). These glands secrete a yellowish-colored substance known as earwax or **cerumen**. See Figure 6-3 for an illustration of the anatomy of the ear.

The middle ear, or "tympanic cavity," contains three tiny **auditory ossicles** (bones), which include the **malleus** (which resembles a hammer), the **incus** (which resembles an anvil), and the **stapes** (which resembles a stirrup). The **Eustachian tube** (**auditory tube**) connects the middle ear to the nasopharynx (throat), and serves to equalize pressure between the outer and middle ear. The middle ear is separated from the inner ear by the **oval window**, an opening in the wall of the tympanic cavity.

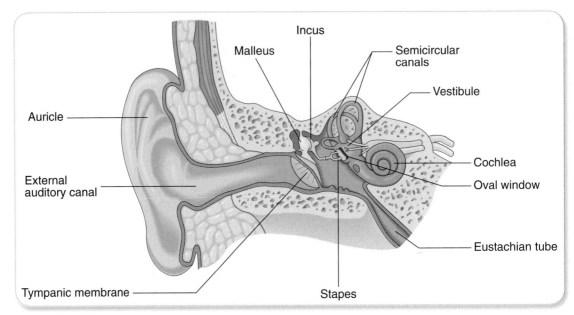

Incus

Malleus

Semicircular canals

Vestibule

Auricle

External auditory canal

Cochlea

Oval window

Eustachian tube

Tympanic membrane

Stapes

Figure 6-3 Structures of the ear.

The inner ear, because of its complex shape, is described as a **labyrinth**, which means "maze." The **vestibule** (central portion) contains the **utricle** and **saccule**, which aid in maintaining balance. These chambers each have tiny structures called **macula** that contain hair cells serving as sensory receptors. The organs of **static equilibrium** maintain stability and posture when the head and body remain still. The organs of **dynamic equilibrium** detect when the head and body change position, aiding in maintaining balance.

A snail-shaped, bony structure (the **cochlea**), contains auditory fluids (the *endolymph* and *perilymph*) that aid in sound vibration transmissions. A slight swelling at the end of the canal of the osseous portion of the ear is called the **ampulla**, which houses sensory organs called **crista ampulares**. These are similar to the macula, with hair cells that act as sensors.

The true organ of hearing (the **organ of Corti**, or **spiral organ**), is housed within the cochlea. The **semicircular canals**, behind the vestibule, help to maintain balance. The lower compartment of the cochlea extends to a membrane-covered opening in the inner ear wall called the **round window**.

GENERAL TERMINOLOGY RELATED TO THE EYES AND EARS

The following are commonly used terms that relate to the eyes.

Word	Pronunciation	Definition
aqueous humor	AK-wee-us HYOO-mer	watery; as in the fluid found in the eye
choroid	KOR-oyd	thin posterior membrane in the middle layer of the eye
cones	KOHNZ	specialized receptor cells in the retina that perceive color and bright light
corneal	KOR-nee-al	relating to the cornea of the eye
emmetropia	em-eh-TROH-pee-ah	normal vision, with direct retinal focus
eyelashes	EYE-lah-shes	a group of hairs protruding from the end of each eyelid; they help to keep foreign particles from entering the eye
eyelid	EYE-lid	a moveable covering of skin over each eye
fovea	FOH-vee-ah	small depression in the center of the macula; has the greatest visual acuity, and lies directly opposite to the pupil
iris	EYE-ris	colored ring of tissue with muscles that contract or relax to change the size of the pupil at its center
lacrimal gland	LAK-rim-al	the gland located near the superior–lateral aspect that produces and releases tears through lacrimal ducts
lens	LENZ	a colorless, flexible, transparent body behind the body
miosis	my-OH-sis	constriction of the iris muscle to decrease pupil size and limit amounts of light entering the eye
mydriasis	mid-RYE-ah-sis	relaxation of the iris muscle to increase pupil size and increase amounts of light entering the eye
ophthalmologist	off-thal-MALL-oh-jist	a physician who specializes in the treatment of eye diseases and disorders; ophthalmologists are able to perform eye surgeries if required
ophthalmology	off-thal-MALL-oh-jee	the study of eye diseases and disorders
optic	OP-tik	relating to the eyes or to eyesight
optometrist	op-TAW-meh-trist	a health professional who specializes in testing eyes for visual acuity, and prescribing corrective lenses; optometrists cannot perform eye surgeries
pupil	PYOO-pil	the black circular center of the eye; it opens and closes when muscles in the iris expand and contract in response to light
refraction	ree-FRAK-shun	the process of bending light rays
retina	REH-tih-nuh	the sensitive membrane in the interior layer of the eye; it decodes light waves and transmits information to the brain
rods	RODZ	specialized receptor cells in the retina that perceive black to white shades
sclera	SKLEH-ruh	a thick, tough membrane in the outer eye layer
uvea	YOO-vee-uh	the region of the eye containing the iris, choroid membrane, and ciliary bodies
vitreous humor	VIT-ree-us HYOO-mer	clear, gel-like substance that fills the eye's posterior cavity

The following are commonly used terms that relate to the ears.

Word	Pronunciation	Definition
acoustic	ah-KOOS-tik	relating to hearing or sound
audiogram	AW-dee-oh-gram	a test designed to reveal hearing loss
auditory ossicles	AW-dih-tor-ee OS-ih-kulz	three specially shaped bones in the middle ear that anchor the eardrum to the tympanic cavity and transmit vibrations to the inner ear
auricle	AW-rih-kul	a funnel-like structure leading from the external ear to the external auditory meatus; also called the "pinna"
cochlea	KOK-lee-uh	a snail-shaped structure in the inner ear that contains the organ of Corti
endolymph	EN-doh-limf	fluid inside the membranous labyrinth of the ear
Eustachian tube	YOO-stay-shun TOOB	the tube that connects the middle ear to the nasopharynx and equalizes pressure between the outer and middle ear
incus	ING-kus	one of the three ossicles of the middle ear
labyrinth	LAB-ih-rinth	the inner ear, named for its complex, maze-like structure
malleus	MAH-lee-us	one of the three auditory ossicles; also known as the "hammer"
membranous labyrinth	MEM-brah-nus LAB-ih-rinth	one of the two tubes that make up the semicircular canals of each ear
myringoplasty	mir-IN-goh-plas-tee	surgical repair of the eardrum to correct hearing loss
myringotomy	mir-in-GOT-oh-mee	surgical incision of the tympanic membrane, performed to drain the middle ear cavity or to insert a tube into the tympanic membrane for drainage
otoliths	OH-toh-liths	small calcifications in the inner ear that help to maintain balance
purulent	PEWR-yoo-lent	containing pus as a result of infection
salpingoscope	sal-PING-goh-skohp	a device used to examine the nasopharynx and Eustachian tube
serous	SEER-us	relating to any clear bodily fluid
stapedectomy	stay-pee-DEK-toh-mee	surgical removal of the stapes and insertion of a graft and prosthesis, designed to improve hearing
stapes	STAY-peez	one of the three auditory ossicles
tympanic membrane	tim-PAH-nik MEM-brayn	the eardrum
vestibule	VES-tih-byool	the chamber of the inner ear that contains some of the receptors needed for equilibrium
vestibulocochlear nerve	ves-tih-byoo-loh-KOK-lee-ar NERV	the nerve that transmits impulses for hearing and equilibrium from the ear to the brain

PATHOLOGICAL CONDITIONS OF THE EYES

The following are common disorders and conditions related to the eyes.

Amblyopia – reduced vision in an eye that is not correctable by a manifest refraction, and having no obvious pathologic or structural cause

Aphakia – absence of a lens, due to removal of a cataract

Asthenopia – a condition in which the eyes tire easily because of weakness of the ocular or ciliary muscles; also called *eyestrain*

Astigmatism – inability to focus, resulting in blurred vision; due to an abnormally shaped cornea

Blepharitis – inflammation or infection of the eyelids, with redness, crusting, and scales at the bases of the eyelids

Blepharoptosis (ptosis) – drooping of the upper eyelid due to excessive fat or tissue sagging that is caused by aging; also may be a form of disease that affects the muscles or nerves, such as myasthenia gravis or stroke (Figure 6-4)

Blindness – a condition of complete or partial loss of vision

Cataract – a clouding of the lens causing loss of normal transparency and the altering of vision (Figure 6-5); protein molecules in the lens begin to clump together in this condition, which is commonly caused by aging, sun exposure, eye trauma, smoking, and some medications

Color blindness – a genetic condition in which the cones, particularly those that perceive the colors green and red, are absent or do not contain enough visual pigment to respond to the light from objects of these colors

Conjunctivitis – inflammation of the mucous membranes lining the eyelids and covering the front part of the eyeballs; it usually creates an itching sensation in the eyes

Dacryocystitis – an inflammation of a lacrimal gland

Diabetic retinopathy – a chronic, progressive condition in which new, fragile retinal blood vessels are formed in patients with uncontrolled diabetes mellitus; leaking microaneurysms form dried fluid deposits (exudates) on the retina

Diplopia – double vision, caused by each eye focusing separately

Ectropion – weakening of connective tissue in the lower eyelid in older patients, causing it to turn outward (Figure 6-6)

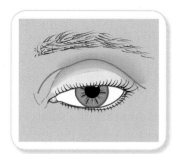

Figure 6-4 Blepharoptosis.

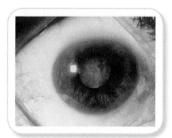

Figure 6-5 Cataract. *Courtesy of the National Eye Institute, NIH*

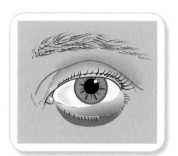

Figure 6-6 Ectropion.

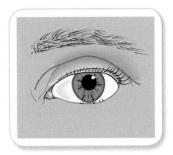

Figure 6-7 Entropion.

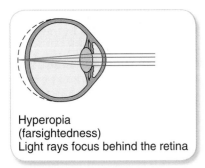

Figure 6-8 Hordeolum (stye).

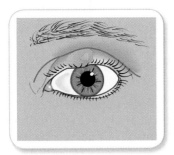

Hyperopia
(farsightedness)
Light rays focus behind the retina

Figure 6-9 Hyperopia (farsightedness).

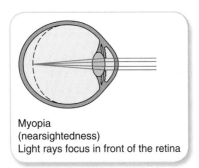

Myopia
(nearsightedness)
Light rays focus in front of the retina

Figure 6-10 Myopia (nearsightedness).

Entropion – weakening of the muscle in the lower eyelid in older patients, causing it to turn inward (Figure 6-7)

Exophthalmos – pronounced outward bulging of the anterior eye surface, causing a startled or staring expression; usually caused by hyperthyroidism

Esotropia – "crosseye;" turning inward of one eye toward the other

Exotropia – "walleye;" turning outward of one eye from the other; a type of strabismus in which the visual axes diverge

Glaucoma – increased intraocular pressure because of inability of the aqueous humor to circulate freely; can progress to blindness

Hemianopia – loss of vision in one half of the visual field, affecting one or both eyes

Hordeolum (stye) – inflammation and infection of a sebaceous gland of the eyelid (Figure 6-8)

Hyperopia – farsightedness; a refractive error of the lens causing inability to focus on near images; caused by a shorter-than-normal eyeball or abnormal lens function (Figure 6-9)

Keratitis – inflammation of the cornea that can cause scarring

Macular degeneration – the breakdown of macular tissue, which leads to loss of central vision (the vision we use for reading, driving, and watching television); some specific conditions within the eye may affect vision (for example, papilledema or edema of the optic disk)

Miosis – abnormal contraction of the pupils

Mydriasis – abnormal dilation of the pupils

Myopia – nearsightedness; a refractive error resulting in impaired distant vision (because the eyeball is longer than normal); see Figure 6-10

Nyctalopia – night blindness; the inability to see well in dim light or at night, often due to a lack of vitamin A

Nystagmus – involuntary, erratic eye movements; may be caused by alcohol, drugs, lesions, congenital abnormalities, nerve injury, or abnormal retinal development

Ophthalmopathy – any eye disease

Papilledema – inflammation and edema of the optic disk caused by increased intracranial pressure from a brain tumor or head trauma; also known as a "choked disk"

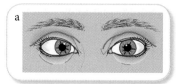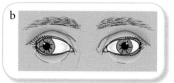

Figure 6-11 Strabismus (a) convergent (b) divergent.

Photophobia – an extreme sensitivity to light, sometimes as a result of a disease

Presbyopia – "old eye"; the loss of flexibility of the lens with blurry near vision and loss of accommodation

Retinal detachment – separation of the retina from the choroid layer beneath it that can be caused by head trauma; in diabetic patients, hemorrhage of the fragile retinal blood vessels can separate the layers

Retinitis pigmentosa – a progressive, inherited disorder, usually accompanied by scarring on the retina

Retinopathy – any non-inflammatory disease of the retina

Scotoma – a temporary or permanent visual field defect in one or both eyes

Strabismus – deviation of one or both eyes medially or laterally (Figure 6-11)

Trachoma – a chronic infectious disease caused by the bacterium *Chlamydia trachomatis*; a significant cause of blindness, and endemic to hot, dry, poverty-ridden areas

Uveitis – inflammation or infection of the uveal tract (iris, ciliary body, and choroid)

PATHOLOGICAL CONDITIONS OF THE EARS

The following are common disorders and conditions of the ears.

Acoustic neuroma – a tumor of the eighth cranial nerve, commonly causing hearing loss

Anacusis – a total loss of hearing

Cholesteatoma – a slow-growing epithelial cystic mass or sac (of cell debris and cholesterol) found in the middle ear

Conductive hearing loss – hearing impairment that results from blockage of sound transmission to the inner ear

Deafness – a partial or total hearing loss

Impacted cerumen – an excessive accumulation of earwax from the glands of the external ear canal that can impede hearing

Labyrinthitis – inflammation or infection of the inner ear's labyrinth (which is important for equilibrium and balance)

Mastoiditis – inflammation of the mastoid process, usually due to acute middle ear infection

Meniere's disease – edema of the semicircular canals with destruction of the cochlea, causing hearing loss and vertigo; can be caused by head trauma or middle ear infections

Myringitis (or tympanitis) – an inflammation of the eardrum

Otalgia – ear pain, earache, or otodynia that can interfere with hearing

Otitis externa – inflammation of the external auditory canal, also known as "swimmer's ear"

Otitis media – inflammation of the middle ear with accumulation of serous (watery) or mucoid fluid

Otomycosis – fungal infection of the outer ear canal

Otorrhagia – bleeding in the ear

Otorrhea – drainage of serous fluid or pus from the ear

Otosclerosis – abnormal formation of bone in the inner ear, particularly between the stapes and the oval window; the stapes becomes immovable, causing conductive hearing loss

Perforation of the tympanic membrane – rupture of the eardrum due to excessive pressure or infection; unequal air pressure in the middle ear, due to extreme altitudes or depths, can rupture the tympanic membrane

Presbycusis – loss of hearing caused by aging

Tinnitus – sounds (buzzing or ringing) that are heard in one or both ears, even in a quiet environment

Vertigo – an illusion of movement, as of the body moving in space or of the environment moving around the body; gives the sensation of spinning or swaying while the body is actually stationary

ABBREVIATIONS RELATED TO THE EYES AND EARS

The following are commonly used abbreviations that relate to the eyes.

Abbreviation	Meaning
acc.	accommodation
AMD	age-related macular degeneration
AS, AST	astigmatism
CC	with correction (with glasses)
EOM	extraocular movements
ERG	electroretinogram
HEENT	head, eyes, ears, nose, and throat
ICCE	intracapsular cataract extraction
IOL	Intraocular lens
IOP	Intraocular pressure
LTK	laser thermal keratoplasty
NV	near vision
O.D.	right eye (*ocular dexter*)
O.S.	left eye (*ocular sinestra*)
O.U.	each eye (*oculus uterque*)
Pr	presbyopia
PRK	photorefractive keratectomy
ROP	retinopathy of prematurity
RP	retinitis pigmentosa
VA	visual acuity
VF	visual field
XT	exotropia

The following are commonly used abbreviations related to the ears.

Abbreviation	Meaning
ABR	auditory brainstem response
A.D.	right ear (*auris dextra*)
A.S.	left ear (*auris sinestra*)
A.U.	each ear (*auris uterque*), both ears (*auris unitas*)
BOM	bilateral otitis media
dB, db	decibel
EAC	external auditory canal
ENT	ears, nose, and throat
Hz	hertz
PE	polyethylene (tube)

(continues)

Abbreviation	Meaning
PTS	permanent threshold shift
SOM	serous otitis media
T&A	tonsillectomy and adenoidectomy
TM	tympanic membrane
URI	upper respiratory infection

MEDICATIONS USED TO TREAT EYE AND EAR DISORDERS

The following are common medications used for eye disorders.

Drug Class	Generic Name	Pronunciation for Generic Name	Trade Name	Use
antihistamine / mast-cell stabilizer	azelastine	ah-ZEL-as-teen	Astelin®	conjunctivitis
fluoroquinolone antibiotic	levofloxacin	lev-oh-FLOK-sah-sin	Levaquin®	
macrolide antibiotic	erythromycin	eh-RITH-roh-my-sin	(various)	
beta₁ receptor blocker sympathomimetic	betaxolol apraclonidine	beh-TAK-so-lol ap-rah-KLON-ih-deen	Betoptic® Iopidine®	glaucoma
tropane (nitrogenous) alkaloid	atropine	AT-roh-peen	Atropair®, Atropen®, Atropinol®	to dilate the pupils (mydriatics)

The following medications are commonly used for ear conditions.

Drug Class	Generic Name	Pronunciation for Generic Name	Trade Name	Use
anesthetic	benzocaine	BEN-zoh-kayn	Americaine®	otitis media; swimmer's ear; otitis externa
antibiotic	amoxicillin	ah-MOK-sih-sil-lin	Augmentin®	otitis media
antibiotic (combination)	trimethoprim-sulfamethoxazole	try-METH-oh-prim sul-fah-meh-THOK-sa-zol	Bactrim®, Septra®	otitis media
antimicrobial	chloramphenicol	klor-am-FEH-nih-kol	Chloromycetin®	infections of the external auditory canal

DRUG TERMINOLOGY FOR THE EYES AND EARS

The following are common types of drugs used for eye conditions.

Drug	Pronunciation	Use
adrenergics	ad-DREH-ner-jiks	glaucoma
alpha agonists	AL-fa AG-oh-nists	glaucoma
beta blockers	BAY-ta blockers	glaucoma
carbonic anhydrase inhibitors	kar-BON-ik an-HY-drace inhibitors	glaucoma
cholinergics (miotics)	koh-lih-NER-jiks (my-OT-iks)	glaucoma
H_1-receptor antagonists	—	conjunctivitis
mast-cell stabilizers	—	conjunctivitis
mydriatics	mih-dree-AT-iks	pupil dilation; cataract (rarely); some types of glaucoma
NSAIDS	—	conjunctivitis
prostaglandin analogs	pros-tah-GLAN-din analogs	glaucoma

The following are common types of drugs used for ear conditions.

Drug	Pronunciation	Use
antihistamine	an-tie-HIS-tah-meen	allergic conditions
corticosteroid	kor-tih-koh-STAIR-oid	allergic conditions
cromolyn sodium	KROH-moh-lin SOH-dee-um	allergic conditions
decongestant	dee-con-JES-tent	allergic conditions

REVIEW EXERCISES

Multiple Choice

Select the best answer and write the letter of your choice to the left of each number.

1. The highest concentration of cone cells is located within the:

   A. macula lutea
   B. optic nerve
   C. lens
   D. iris

2. The ciliary body contains a muscle that controls the shape of the lens. This process is known as:

   A. hemianopia
   B. miosis
   C. accommodation
   D. myopia

3. Which of the following terms means "night blindness"?

   A. myopia
   B. hyperopia
   C. hemianopia
   D. nyctalopia

4. Deviation of one or both eyes medially or laterally is called:

   A. scotoma
   B. strabismus
   C. nystagmus
   D. hyperopia

5. Which of the following ear bones is attached to the oval window?

   A. stapes
   B. incus
   C. malleus
   D. cochlea

6. Cholesteatoma is a slow-growing epithelial cystic mass found in which of the following?

   A. the inner ear
   B. the middle ear
   C. the iris
   D. the macula lutea

7. Edema of the semicircular canals with destruction of the inner ear, causing hearing loss, is called:

   A. conductive hearing loss
   B. acoustic neuroma
   C. otitis media
   D. Meniere's disease

8. An inflammation or redness of the sclera and the underside of the eyelid is called:

   A. blepharitis
   B. conjunctivitis
   C. retinitis
   D. keratitis

9. The eardrum is also called the:

   A. utricle
   B. auditory tube
   C. saccule
   D. tympanic membrane

10. Loss of hearing caused by aging is referred to as:

    A. presbycusis
    B. vertigo
    C. labyrinthitis
    D. conductive hearing loss

11. Which of the following terms refers to a temporary or permanent visual field defect in one or both eyes?

    A. retinal detachment
    B. papilledema
    C. strabismus
    D. scotoma

12. An abnormal dilation of the pupils of the eyes is referred to as:

    A. miosis
    B. mydriasis
    C. keratosis
    D. hyperopia

13. The middle ear is also called the:

    A. Eustachian tube
    B. auditory canal
    C. tympanic cavity
    D. auditory tube

14. Endolymph is located in which of the following parts of the ear?

    A. cochlea
    B. ampulla
    C. organ of Corti
    D. spiral organ

15. Uveitis is an inflammation or infection of the ciliary body, choroid, and _____.

    A. lens
    B. iris
    C. retina
    D. lacrimal gland

Fill in the Blank

Use your knowledge of medical terminology to insert the correct term from the list below into the appropriate statement.

labyrinth	nystagmus	astigmatism
cochlear	cornea	ptosis
retina	pupil	entropion
diplopia	vitreous humor	stye
exotropia	choroid	strabismus

1. A _____ is also called a "hordeolum."

2. Weakening of the muscle in the lower eyelid in older patients causing it to turn inward is referred to as _____.

3. The term _____ relates to the labyrinth of the ear.

4. An involuntary, rhythmic jerking of the eye in different directions is known as _____.

5. The circular orifice in the center of the iris where light rays enter the eye is referred to as the _____.

6. The fluid component of the clear, jelly-like substance filling the interior of the eyeball between the lens and retina is called _____.

7. The _____ is the transparent portion at the front of the eye that covers the iris and anterior chamber.

8. A turning outward of one eye from the other is referred to as _____.

9. Double vision is also called _____.

10. _____ is an inability to focus due to an abnormally shaped cornea.

Labeling – The Structures of the Eye

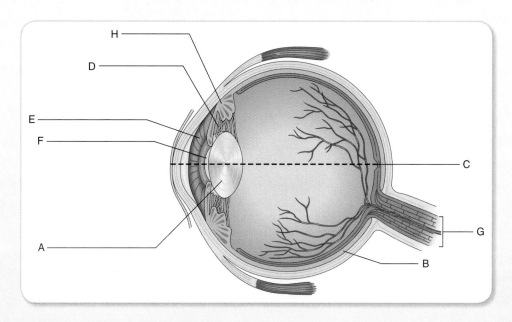

Write in the eye structure below that corresponds with each letter on the figure above.

A. _____

B. _____

C. _____

D. _____

E. _____

F. _____

G. _____

H. _____

True / False

Identify each of the following questions as true or false by placing a "T" or "F" on the line beside each number.

_____ **1.** Amoxicillin is used for the treatment of otitis media.

_____ **2.** Corticosteroids and cromolyn sodium are used for the treatment of presbycusis.

_____ **3.** Myringoplasty is a surgical incision of the tympanic membrane.

_____ **4.** A test designed to reveal hearing loss is called an *audiogram.*

_____ **5.** A fungal infection of the outer ear canal is referred to as "otalgia."

_____ **6.** Drooping of the upper eyelid from excessive fat or sagging of the tissues due to age is known as "ptosis."

_____ **7.** Optometrists cannot perform eye surgeries.

_____ **8.** An agent that causes the pupils to dilate is called a *miotic.*

_____ **9.** A genetic condition in the cones, particularly affecting the colors green or red, is called "conjunctivitis."

_____ **10.** Bulging of the anterior surface of the eye is known as "exophthalmos."

Labeling – The Structures of the Ear

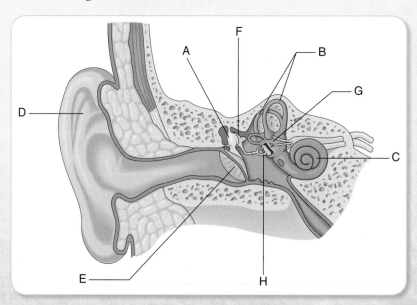

Write in the ear structure below that corresponds with each letter on the figure above.

A. _____

B. _____

C. _____

D. _____

E. _____

F. _____

G. _____

H. _____

Definitions

Define each of the following words in one sentence.

1. eyelashes: _____

2. choroid: _____

3. corneal: _____

4. miosis: _____

5. cataract: _____

6. hordeolum: _____

7. otalgia: _____

8. purulent: _____

9. myringoplasty: _____

10. acoustic: _____

Abbreviations

Write the full meaning of each abbreviation:

Abbreviation	Meaning
1. A.D.	_____
2. O.S.	_____
3. RP	_____
4. TM	_____
5. EAC	_____
6. O.U.	_____
7. AST	_____

8. Hz   _____

9. SOM   _____

10. BOM   _____

Matching – Terms and Definitions

Match the following terms with their definitions by placing the matching letter on the line to the left of each number.

_____ 1. otorrhea

_____ 2. tinnitus

_____ 3. emmetropia

_____ 4. scotoma

_____ 5. otalgia

_____ 6. vestibule

_____ 7. salpingoscope

_____ 8. photophobia

_____ 9. hemianopia

_____ 10. hyperopia

A. normal vision with direct retinal focus

B. blindness in one half of the visual field

C. farsightedness

D. abnormal sensitivity or intolerance to light

E. a device used to examine the nasopharynx and Eustachian tube

F. visual field defect

G. earache

H. located in the inner ear

I. infected drainage from the middle ear

J. a ringing noise in the ear

Spelling

Circle the correct spelling from each pairing of words.

1. astigmatizm   astigmatism

2. dacryocystitis   dacreocystitis

3. poupil   pupil

4. uevea   uvea

5. vitreous   vitrous

6. miosis   myosis

7. nistagmus   nystagmus

8. emetropia   emmetropia

9. cholesteatoma   cholestetoma

10. otorhea   otorrhea

Nervous System

OBJECTIVES

Upon completion of this chapter, the reader should be able to:

1. Describe the functions of the nervous system.

2. List the subdivisions of the nervous system.

3. Identify the major structures of the brain.

4. List the cranial nerves and their numbers.

5. Define, pronounce, and spell the diseases and disorders of the nervous system.

6. Interpret the terms that are signified by the abbreviations presented in this chapter.

7. Recognize common pharmacological agents used in treating disorders of the nervous system.

8. Describe the common types of drugs used for nervous system conditions.

STRUCTURE AND FUNCTION OF THE NERVOUS SYSTEM

The nervous system is the most complex system in the body. It plays a role in nearly every function and acts as the primary means of self-protection. The nervous system consists of the brain, spinal cord, and nerves. It works with the endocrine system to coordinate and control all body activities (Figure 7-1).

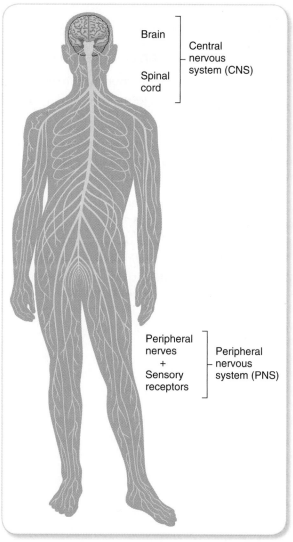

Figure 7-1 The central and peripheral nervous systems.

The nervous system has two primary divisions: the **central nervous system (CNS)**, and the **peripheral nervous system (PNS)**. The PNS consists of 12 pairs of cranial nerves and 31 pairs of spinal nerves. The PNS is separated into two divisions: the *somatic nervous system* (which is under voluntary control), and the **autonomic nervous system (ANS)**. The **parasympathetic nerves** regulate other involuntary functions that complement those of the sympathetic nerves. Figure 7-2 summarizes the divisions of the nervous system.

Neurons (nerve cells) receive stimuli and transmit impulses to other neurons, or to receptors in other organs. Each neuron consists of a cell body and two types of extensions, called *dendrites* and *axons*. Dendrites are short, highly branched extensions of the neuron's cell body. They conduct impulses toward the cell body. A single axon arises from the cell body and carries impulses away from the cell body (Figure 7-3).

The nervous system has three general functions: sensory, integrative, and motor. The **sensory** function involves the use of receptors that detect (sense) changes in internal and external body

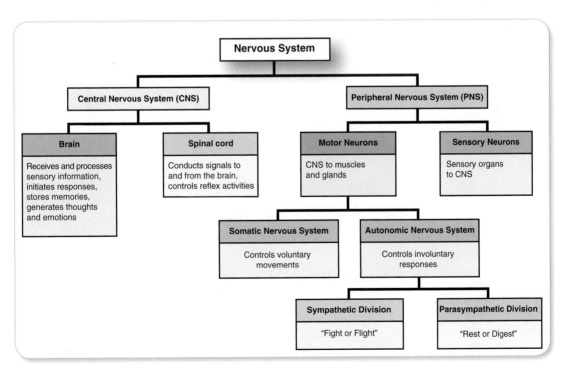

Figure 7-2 Divisions of the nervous system.

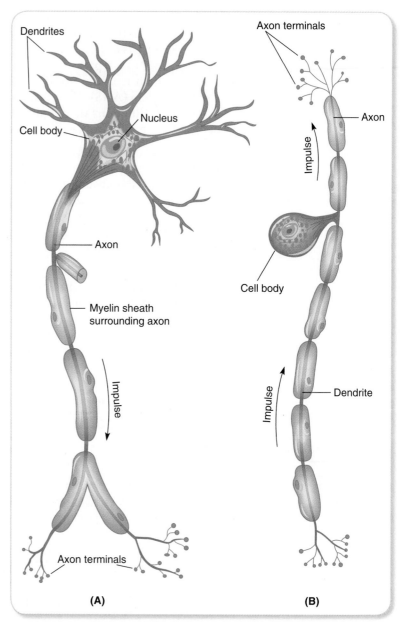

Figure 7-3 Structure of a neuron (a) motor (b) sensory.

conditions to regulate homeostasis, the condition of balance. The integrative function coordinates the sensory information with internal activity and motor function. Motor function implies skeletal muscle activity in which muscles respond when they are stimulated by motor impulses.

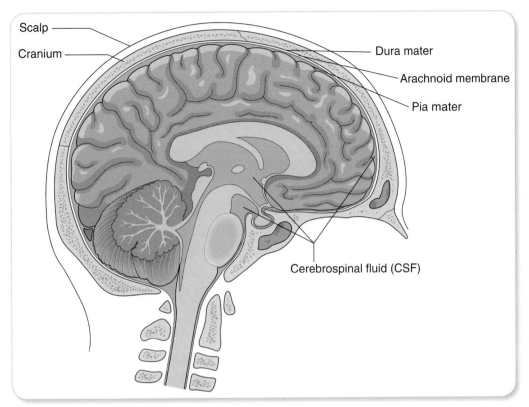

Scalp

Cranium

Dura mater

Arachnoid membrane

Pia mater

Cerebrospinal fluid (CSF)

Figure 7-4 Protective coverings of the brain.

The brain and spinal cord are protected by surrounding bone tissue, three membranes called *meninges*, cerebrospinal fluid (CSF), dura mater, and pia mater (Figure 7-4).

The brain is the major portion of the central nervous system. The **cerebrum** is the largest part of the brain, consisting of two cerebral hemispheres connected by the **corpus callosum**, which is composed of nerve fibers. The cerebrum controls the skeletal muscles, interprets general senses (such as temperature, pain, and touch), and contains centers for sight and hearing. Intellect, memory, and emotional reactions also take place in the cerebrum. The **cerebellum** is the second-largest region of the brain. It is located under the posterior portion of the cerebrum. It assists in coordination of skeletal muscles and in maintaining balance.

The **diencephalon**, located between the cerebrum and midbrain, contains the thalamus, hypothalamus, and pineal gland. The *brain stem* (sometimes written "*brainstem*") is the stem-like portion of the brain that connects with the spinal cord and contains the midbrain, pons, and medulla oblongata. Cranial nerves originate in the brain stem (Figure 7-5). The 10 pairs of the 12 cranial nerves arise from the brain stem, except for the first pair. Cranial nerves are numbered with Roman numerals (Table 7-1).

TABLE 7-1 Cranial Nerves

Cranial Nerve and Number	Pronunciation	Function
I – olfactory nerve	ol-FAK-toh-ree	controls the sense of smell
II – optic nerve	OP-tik	controls the sense of vision
III – oculomotor nerve	ok-yoo-loh-MO-tor	moves the eye muscles
IV – trochlear nerve	TROK-lee-ar	controls a specific eyeball muscle
V – trigeminal nerve	try-JEM-ih-nal	controls chewing and carries impulses from the face
VI – abducens nerve	ab-DOO-sens	controls a specific eyeball muscle
VII – facial nerve	FAY-shal	partially controls the sense of taste, and controls facial expression muscles as well as tear and salivary glands
VIII – vestibulocochlear nerve (also called *acoustic* or *auditory* nerve)	ves-tib-yoo-loh-KOK-lee-ar	controls the sense of hearing as well as balance (equilibrium)
IX – glossopharyngeal nerve	glos-o-fah-RIN-jee-al	controls the sense of taste as well as stimulates the parotid salivary gland; it partly controls swallowing
X – vagus nerve	VAY-gus	controls digestive secretions, and supplies most thorax and abdominal organs
XI – spinal accessory nerve	ak-SES-oh-ree	controls the neck muscles
XII – hypoglossal nerve	hy-poh-GLOS-al	controls the tongue muscles

The autonomic nervous system is the portion of the peripheral nervous system that functions independently (autonomously) and continuously without conscious effort. This system controls visceral functions by regulating the actions of smooth muscles, cardiac muscles, and glands. It regulates heart rate, blood pressure, breathing rate, and body temperature. Portions of the autonomic nervous system respond to emotional stress and prepare the body to meet the demands of strenuous physical activity.

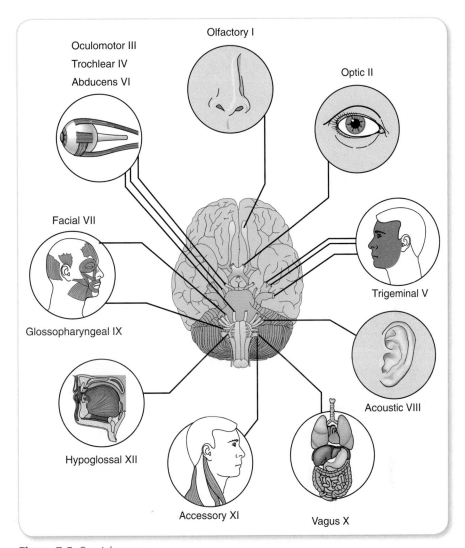

Figure 7-5 Cranial nerves.

The autonomic nervous system has two subdivisions: the sympathetic and parasympathetic nervous systems. The **sympathetic nervous system (SNS)** prepares the body for stressful and emergency conditions, resulting in what is frequently called the *fight or flight* response. The parasympathetic nervous system (PSNS) returns the body to normal after a response to stress (Figures 7-6A and 7-6B).

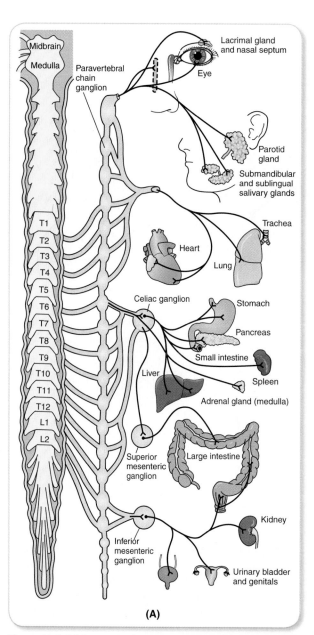

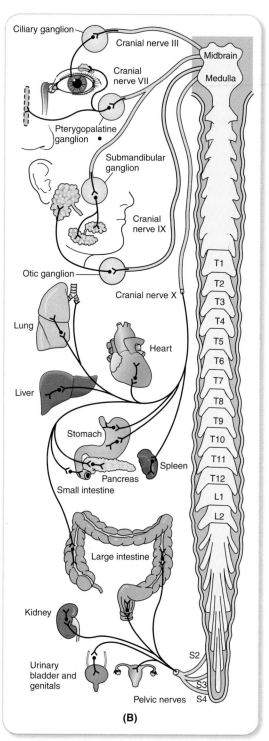

Figure 7-6 (a) Sympathetic nervous system (b) Parasympathetic nervous system.

GENERAL TERMINOLOGY RELATED TO THE NERVOUS SYSTEM

The following are common terms that relate to the nervous system.

Term	Pronunciation	Definition
analgesia	an-al-JEE-zee-ah	loss of sensation of pain by interruption of the sensory pathway to the brain
anesthesia	an-ess-THEE-zee-ah	lacking sensation or feeling; anesthesia is used for surgeries and other medical procedures
astrocyte	ASS-troh-sight	star-shaped glial cells in the brain; also called *astroglia*
Axon	AK-son	a nerve fiber; a long, slender projection of a neuron that conducts electrical impulses away from the cell body
Brain	BRAYN	the nervous tissue contained within the cranium; consists of the cerebrum, diencephalon, brain stem, and cerebellum
brain stem	BRAYN stem	the lower part of the brain, which adjoins the spinal cord; consists of the midbrain, pons, and medulla oblongata
cerebellum	ser-eh-BELL-um	the region at the base of the brain that plays an important part in sensory regulation and motor control
cerebral cortex	seh-REE-bral COR-teks	the brain structure that plays a key role in many brain functions; its outermost layer is referred to as the "gray matter"
cerebrospinal fluid	ser-eh-broh-SPY-nal FLOO-id	the clear fluid within the subarachnoid space and ventricles around and inside the brain
cerebrum	seh-REE-brum	the largest, uppermost region of the brain, responsible for many brain activities; also called the *telencephalon* or *forebrain*
Corpus callosum	KOR-pus kah-LOH-sum	white matter (myelinated tissue) composed of nerve fibers that connect the cerebral hemispheres
Cranial nerves	KRAY-nee-al NERVZ	the 12 pairs of nerves that are connected to the brain
craniotomy	kray-nee-OTT-oh-mee	a surgical operation to access the brain by removing a "bone flap" from the skull
dendrite	DEN-dryt	a fiber of a neuron that conducts impulses toward the cell body
diencephalon	dye-en-SEFF-ah-lon	the part of the brain that contains the thalamus, hypothalamus, and pituitary gland; located between the cerebrum and the brain stem
dura mater	DOO-rah MAH-ter	the strong, fibrous outermost layer of the meninges

(continues)

Term	Pronunciation	Definition
epidural space	ep-ih-DOO-ral space	the space outside the spine's dura mater, within the spinal canal, that is formed by the vertebrae
fontanelle (fontanel)	fon-tah-NELL	a soft spot on an infant's skull that allows the skull to flex during the birth process; by age two, the skull fuses completely
ganglion	GANG-lee-on	a collection of nerve cell bodies outside the CNS
gray matter	GRAY MAH-ter	unmyelinated tissue of the nervous system
Gyrus	JY-rus	a raised convolution of the surface of the cerebrum
hypothalamus	high-poh-THAL-ah-mus	the brain region located below the thalamus, just above the brain stem, that is responsible for certain metabolic processes and other ANS activities
medulla oblongata	meh-DOO-lah ob-lon-GAH-tah	the lower part of the brain stem that is continuous with the spinal cord
melatonin	meh-luh-TOH-nin	a natural hormone produced by the pineal body that helps to regulate puberty, the menstrual cycle, and many other body functions
meninges	men-IN-jeez	the three membranes that envelop the brain and spinal cord
microglia	my-KROG-lee-ah	the glial cells of the immune system that can engulf various substances
midbrain	MID-brain	the middle of the three vesicles arising from the neural tube; also called the *mesencephalon*; considered part of the brain stem
myelin	MY-eh-lin	a whitish, fatty substance that surrounds certain axons of the nervous system
neuroglia	noo-ROG-lee-uh	the support cells of the nervous system; also called *glial cells*
neurologist	noo-ROL-oh-jist	physician who specializes in neurology
Neuron	NOO-ron	the basic unit of the nervous system
neurotransmitter	noo-roh-TRANS-mit-ter	a chemical that transmits signals between neurons and other cells
Nerve	NERV	a bundle of nerve cell fibers outside the CNS
parasympathetic nerves	pair-ah-SIM-pah-theh-tik NERVS	nerves that regulate involuntary functions that complement those of the sympathetic nerves
Parasympathomimetic	pair-ah-sim-pah-tho-mih-MET-ik	stimulating or mimicking the actions of the (PSNS); also called *cholinergics*
phagocytosis	fag-oh-sign-TOH-sis	the process of engulfing solid particles by the cell membrane

pia mater	PEE-uh MAH-ter	the innermost layer of the meninges
pineal body (gland)	PAHY-nee-uhl BAH-dee (GLAND)	the small endocrine gland in the brain that extends from the diencephalon and produces melatonin
Plexus	PLEK-sus	a "nerve net" consisting of the joining of the processes of neurons
Pons	PONZ	a structure on the brain stem that relays sensory information between the cerebrum and cerebellum
receptor	ree-SEP-tor	any sensory structure that produces a nerve impulse
Reflex	REE-fleks	a simple, rapid, and automatic response to a stimulus
sensory	SEN-soh-ree	the type of nerve function involving the use of receptors that sense changes in body conditions to regulate homeostasis
somatic nervous system	soh-MAH-tik NER-vus SIS-tem	the division of the nervous system that controls skeletal (voluntary) muscles
spinal cord	SPY-nul KORD	the nervous tissue contained within the spinal column; extends from the medulla oblongata to the second lumbar vertebra
Sulcus	SUL-kus	a shallow furrow or groove, as on the surface of the cerebrum
sympathetic nervous system	sim-pah-theh-tik NER-vus SIS-tem	the part of the ANS that becomes more active during times of stress; its actions comprise the "fight or flight" response
sympathomimetic	sim-pah-thoh-mih-MET-ik	mimicking the effects of epinephrine and norepinephrine; this raises the blood pressure
synapses	SIH-nap-sees	the spaces that exist between nerves
thalamus	THAL-ah-mus	the main part of the diencephalon; plays major roles in processing and relaying sensory information
ventricle	VEN-trih-kul	a small cavity in the brain in which CSF is produced
visceral nervous system	VIH-seh-rul NER-vus SIS-tem	the autonomic nervous system
White matter	WYT MAH-ter	myelinated tissue of the nervous system

PATHOLOGICAL CONDITIONS

The following are pathological conditions of the nervous system.

Absence seizure – a small "petit mal" seizure that lasts a few seconds, with a sudden, temporary loss of consciousness

Agraphia – inability to convert thoughts into writing, not caused by intellectual impairment

Alzheimer's disease – the most common cause of dementia; a degenerative and terminal disease occurring most prevalently in people over age 65

Amyotrophic lateral sclerosis – a progressive, often fatal, neurodegenerative disease in the CNS, causing inability to control voluntary muscle movement

Anencephaly – congenital defective development of the brain in which a neural tube defect results in the absence of most of the brain, skull, and scalp

Aneurysm – a localized, blood-filled bulge of a blood vessel due to disease or weakening of the vessel wall

Aphasia – a loss of ability to produce or comprehend language due to brain injury

Ataxia – gross incoordination of muscle movements

Aura – a perceptual disturbance that may occur before a migraine headache or an epileptic seizure

Bell's palsy – paralysis of the facial nerve that results in lack of control of the facial muscles on the affected side; usually unilateral

Bradykinesia – slowness in the ability to execute movements

Cephalalgia – a headache; also known as *cephalgia*

Cerebral concussion – a mild brain injury that can cause a transient loss of brain function; can also cause physical and emotional symptoms

Cerebral contusion – a bruising of the brain tissue caused by small blood vessel leaks

Cerebral palsy – a group of permanent, non-progressive brain conditions or lesions present at birth, or shortly thereafter, that cause physical disability including lack of voluntary muscle control

Cerebrovascular accident – an abnormal condition of the brain characterized by rapidly decreasing brain functions because of disturbed blood flow to the brain; also called *stroke* or *brain attack*

Cluster headache – a neurological disease causing immense pain that occurs periodically, often after falling asleep

Dementia – progressive decline in cognitive function due to brain damage or disease (beyond normal aging)

Dyslexia – a learning disability involving written language

Dysphasia – a language disorder involving speech impairment and inability to comprehend speech

Encephalitis – acute brain inflammation caused by a variety of infections or parasites; can cause brain damage and even death

Epidural hematoma – a buildup of blood between the dura mater and the skull

Epilepsy – a disorder characterized by abnormal electrical activity in the brain that causes changes in consciousness, changes in thought processes, and/or involuntary muscle contractions; manifests itself in many ways depending upon the location, intensity, and extensiveness of the electrical abnormalities

Grand mal seizure – an epileptic seizure characterized by a generalized involuntary muscular contraction and cessation of respiration, followed by tonic and clonic spasms of the muscles; the term *grand mal seizure* is being used less frequently, and *tonic-clonic seizure* is more frequently used

Hemiparesis – partial paralysis of one side of the body

Hemiplegia – a paralytic condition of one-half of the body

Herpes zoster (shingles) – an infection caused by the varicella zoster virus (the same virus that causes chickenpox); the virus may reemerge during times of physical stress or when the immune system is impaired, inflaming nerves in the trunk and abdomen, and causing blisters and severe pain (Figure 7-7)

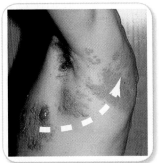

Figure 7-7 Shingles. *Courtesy of Robert A. Silverman, M.D., Clinical Associate Professor, Department of Pediatrics, Georgetown University*

Hydrocephalus – an abnormal accumulation of cerebrospinal fluid in the cavities of the brain; can result in increased intracranial pressure, head enlargement, convulsions, and mental disability

Hyperesthesia – an abnormal increase in sensitivity to sensory stimuli

Hyperkinesis – overactive restlessness in children

Lethargy – fatigue, sluggishness, or inactivity

Meningitis – an inflammation of one or more of the membranes (meninges) that cover the brain and spinal cord; may be caused by viral or bacterial infection

Meningocele – protrusion of the meninges (through a defect in the skull or vertebral column); see Figure 7-8

Meningomyelocele – protrusion of the meninges and spinal cord through a defect in the vertebral column (see Figure 7-9)

Multiple sclerosis (MS) – a nervous system disease affecting the brain and spinal cord that damages the myelin sheath, slowing down or blocking messages between the brain and body; it is degenerative but controllable

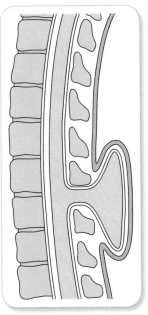

Figure 7-8 Meningocele.

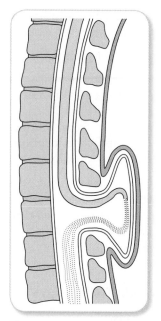

Figure 7-9 Meningomyelocele.

Myasthenia gravis – a chronic, progressive neuromuscular disease that leads to variable muscle weakness and fatigue

Narcolepsy – a neurological condition that can cause periods of random sleep to occur at any time

Neuralgia – a painful disorder of the nerves

Neuritis – general inflammation of the peripheral nervous system

Paraplegia – impairment in motor and sensory function of the lower extremities

Parkinson's disease – a degenerative, slowly progressive CNS deterioration involving the motor nerves; characterized by a stooped posture, a bowed head, a shuffling gait, pill-rolling gestures, a mask-like facial appearance, muffled speech, and difficulty in swallowing

Peripheral neuritis – inflammation of the peripheral nerves

Petit mal seizure – an epileptic seizure characterized by sudden, small seizures with temporary loss of consciousness, lasting only a few seconds; the term *absence seizure* is used more commonly today than *petit mal seizure*

Poliomyelitis – an acute, infectious viral disease that affects the spinal cord and brain motor neurons in receiving stimulation; results in muscular and respiratory paralysis

Quadriplegia – paralysis that affects all four limbs, as well as the trunk, due to spinal cord injury

Reye's syndrome – a metabolic disorder that affects primarily the central nervous system of children and adolescents; usually follows a viral infection and has been associated with the use of aspirin

Sciatica – pain or other symptoms caused by sciatic nerve root compression or irritation

Skull fracture (depressed) – comminuted skull fracture in which broken skull bones are displaced inward, puncturing the brain

Stupor – a loss of cognitive function that causes insensibility; due to a variety of causes

Subdural hematoma – a traumatic brain injury wherein blood gathers between the dura mater and the arachnoid layer of the meninges; can cause increased intracranial pressure

Syncope – sudden loss of consciousness, usually due to a lack of sufficient blood and oxygen in the brain; also called *fainting*

Tetanus – a condition of sustained, strenuous, and involuntary muscle contractions caused by a rapid succession of nerve impulses that come so rapidly that the muscle does not have time to relax between them; a potentially fatal infectious disease caused by *Clostridium tetani*, an organism that secretes a toxin that causes uncontrolled muscle contractions; can be prevented by immunization

Trigeminal neuralgia (tic douloureux) – a neuropathic disorder of the trigeminal nerve that causes short periods of severe unilateral pain radiating through the scalp, forehead, eyes, lips, nose, and jaw

ABBREVIATIONS

The following are common abbreviations that relate to the nervous system.

Abbreviation	Meaning
ACh	acetylcholine
AD	Alzheimer's disease
ADHD	attention deficit–hyperactivity disorder
ALS	amyotrophic lateral sclerosis
ANS	autonomic nervous system
CNS	central nervous system
CP	cerebral palsy
CSF	cerebrospinal fluid
CVA	cerebrovascular accident (stroke)
CVD	cerebrovascular disease
DTR	deep tendon reflexes
ICP	intracranial pressure
LOC	level of consciousness
LP	lumbar puncture
MRI scan	magnetic resonance imaging scan
MS	multiple sclerosis
OCD	obsessive-compulsive disorder
PD	Parkinson's disease
PET scan	positron emission tomography scan
PNS	peripheral nervous system
PTSD	post-traumatic stress disorder
REM	rapid eye movement (during sleep)
SNS	somatic nervous system
TIA	transient ischemic attack

MEDICATIONS USED TO TREAT NERVOUS SYSTEM DISORDERS

The following are common medications used for nervous system disorders.

Drug Class	Generic Name	Pronunciation for Generic Name	Trade Name	Use
Analgesics	acetaminophen	ah-see-ta-MIN-o-fen	Tylenol®	to relieve pain
	codeine	KO-deen	(various)	
	hydrocodone	hy-droh-KO-doan	Vicodin®	
	meperidine	meh-PAIR-ih-deen	Demerol®	
	morphine	MOR-feen	(various)	
	oxycodone	ok-see-KO-doan	(various)	
Anesthetics	droperidol	dro-PAIR-ih-dall	Inapsine®	to reduce or eliminate the perception of sensation
	lidocaine	LY-doh-kayn	Xylocaine®	
	midazolam	mih-DAY-zo-lam	Versed®	
	procaine	PRO-kayn	Novocain®	
	propofol	PRO-poh-fol	Diprivan®	
	thiopental	thy-oh-PEN-tall	Pentothal®	
antianxiety drugs (psychotropics)	alprazolam	al-PRAZ-oh-lam	Xanax®	to reduce or eliminate anxiety
	diazepam	dy-AZ-eh-pam	Valium®	
	lorazepam	lor-AZ-eh-pam	Ativan®	
Anticonvulsants	diazepam	dy-AZ-eh-pam	Valium®	to prevent or relieve convulsions
	phenobarbital	fee-no-BAR-bih-tall	Solfoton®, Luminal®	
	phenytoin	FEN-ih-toyn	Dilantin®	
	primidone	PRIH-mih-doan	Mysoline®	
Antidepressants	fluoxetine	floo-OX-eh-teen	Prozac®	to prevent or relieve depression
	paroxetine	pah-ROX-eh-teen	Paxil®	
	sertraline	SER-trah-leen	Zoloft®	
	venlafaxine	VEN-lah-fax-een	Effexor®	
antipsychotics	chlorpromazine	klor-PRO-mah-zeen	Thorazine®	to treat psychoses
	haloperidol	hal-oh-PAIR-ih-dol	Haldol®	
	lithium	LITH-ee-um	Lithotabs®	
hypnotics (sedatives)	chloral hydrate	KLOR-al HY-drayt	Aquachloral®	to reduce activity and excitement; used for short-term treatment of insomnia
	diphenhydramine	dy-fen-HY-drah-meen	Benadryl®, Nytol®	
	lorazepam	lor-AZ-eh-pam	Ativan®	
	pentobarbital	pen-toh-BAR-bih-tall	Nembutal®	
	secobarbital	see-koh-BAR-bih-tall	Seconal®	
	zolpidem	ZOHL-pih-dem	Ambien®	

| major tranquilizers | chlorpromazine haloperidol lithium | klor-PRO-mah-zeen hal-oh-PAIR-ih-dol LITH-ee-um | Thorazine® Haldol® Lithotabs® | to calm, soothe, and prevent psychotic behavior |
| minor tranquilizers | alprazolam diazepam lorazepam | al-PRAZ-oh-lam dy-AZ-eh-pam lor-AZ-eh-pam | Xanax® Valium® Ativan® | to calm, soothe, and prevent anxiety |

DRUG TERMINOLOGY

The following are common types of drugs used for nervous system conditions.

Drug Type	Pronunciation	Definition
Analgesics	an-al-JEE-ziks	agents that relieve pain
Anesthetics	an-ess-THET-icks	agents that block the perception of sensation
Anticonvulsants	an-tie-con-VUL-sants	agents that prevent or relieve seizures or convulsions
Antidepressants	an-tie-dee-PRESS-ants	agents that prevent or relieve depression
Antipsychotics	an-tie-sy-KOT-icks	agents that are effective in the treatment of psychoses, including schizophrenia, bipolar disorder, mania, and delusions
Hypnotics	hip-NOT-icks	agents that induce sleep, which may also be used for surgical anesthesia; also known as *sedatives*
Psychotropics	sy-koh-TROH-pics	agents that change mood, perception, behavior, and consciousness; also known as *antianxiety drugs*
tranquilizers, major	TRANK-wil-eye-zers, major	agents that have a calm, soothing effect and are often used to treat mental illness; also known as *antipsychotic agents*
tranquilizers, minor	TRANK-wil-eye-zers, minor	agents that have a calm, soothing effect; used to decrease anxiety or induce sleep; can be used as general anesthetics

REVIEW EXERCISES

Multiple Choice

Select the best answer and write the letter of your choice to the left of each number.

1. The cerebral hemispheres are covered by a thin layer of gray matter that is referred to as:

   A. cerebellum
   B. cerebral cortex
   C. basal ganglia
   D. occipital lobe

2. Long, slender nerve fibers that conduct electrical impulses from the cell body of a neuron are called:

   A. dendrites
   B. myelin sheaths
   C. synapses
   D. axons

3. Which of the following is the main part of the diencephalon?

   A. sulci
   B. pons
   C. thalamus
   D. pia mater

4. Which of the following is the outermost layer of meninges?

   A. dura mater
   B. pia mater
   C. arachnoid membrane
   D. myelin sheath

5. Cranial nerve number VII is referred to as the:

   A. optic nerve
   B. facial nerve
   C. vestibulocochlear nerve
   D. vagus nerve

6. A neurological condition that can cause periods of random sleep to occur at any time is known as:

   A. neuralgia
   B. neuroglia
   C. paraplegia
   D. narcolepsy

7. A congenital neural tube defect that results in the absence of most of the brain and skull is referred to as:

   A. encephalitis
   B. cerebrovascular accident
   C. anencephaly
   D. cerebral palsy

8. Which of the following terms means blood gathering between the dura mater and the arachnoid layer of the meninges?

   A. subdural hematoma
   B. epidural hematoma
   C. intracranial hematoma
   D. malignant hemorrhage

9. A chronic, progressive neuromuscular disease that leads to variable muscle weakness and fatigue is called:

   A. myasthenia gravis
   B. multiple sclerosis
   C. Parkinson's disease
   D. petit mal seizure

10. *Tic douloureux* is referred to as:

    A. Reye's syndrome
    B. Tay-Sachs disease
    C. trigeminal neuralgia
    D. petit mal seizure

11. Which of the following agents is a hypnotic?

    A. chlorpromazine
    B. lithium
    C. sertraline
    D. lorazepam

12. An agent that is effective in the treatment of schizophrenia is referred to as:

    A. an antidepressant
    B. an antipsychotic
    C. an anticonvulsant
    D. an anesthetic

13. Which of the following cranial nerves controls digestive secretions and supplies most thorax and abdominal organs?

    A. olfactory nerve
    B. trochlear nerve
    C. glossopharyngeal nerve
    D. vagus nerve

14. Which of the following prefixes pertains to the spinal cord?

    A. encephal/o
    B. myel/o
    C. kinest/o
    D. neur/o

15. Inability to convert thoughts into writing that is not caused by intellectual impairment is known as:

    A. dysphasia
    B. dyslexia
    C. agraphia
    D. alexia

Fill in the Blank

Use your knowledge of medical terminology to insert the correct term from the list below.

craniotomy	fontanelle	aneurysm
dyslexia	pons	alexia
lethargy	plexus	astrocyte
microglia	stupor	agnosia
dementia	midbrain	paraplegia

1. _____ means the loss of mental ability to understand sensory stimuli, usually caused by brain injury or illness.

2. A group of nerve cells that are involved with the immune system and engulf various substances are referred to as _____.

3. A learning disability involving written language is called _____.

4. _____ means a loss of cognitive function that causes insensibility due to a variety of causes.

5. A "nerve net" consisting of the joining of the processes of neurons is called a(n) _____.

6. _____ is a term that means fatigue or sluggishness.

7. A structure on the brain stem that relays sensory information between the cerebrum and cerebellum is referred to as the _____.

8. A(n) _____ is a surgical operation performed to access the brain by removing a "bone flap" from the skull.

9. Impairment in motor and sensory function of the lower extremities is referred to as _____.

10. _____ means a localized, blood-filled bulge of a blood vessel due to disease or weakening of the vessel wall.

Labeling – The Neuron

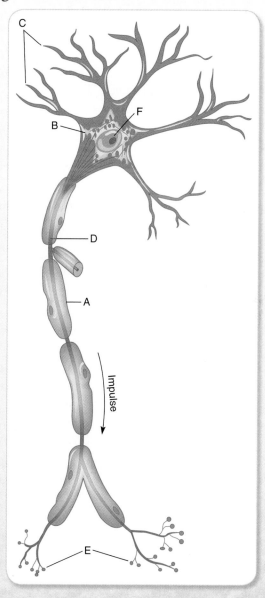

Write in the term below that corresponds with each letter on the figure above.

A. _____

B. _____

C. _____

D. _____

E. _____

F. _____

True / False

Identify each of the following statements as true or false by placing a "T" or "F" on the line beside each number.

_____ 1. Tranquilizers are administered to relieve pain and prevent seizures.

_____ 2. Chemical substances that transmit impulses over synapses are known as *neurotransmitters.*

_____ 3. The pons is a part of the brain stem located between the midbrain and spinal cord.

_____ 4. The pineal gland in the brain produces melanin.

_____ 5. Sulci are elevations on the surface of the brain that surround the gyri.

_____ 6. The olfactory nerve controls the sense of smell.

_____ 7. A neurological disorder causing loss of ability to execute learned and intentional movements is referred to as *apraxia.*

_____ 8. Loss of mental ability to understand sensory stimuli usually caused by brain injury or illness is referred to as *alexia.*

_____ 9. Partial paralysis of one side of the body is known as *hemiplegia.*

_____10. Dementia is a progressive decline in cognitive function due to brain damage or disease.

Labeling – The Brain

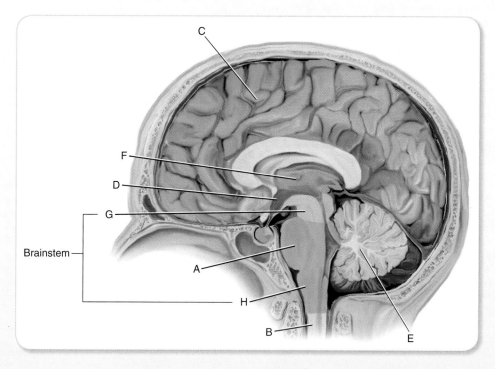

Write in the term below that corresponds with each letter on the figure above.

A. _____

B. _____

C. _____

D. _____

E. _____

F. _____

G. _____

H. _____

Definitions

Define each of the following words in one sentence.

1. anencephaly: _____

2. astrocyte: _____

3. diencephalon: _____

4. medulla oblongata: _____

5. myelin sheath: _____

6. neuron: _____

7. pineal body: _____

8. synapses: _____

9. cerebellum: _____

10. corpus callosum: _____

Abbreviations

Write the full meaning of each abbreviation.

Abbreviation	Meaning
1. ACh	_____
2. ALS	_____
3. CSF	_____
4. AD	_____
5. CVA	_____
6. LP	_____
7. MRI	_____
8. MS	_____
9. PET	_____
10. PNS	_____

Matching – Terms and Definitions

Match each term with its correct definition by placing the corresponding letter on the line to its left.

_____ 1. aura

_____ 2. dementia

_____ 3. sciatica

_____ 4. syncope

_____ 5. stupor

_____ 6. paraplegia

_____ 7. cephalgia

A. fainting; a sudden loss of consciousness

B. a painful disorder of the nerves

C. a perceptual disturbance that may occur before a migraine headache or an epileptic seizure

D. a headache; also known as *cephalalgia*

_____ **8.** hydrocephalus

_____ **9.** neuralgia

_____**10.** analgesia

E. progressive decline in cognitive function due to brain damage or disease (beyond normal aging)

F. loss of sensation of pain by interruption of the sensory pathway to the brain

G. a loss of cognitive function that causes insensibility

H. pain or other symptoms caused by sciatic nerve root compression or irritation

I. an abnormal accumulation of cerebrospinal fluid in the cavities of the brain

J. impairment in motor and sensory function of the lower extremities

Spelling

Circle the correct spelling from each pairing of words.

1. atacia   ataxia

2. aneurysm   anurysm

3. cerebelum   cerebellum

4. anesthesia   anestesia

5. astrocite   astrocyte

6. bradykenesia   bradykinesia

7. dyslexia   dislexia

8. dementia   dimentia

9. corpus calosum   corpus callosum

10. melatonin   mellatonin

Endocrine System

OBJECTIVES

Upon completion of this chapter, the reader should be able to:

1. Name the glands that comprise the endocrine system.
2. Identify the differences among diabetes mellitus, diabetes insipidus, and gestational diabetes.
3. List the nine endocrine glands that are discussed in this chapter.
4. Define, pronounce, and spell the hormones that are secreted by the pituitary gland.
5. List five hormones of the adrenal glands.
6. Interpret the meaning of abbreviations presented in this chapter.
7. Define, pronounce, and spell the diseases and disorders of the endocrine system.
8. Recognize common pharmacological agents used in treating disorders of the endocrine system.

STRUCTURE AND FUNCTION OF THE ENDOCRINE SYSTEM

The endocrine system is made up of glands that secrete hormones and control how specific body organs work. Hormones regulate many intricate body functions, and are often transported in the blood to target cells that contain specific receptor proteins for the hormones. The ductless glands of the endocrine system secrete their hormones directly onto a structure's surface rather than through ducts.

The endocrine system is composed of several organs (Figure 8-1). These organs include:

- pituitary gland, with the connection to the hypothalamus
- pineal gland
- thyroid gland
- parathyroid glands
- thymus gland
- adrenal glands
- pancreas
- testes and ovaries

The endocrine glands and their functions are as follows:

- *hypothalamus* – releases TRH, CRH, GnRH, and GHRH, and controls the release of anterior pituitary hormones
- *pituitary* – The pituitary gland includes the anterior and posterior pituitary. The posterior pituitary (**neurohypophysis**) stores and releases hormones that are actually produced by the hypothalamus, whereas the anterior pituitary (**adenohypophysis**) produces and secretes its own hormones. The anterior pituitary, however, is regulated by hormones secreted by the hypothalamus, as well as by feedback from the target gland hormones (Figure 8-2).
- The **pituitary gland**, or *hypophysis*, is located in the brain. It is attached to the hypothalamus by a stalk-like structure called the *infundibulum*. The pituitary gland is roughly the size of a pea and is also called the "master gland."
- **anterior pituitary** – The hormones secreted by the anterior pituitary are called **trophic hormones**. They are as follows:
  1. **growth hormone** (**GH**, or **somatotropin**) – promotes overall tissue and organ growth

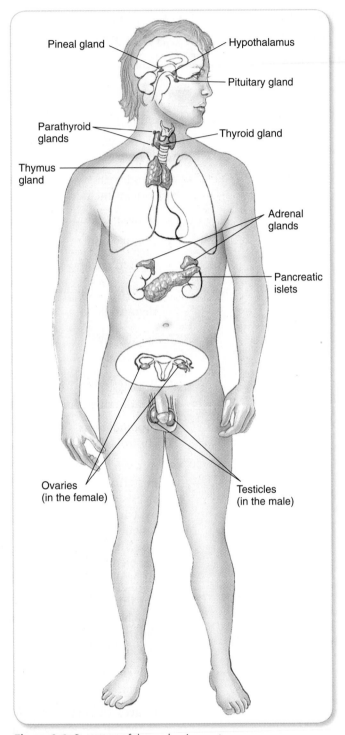

Figure 8-1 Structure of the endocrine system.

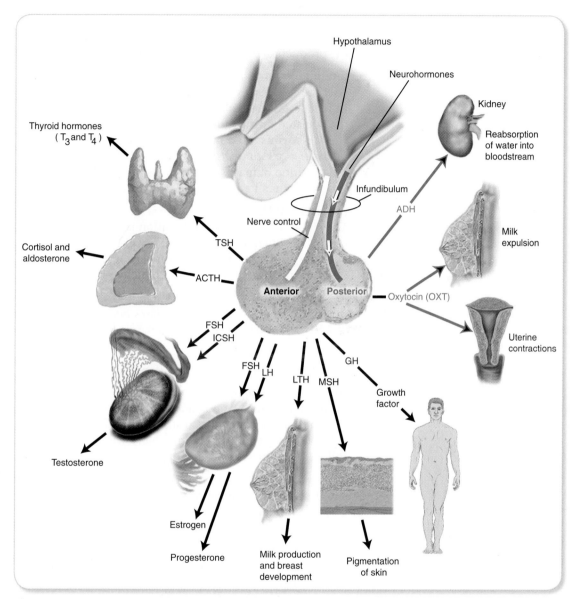

Figure 8-2 Hormones secreted by the pituitary gland.

2. **thyroid-stimulating hormone** (**TSH**, or **thyrotropin**) – stimulates the thyroid gland to produce and secrete thyroxine

3. **adrenocorticotropic hormone** (**ACTH**, or **corticotropin**) – stimulates the adrenal cortex to secrete the glucocorticoids, such as hydrocortisone (cortisol)

4. **follicle-stimulating hormone** (**FSH**, or **folliculotropin**) – stimulates the growth of ovarian follicles in females, and the production of sperm cells in the testes of males

5. **luteinizing hormone** (**LH**, or **luteotropin**) – LH and FSH are collectively called **gonadotropic hormones**. In females, LH stimulates ovulation and the conversion of the ovulated ovarian follicle into an endocrine structure called a **corpus luteum**. In males, LH is sometimes called *interstitial cell stimulating hormone,* or *ICSH*; it stimulates the secretion of male sex hormones (mainly testosterone) from the interstitial cells (Leydig cells) in the testes.

6. **prolactin** (**PRL**) – This hormone is secreted in both males and females. Its best known function is the stimulation of milk production by the mammary glands of women after the birth of a baby. Prolactin plays a supporting role in the regulation of the male reproductive system by the gonadotropins (FSH and LH).

- **posterior pituitary** – stores and releases two hormones, both of which are produced in the hypothalamus

  1. **antidiuretic hormone** (**ADH**) – stimulates water retention by the kidneys so that less water is excreted in the urine

  2. **oxytocin** – In females, oxytocin stimulates contractions of the uterus during labor, and for this reason is needed for childbirth. Oxytocin also stimulates contractions of the mammary gland alveoli and ducts, which result in the milk-ejection reflex in a lactating woman.

- *pineal gland* – The **pineal gland** is located deep within the brain. It secretes the hormone **melatonin**, the production of which is influenced by light–dark cycles. The secretion of melatonin increases at night and decreases during daylight.

- *thyroid* – releases thyroid hormones (which increase metabolic rate and are essential for normal growth and nerve development) and calcitonin (which decreases plasma calcium concentrations)

- *parathyroid* – releases parathyroid hormone, which regulates the exchange of calcium between blood and bones, as well as increasing calcium levels in the blood

- *thymus* – releases thymosin, which enhances proliferation and function of T-lymphocytes

- *adrenal glands* – These glands consist of the adrenal cortex and adrenal medulla, which are structurally and functionally different. The adrenal medulla secretes **catecholamine** hormones, which complement the sympathetic nervous system in the "fight or flight" reaction. The adrenal cortex secretes steroid hormones that participate in the regulation of mineral and energy balance.

- *adrenal cortex* – releases aldosterone (which increases sodium reabsorption and potassium secretion in kidney tubules), cortisol (which increases blood glucose at the expense of protein and fat stores, and contributes to stress adaptation), and androgens (which are responsible for development of secondary sex characteristics)

- *adrenal medulla* – releases epinephrine (which increases blood pressure and heart rate) and norepinephrine (which reinforces the sympathetic nervous system)

- *pancreas* – The pancreas is a mixed gland. It contains both exocrine and endocrine glands. The endocrine portion of the pancreas is composed of clusters of cells called the **pancreatic islets**. This portion secretes **insulin** and **glucagon**. Insulin promotes cellular uptake, is required for cellular metabolism of nutrients, and decreases blood sugar levels. Glucagon stimulates the liver to release glucose and increase blood sugar levels.

- *ovaries* – release estrogens (which promote follicular development, secondary sex characteristics, uterine growth, and breast growth) and progesterone (which prepares the uterus for pregnancy)

- *testes* – release testosterone, which stimulates production and maturation of spermata, and promotes the development of secondary sex characteristics

GENERAL TERMINOLOGY RELATED TO THE ENDOCRINE SYSTEM

The following are common terms that relate to the endocrine system.

Term	Pronunciation	Definition
Adenohypophysis	ad-eh-noh-high-POFF-ih-sis	the anterior pituitary gland, which regulates stress, growth, and reproduction
Aldosterone	al-DOSS-ter-ohn	an adrenal cortex hormone that causes the kidneys to retain sodium and water
Androgen	AN-droh-jen	a male steroid hormone that increases male (masculine) characteristics

(continues)

Term	Pronunciation	Definition
Antidiuretic	an-tie-dye-yoo-RET-ik	an agent that controls body water balance by affecting the kidneys and reducing urine output
Calcitonin	kal-sih-TOH-nin	a thyroid hormone that lowers plasma calcium and phosphate ion levels by inhibiting bone resorption and increasing renal excretion of phosphate and calcium
catecholamine	kah-teh-KOH-lah-min	one of a group of chemicals produced in nervous tissue that regulates a wide range of functions; the most common catecholamines are epinephrine and norepinephrine
Cortex	COR-tex	the outermost, superficial layer of an organ
endocrinologist	en-doh-krin-ALL-oh-jist	a doctor who specializes in diseases and disorders of the endocrine system
endocrinology	en-doh-krin-ALL-oh-jee	the study of endocrine system diseases and disorders
Epinephrine	ep-ih-NEF-rin	an adrenal medulla hormone and neurotransmitter that responds to stress by rapidly preparing the body for action
Estrogen	ESS-troh-jen	the primary type of female sex hormone; important in development of secondary sex characteristics
Glucagon	GLOO-kah-gon	a pancreatic hormone (from the alpha cells) that elevates blood glucose
Gonads	GOH-nadz	the sex glands (in the female, the gonads are the ovaries; in the male, they are the testes)
growth hormone	GROWTH HOR-moan	the hormone that regulates the growth of bone, muscle, and other body tissues
hypothalamus	hy-poh-THAL-ah-mus	an area at the central underside of the brain that produces and releases hormones
Insulin	IN-soo-lin	the pancreatic hormone (from the beta cells) that lowers blood glucose
Medulla	meh-DULL-lah	the inner core of an organ or structure
neurohypophysis	noo-roh-hy-PAW-fih-sis	the posterior pituitary, which stores and releases hormones
norepinephrine	nor-ep-ih-NEH-frin	the adrenal medulla hormone and neurotransmitter that increases heart rate, blood pressure, and blood glucose levels in response to stress
Oxytocin	ok-see-TOH-sin	the posterior pituitary gland hormone that stimulates contractions during labor and milk ejection from the breasts
pancreatic islets	PANG-kree-ah-tik EYE-lets	the areas of the pancreas with endocrine function that control blood sugar levels and the metabolism of glucose

parathormone	pah-ruh-THOR-moan	the hormone which regulates blood calcium and phosphorus ion levels; also called *parathyroid hormone*
pineal gland	PY-nee-uhl GLAND	a pinecone-shaped organ in the brain that secretes melatonin, which influences sexual maturation and the circadian cycle
pituitary gland	pih-TOO-ih-tair-ee GLAND	the master gland that orchestrates endocrine function; also called the *hypophysis*
progesterone	proh-JESS-ter-ohn	a hormone secreted by the ovaries (as well as the placenta) that prepares the uterus for pregnancy and causes development of the breasts
somatotropic hormone	soh-mat-oh-TROH-pik HOR-moan	growth hormone; secreted from the anterior pituitary gland, it promotes growth and cell reproduction
Thymosin	thy-MOH-sin	another thymus hormone that stimulates T-cell production involved in immune responses
thyroid gland	THY-royd GLAND	the gland that secretes thyroid hormone
Thyroxine	thy-ROCK-sin	a thyroid hormone that helps maintain normal body metabolism; also known as "T_4"

PATHOLOGICAL CONDITIONS

The following are pathological conditions of the endocrine system.

Acromegaly – a disorder marked by progressive enlargement of the head, face, hands, and feet due to excessive secretion of growth hormone

Addison's disease – failure of the adrenal cortex to secrete enough corticoids; symptoms include weakness, weight loss, hypotension, GI disturbances, and pigmentation changes

Cretinism – a congenital birth condition mostly characterized by dwarfism and slowed mental development

Cushing's syndrome – a disorder resulting from increased adrenocortical secretion of cortisol, due to a tumor of the adrenal cortex, or excessive administration of steroids; characterized by obesity of the trunk, "moon face," acne, abdominal striae, hypertension, diabetes mellitus, hypertension, psychiatric disturbance, osteoporosis, amenorrhea, and hirsuitism

Diabetes insipidus – chronic excretion of very large amounts of pale urine of low specific gravity, causing dehydration and extreme thirst; ordinarily results from inadequate output of pituitary antidiuretic hormone

Diabetes mellitus – a metabolic disease in which carbohydrate use is reduced, and that of lipids and proteins is enhanced; caused by an absolute or relative deficiency in insulin

Diabetic retinopathy – retinal changes occurring in diabetes of long duration, marked by hemorrhages, micro-aneurysms, and sharply defined waxy deposits

Dwarfism – a condition of extremely small size due to deficiency of GH; also known as *congenital hypopituitarism*

Exophthalmia – a condition of extreme outward protrusion of the eyeballs, commonly caused by Graves' disease

Gestational diabetes – diabetes that develops during pregnancy in women who were not previously diabetics; usually subsides after delivery

Gigantism – a condition of abnormal size or overgrowth of the entire body, due to hypersecretion of GH before puberty

Goiter (simple; nontoxic) – a chronic enlargement of the thyroid gland, not due to a neoplasm, occurring endemically in certain locations, where the soil is low in iodine

Glycosuria – above-average amounts of glucose in the urine, often because of diabetes

Goiter – a swelling of the neck because of an enlarged thyroid gland

Graves' disease – toxic goiter characterized by diffuse hyperplasia of the thyroid gland; a form of hyperthyroidism; exophthalmia is a common component of this disease

Hashimoto disease – an autoimmune disease that causes an inflamed thyroid gland

Hirsuitism – excessive hair growth on a female's face or body that may signify an androgen level disorder

Hypercalcemia – elevated blood calcium level, often due to other disorders or conditions

Hyperglycemia – elevated blood sugar level, commonly related to diabetes

Hypergonadism – excessive secretion of gonadal hormones

Hyperinsulinism – an excessive amount of insulin, resulting in hypoglycemia

Hyperkalemia – higher-than-normal levels of potassium in the blood

Hypernatremia – higher-than-normal levels of sodium in the blood

Hyperparathyroidism – a condition due to an increase in the secretion of the parathyroids, causing elevated serum calcium, low levels of calcium in the bones, and low levels of phosphate (a phosphorus salt) in the blood

Hyperpituitarism – overproduction of anterior pituitary gland hormones

Hyperthyroidism – overproduction of thyroid hormones from the thyroid gland

Hypocalcemia – lower-than-normal levels of calcium in the blood

Hypoglycemia – lower-than-normal levels of glucose in the blood

Hypokalemia – lower-than-normal levels of potassium in the blood

Hyponatremia – lower-than-normal levels of sodium in the blood

Hypoparathyroidism – a condition caused by lack of secretion of parathyroid hormones, with low serum calcium, tetany, and, occasionally, increased bone density

Hypopituitarism – a condition resulting from diminished activity of the anterior lobe of the pituitary, with inadequate secretion of one or more anterior pituitary hormones

Hypothyroidism – low levels of thyroid hormone, leading to clinical manifestations of thyroid insufficiency, including somnolence, dryness of skin, loss of hair, subnormal temperature, hoarseness, muscle weakness, and occasionally, myxedema

Insulin resistance syndrome – a condition in which the receptors on body cells show resistance and do not allow insulin to bring glucose into the cells to be metabolized; in this condition, the pancreas secretes large amounts of insulin

Insulin shock – acute hypoglycemia, usually caused by insulin overdosage; can lead to coma

Myxedema – severe adult hypothyroidism; signified by skin changes, slow metabolism, and mental deterioration

Pancreatitis – destructive inflammation of the pancreas that may be chronic or acute; marked by severe abdominal pain, nausea, and vomiting

Pheochromocytoma – adrenal medulla tumor that produces oversecretion of epinephrine and norepinephrine; leads to hypertension, heart palpitations, anxiety, headache, weight loss, and excessive sweating

Polydipsia – excessive or abnormal thirst

Polyphagia – excessive or abnormal appetite

Polyuria – excessive urine secretion, often because of diabetes

Thyroiditis – chronic thyroid gland inflammation leading to thyroid gland enlargement; most often caused by antibodies attacking the thyroid gland

Thyrotoxicosis – the condition produced by excessive quantities of thyroid hormone; also called *thyroid storm*

Virilism – development of male secondary sex characteristics in a female

ABBREVIATIONS

The following are common abbreviations that relate to the endocrine system.

Abbreviation	Meaning
ACTH	adrenocorticotropic hormone
ADH	antidiuretic hormone
BMR	basal metabolic rate
BUN	blood urea nitrogen
Ca^{++}	calcium ion
CT	calcitonin
DI	diabetes insipidus
DM	diabetes mellitus
E	epinephrine
FBS	fasting blood sugar
FSH	follicle-stimulating hormone
GDM	gestational diabetes mellitus
GH	growth hormone
GTT	glucose tolerance test
HbA1c	hemoglobin A1C
hGH	human growth hormone; somatotropin
IDDM	insulin-dependent diabetes mellitus

IRS	insulin resistance syndrome
K^+	potassium ion
LH	luteinizing hormone
LTH	lactogenic hormone
MSH	melanocyte-stimulating hormone
Na^+	sodium ion
NE	norepinephrine
NIDDM	non-insulin-dependent diabetes mellitus
OGTT	oral glucose tolerance test
OT	oxytocin
OXT	oxytocin
PBI	protein-bound iodine
PRL	prolactin
PTH	parathyroid hormone
RAI	radioactive iodine
RAIU	radioactive iodine uptake
T_3	triiodothyronine
T_4	thyroxine (tetraiodothyronine)
TFT	thyroid function test
TSH	thyroid-stimulating hormone

MEDICATIONS USED TO TREAT ENDOCRINE SYSTEM DISORDERS

The following are common medications used for endocrine system disorders.

Generic Name	Trade Name	Drug Class	Use
chlorpropamide	Diabinese®	antihyperglycemics	to lower blood glucose, or to increase insulin sensitivity
glyburide	Diabeta®, Micronase®		
insulin	Humulin®, Novolin®		
pioglitazone	Actos®		
rosiglitazone	Avandia®		
glucagon	Glucagon® Diagnostic Kit®	antihypoglycemics	to prevent or relieve insulin reaction or hypoglycemia

(continues)

Generic Name	Trade Name	Drug Class	Use
somatotropin	Humatrope®, Nutropin®	human growth hormone	to increase growth in cases of less-than-normal height
dexamethasone methylprednisolone prednisone	Decadron®, Cortastat® Medrol® Cortan®, Deltasone®	steroids	to increase growth or relieve symptoms of various diseases, including inflammatory conditions (such as arthritis) and cancer

DRUG TERMINOLOGY

The following are common types of drugs used for endocrine system conditions.

Drug Type	Pronunciation	Definition
Antihyperglycemics	an-tee-hy-per-gly-SEE-miks	agents that counteract high levels of blood glucose
Antihypoglycemics	an-tee-hy-poh-gly-SEE-miks	agents that counteract low levels of blood glucose
Hormone replacement therapy (HRT)	—	the use of natural or synthetic hormones to replace low levels of hormones required by the body
human growth hormone	—	naturally occurring substance made by the human body that promotes growth
Hypoglycemics	hy-poh-gly-SEE-miks	agents that lower the level of glucose in the blood
radioactive iodine therapy	—	a treatment used to eliminate thyroid tumors; it can destroy thyroid gland tissue or thyroid cancer
Steroids	STAIR-oydz	hormones or chemical substances commonly used to increase relieve symptoms of various diseases, especially inflammatory conditions (such as arthritis) and cancer

Review Exercises

Multiple Choice

Select the best answer and write the letter of your choice to the left of each number.

1. Excess secretion of growth hormone during adulthood will cause:

   A. dwarfism
   B. gigantism
   C. acromegaly
   D. cretinism

2. Which of the following hormones is released from the posterior pituitary gland?

   A. prolactin
   B. growth hormone
   C. cortisol
   D. antidiuretic hormone

3. Elevated levels of calcium ions in the blood stimulate the secretion of the hormone:

   A. calcitonin
   B. thyroid hormone
   C. growth hormone
   D. testosterone

4. A male steroid hormone that increases male characteristics is referred to as:

   A. epinephrine
   B. estrogen
   C. androgen
   D. aldosterone

5. Higher-than-normal levels of potassium in the blood signify a condition called:

   A. hypernatremia
   B. hyperkalemia
   C. hypercalcemia
   D. hyperglycemia

6. Which of the following hormones stimulates T-lymphocytes to cause immunity?

   A. oxytocin
   B. insulin
   C. testosterone
   D. thymosin

7. Which of the following hormones is released by the adrenal medulla?

   A. norepinephrine
   B. insulin
   C. thymosin
   D. cortisol

8. Which of the following conditions may be caused by an increase in secretion of cortisol?

   A. dwarfism
   B. diabetes insipidus
   C. acromegaly
   D. Cushing's syndrome

9. Which of the following consists of an abnormal overgrowth of the entire body due to hypersecretion of growth hormone before puberty?

   A. Graves' disease
   B. gestational diabetes
   C. gigantism
   D. goiter

10. Which of the following is also called *thyroid storm*?

    A. thyroiditis
    B. thyrotoxicosis
    C. pheochromocytoma
    D. hypothyroidism

11. Which of the following endocrine glands releases calcitonin?

    A. parathyroid
    B. hypothalamus
    C. thymus
    D. thyroid

12. Which of the following glands produces aldosterone?

    A. testes
    B. pancreas
    C. adrenal cortex
    D. ovaries

13. Excessive hair growth in women signifies a condition called:

    A. hirsuitism
    B. myxedema
    C. acromegaly
    D. pheochromocytoma

14. Oversecretion of epinephrine and norepinephrine due to a tumor of the adrenal medulla may cause:

    A. pheochromocytoma
    B. myxedema
    C. dwarfism
    D. hirsuitism

15. Which of the following agents may lower the level of blood glucose?

    A. hypoglycemics
    B. glucagon
    C. somatotropin
    D. glycogen

Fill in the Blank

Use your knowledge of medical terminology to insert the correct term from the list below.

thyroid gland	anterior pituitary	epinephrine
thymus gland	pineal gland	cretinism
glycosuria	adrenal cortex	myxedema
ovaries	testes	estrogen
aldosterone	posterior pituitary	pancreas

1. A hormone that causes the kidneys to retain sodium and water is known as _____.

2. Thymosin is the only hormone that is secreted from the _____ gland.

3. Growth hormone is produced from the _____ gland.

4. The medulla of the adrenal gland releases _____.

5. A congenital birth condition mostly characterized by dwarfism and slowed mental development is called _____.

6. Calcitonin is released by the _____.

7. Diabetes mellitus is caused by an insufficiency of insulin from the _____.

8. Severe adult hypothyroidism is referred to as _____.

9. Oxytocin is secreted by the _____ gland.

10. Cushing's syndrome is a disorder resulting from increased secretion of cortisol from the _____.

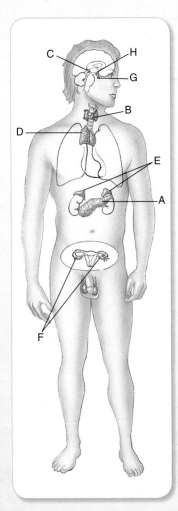

Labeling – The Structures of the Endocrine System

Write in the terms below that correspond with each letter on the figure left.

A. _____

B. _____

C. _____

D. _____

E. _____

F. _____

G. _____

H. _____

True / False

Identify each of the following statements as true or false by placing a "T" or "F" on the line beside each number.

_____ **1.** The adrenal cortex secretes insulin.

_____ **2.** The testes are the primary site of production of estrogen.

_____ **3.** The parathyroid glands cause hypoglycemia.

_____ **4.** The thyroid gland secretes calcitonin.

_____ **5.** The hypothalamus controls and stimulates the anterior pituitary gland.

_____ **6.** Oxytocin is involved in contraction of the uterus during delivery.

_____ **7.** Antidiuretic hormone is secreted by the anterior pituitary gland.

_____ **8.** The hypothalamus releases TRH and CRH.

_____ **9.** A congenital birth condition mostly characterized by dwarfism and slowed mental development is called *hirsuitism*.

_____ **10.** Hyperinsulinism may result in hyperglycemia.

Definitions

Define each of the following words in one sentence.

1. hypernatremia: _____

2. growth hormone: _____

3. hypergonadism: _____

4. endocrinologist: _____

5. androgen: _____

6. hypoglycemia: _____

7. polyphagia: _____

8. goiter: _____

9. glucagon: _____

10. estrogen: _____

Abbreviations

Write the full meaning of each abbreviation.

Abbreviation	Meaning
1. TSH	_____
2. MSH	_____
3. PBI	_____
4. BUN	_____
5. RAI	_____
6. BMR	_____
7. GTT	_____
8. IRS	_____
9. ADH	_____
10. DI	_____

Matching – Terms and Definitions

Match each term with its correct definition by placing the corresponding letter on the line to its left.

_____ 1. adenohypophysis

_____ 2. thymus

_____ 3. gonads

_____ 4. epinephrine

_____ 5. thyroid storm

_____ 6. polyphagia

_____ 7. dwarfism

A. severe adult hypothyroidism

B. excessive appetite

C. the anterior pituitary gland

D. a progressive enlargement of the head, face, hands, and feet due to excessive secretion of growth hormone

_____ **8.** progesterone

_____ **9.** acromegaly

_____**10.** myxedema

E. an extremely small body size due to deficiency of growth hormone

F. a hormone secreted by the ovaries

G. the condition produced by excessive quantities of thyroid hormone

H. the sex glands

I. located in the chest behind the sternum

J. responds to stress by rapidly preparing the body for action

Spelling

Circle the correct spelling from each pairing of words.

1. cretinism   kretinism

2. aldustrone   aldosterone

3. hirsotism   hirsuitism

4. norepinephrine   nurepinephrine

5. jigantism   gigantism

6. pheochromocytoma   pheochromacytoma

7. virilism   viralism

8. kortex   cortex

9. glycosuria   glycozuria

10. oxitocin   oxytocin

Digestive System

OBJECTIVES

Upon completion of this chapter, the reader should be able to:

1. Identify the major structures of the digestive system.
2. Describe the main function of the digestive tract.
3. Explain the accessory organs of the digestive system.
4. Identify at least 10 abbreviations common to the digestive system.
5. Describe the main disorders that affect the stomach and small intestine.
6. Explain the role of the pancreas and liver in digestion.
7. Define, pronounce, and spell the diseases and disorders of the digestive system.
8. Recognize common pharmacological agents used in treating disorders of the digestive system.

STRUCTURE AND FUNCTION OF THE DIGESTIVE SYSTEM

The digestive system is referred to as the *gastrointestinal tract*, the *alimentary canal*, and the *digestive tract*. It takes in food, digests it, and expels wastes. The alimentary canal extends from the mouth to the anus. Several accessory organs secrete substances into the canal that are used in the process of digestion. The alimentary canal includes the mouth, pharynx, esophagus, stomach, small intestine, large intestine, rectum, and anus. The accessory organs include the salivary glands, liver, gallbladder, and pancreas (Figure 9-1).

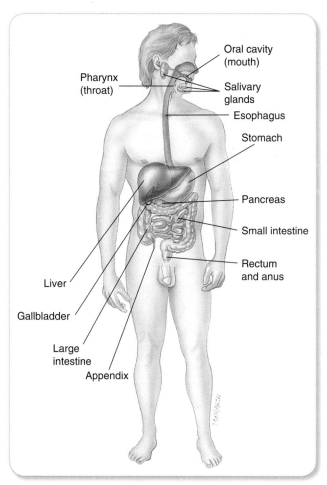

Figure 9-1 Structures of the digestive system.

The digestive organs prepare foods for **absorption** into the bloodstream. The process of breaking down food so that it can be absorbed is known as **digestion**. The process of removing the solid waste from the digestive system is called "elimination." The alimentary canal is a muscular tube about 8 meters long that passes through the body's thoracic and abdominopelvic cavities. The structure of its wall, how it moves food, and its innervation are similar throughout its length.

The mouth receives food and begins digestion by mechanically reducing the size of solid particles and mixing them with saliva. This action is called *mastication*. The lips, cheeks, tongue, and palate surround the mouth, which includes a chamber between the palate and tongue called the *oral cavity* (Figure 9-2).

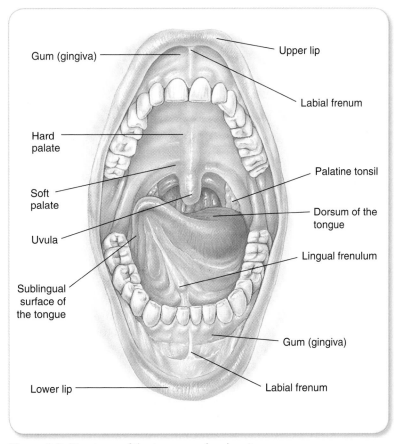

Figure 9-2 Structures of the tongue and oral cavity.

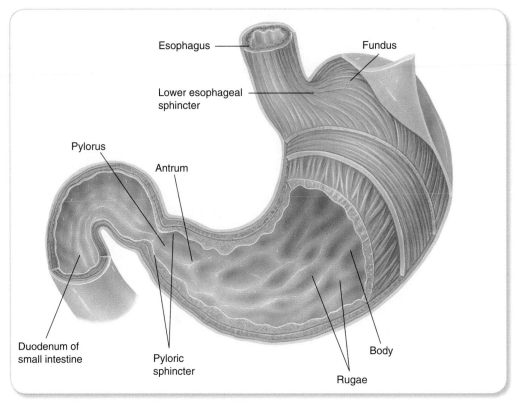

Figure 9-3 Structure of the stomach.

The esophagus is a straight, collapsible tube about 25 centimeters long, which acts as a food passageway from the pharynx to the stomach. The stomach itself is a J-shaped, pouch-like organ that hangs inferior to the diaphragm in the upper left portion of the abdominal cavity, and has a capacity of approximately 1 liter (Figure 9-3). The stomach receives food from the esophagus, mixes the food with gastric juice, initiates protein digestion, carries on limited absorption, and moves food into the small intestine.

The small intestine consists of three portions: the duodenum, the jejunum, and the ileum. The duodenum, which is about 25 centimeters long and 5 centimeters in diameter, is the most fixed portion of the small intestine.

The large intestine is so named because its diameter is greater than that of the small intestine. This portion of the alimentary canal is about 1.5 meters long, and begins in the lower right side of the abdominal cavity, where the ileum joins the cecum. From there, the large intestine ascends on the right side, crosses to the left, and

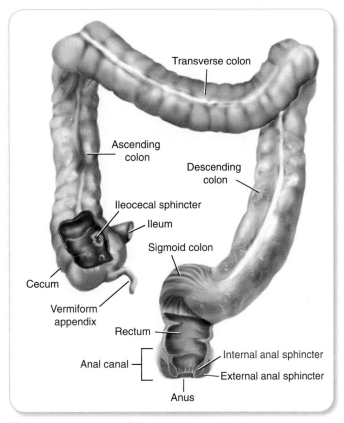

Figure 9-4 Structures of the large intestine.

descends into the pelvis. At its distal end, it opens to the outside of the body at the anus (Figure 9-4).

The accessory organs of digestion are the salivary glands, liver, gallbladder, and pancreas. The pancreas is a "mixed gland," meaning that it has both an endocrine and an exocrine function. Pancreatic juice contains enzymes that digest carbohydrates, fats, and proteins.

The liver is in the upper right quadrant of the abdominal cavity, just inferior to the diaphragm. The average adult liver is the heaviest organ in the body. It weighs about 3 pounds. The liver carries on many important metabolic activities. The only digestive function of the liver is the formation of bile for the emulsification of fats in the small intestine. Bile is stored in the gallbladder, a pear-shaped sac in a depression on the liver's inferior surface (Figure 9-5).

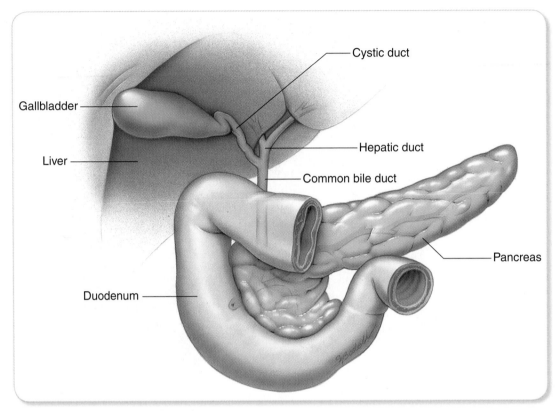

Figure 9-5 The liver, gallbladder, and pancreas.

GENERAL TERMINOLOGY RELATED TO THE DIGESTIVE SYSTEM

The following are common terms that relate to the digestive system.

Term	Pronunciation	Definition
absorption	ab-SORP-shun	the taking up of a substance by cells, tissues, or organs, such as from the digestive tract
adventitia	ad-ven-TIH-shuh	the outermost layer of a structure, composed of connective tissue with collagenous and elastic fibers
alimentary canal	al-ih-MEN-tar-ee-can-NAL	the digestive tract or gastrointestinal tract (which extends from the mouth to the anus)
amino acids	ah-MEE-noh acids	the building blocks of proteins
amylase	AM-ih-lays	a type of enzyme in the saliva that breaks down starch into maltose molecules

antrum	AN-trum	any nearly closed cavity
anus	AY-nus	the external opening of the rectum, through which feces are eliminated from the body
appendix	ah-PEN-diks	an attachment at the end of the large intestine; has no known purpose
bile	BYE-al	a yellow-green fluid secreted from the liver, stored in the gallbladder, which aids in the digestion of lipids
bilirubin	bill-ih-ROO-bin	an orange-yellow excretion in bile that is the breakdown product of normal heme (from hemoglobin) catabolism
bowel	BOW-el	the intestine; the part of the alimentary canal from the pyloric opening of the stomach to the anus
cecum	SEE-kum	a pouch connected to the ascending colon that connects to the vermiform appendix
chyme	KIME	semi-fluid, partly digested food expelled from the stomach into the duodenum
colon	COH-lon	a storage tube for solid wastes, extending from the cecum to the rectum
defecation	deh-feh-KAY-shun	the expelling of feces from the colon and rectum through the anus
deglutition	dee-gloo-TIH-shun	swallowing
diarrhea	dy-uh-REE-uh	the frequent passage of watery bowel movements
digestion	dy-JES-chun	the breaking down of food into an absorbable form
duodenum	doo-OD-eh-num	the hollow first portion of the small intestine, connecting the stomach to the jejunum
emesis	EH-meh-sis	vomiting
enzyme	EN-zime	a substance (usually a protein) that increases the rates of chemical reactions
esophagus	eh-SOF-ah-gus	the "gullet"; a muscular tube through which food passes from the pharynx to the stomach
exocrine gland	EKS-oh-krin gland	a gland that secretes enzymes into ducts
feces	FEE-seez	waste from the digestive tract expelled through the rectum and anus during defecation
gallbladder	GALL-blad-der	the cholecyst; an organ that stores bile and aids in digestion
gastroenterologist	gas-troh-en-ter-ALL-oh-jist	a doctor who specializes in the digestive system and its related disorders
gavage	gah-VAZH	feeding via a tube passed through the nose into the esophagus
gingivae	JIN-jih-vah	the gums; tissue that surrounds the teeth
glucagon	GLOO-kah-gon	an important hormone produced by pancreatic alpha cells involved in carbohydrate metabolism
glucose	GLOO-kohs	a simple sugar (found in fruits and other foods) that is the major source of energy

(continues)

Term	Pronunciation	Definition
glycogen	GLY-koh-jen	a starch (complex sugar) formed from glucose, stored chiefly in the liver that is the major carbohydrate stored in animal cells
hepatocyte	HEP-ah-toh-sight or heh-PAT-oh-sight	a liver cell involved in many normal liver functions; it also begins the formation of bile
hydrochloric acid	high-droh-KOLH-rik-acid	a compound of hydrogen and chlorine that is the major component of gastric acid
ileum	ILL-ee-um	the final section of the small intestine that extends from the jejunum to the cecum
insulin	IN-soo-lin	a hormone secreted by the beta cells in the pancreas in response to increased blood glucose
jejunum	jee-JOO-num	the middle of the small intestine; it connects with the duodenum and ileum
lavage	lah-VAZH	irrigating or washing out an organ for therapeutic reasons
lipase	LIH-pays or LIE-pays	an enzyme that aids in fat digestion and metabolism
liver	LIH-ver	the largest gland (and largest visceral organ) in the body; plays a major role in metabolism, glycogen storage, and detoxification
mastication	mass-tih-KAY-shun	chewing food with the teeth as it is mixed with saliva
mesenteries	MEH-sen-teh-rees	the double peritoneal sheets that hold some of the organs in their proper position in the abdominal cavity
nausea	NAW-zee-uh	an unpleasant sensation in the upper abdomen that often precedes vomiting; typically occurs in digestive upset, motion sickness, and sometimes early pregnancy
palate	PAH-lat	the roof of the mouth
pancreas	PAN-kree-us	an organ located in the abdomen that manufactures insulin and digestive juices
parotid gland	pah-ROT-id gland	the largest of the salivary glands
peristalsis	peh-rih-STAL-sis	the rippling contractions of the muscles in the digestive tract that force food and bile through
pharynx	FAIR-inks	the part of the neck and throat behind the mouth and nasal cavity
pyloric sphincter	py-LOH-rik SFINK-ter	a valvular muscle in the stomach that regulates the passage of food from the pylorus of the stomach into the duodenum
pylorus	py-LOH-rus	the muscle at the juncture of the stomach and the duodenum that controls the flow of stomach contents into the small intestine; is normally closed, but opens to allow the stomach to push partially digested food into the duodenum
rectum	REK-tum	the lower part of the large intestine, which conducts feces out of the body through the anus
rugae	ROO-gay	irregular ridges or folds in the hard palate's mucous membrane lining

saliva	sah-LYE-vuh	the clear fluid secreted by the salivary and mucous glands in the mouth, which helps to begin digestion of food
salivary glands	SAL-ih-vair-ee GLANDZ	glands that secrete saliva into the mouth, aiding in digestion
serosa	seh-ROH-sah	the outermost serous layer of a visceral structure that lies in a body cavity such as the abdomen or thorax
sigmoid colon	SIG-moyd colon	the S-shaped portion of the colon that connects the descending colon to the rectum
sphincter	SFINK-ter	circular muscle fibers that constrict a passage or close a body opening
stomach	STUH-muk	the major organ of digestion, located in the left upper quadrant of the abdomen; lies between the esophagus and the small intestine
triglycerides	try-GLIH-seh-ryds	compounds consisting of a fatty acid and glycerol
upper GI tract	UH-per GEE-EYE TRAKT	the mouth, pharynx, esophagus, and stomach
uvula	YOO-vyoo-lah	cone-shaped process of connective tissue in the mouth that is suspended from the soft palate
villi	VIL-eye	one of many tiny finger-like projections clustered over the entire mucous surface of the small intestine, which aid in absorption

PATHOLOGICAL CONDITIONS

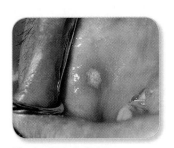

Figure 9-6 Aphthous stomatitis. *Courtesy of Dr. Joseph Konzelman, School of Dentistry, Medical College of Georgia*

The following are pathological conditions of the digestive system.

Achalasia – decreased muscular ability of the lower two-thirds of the esophagus to move food downward, coupled with the inability of the lower esophageal sphincter to relax during swallowing

Aphthous stomatitis – recurrent, painful "canker sores" in the mouth (Figure 9-6)

Appendicitis – an inflammation of the appendix

Ascites – accumulation of fluid in the abdominal cavity; may be caused by cirrhosis of the liver, heart disease, or lymphatic or venous obstruction

Biliary colic – acute abdominal pain caused by gallstones in the bile ducts

Celiac disease – an autoimmune disorder of the small intestine causing nutrient malabsorption because of damaged small-bowel mucosa

Cholecystitis – an inflammation of the gallbladder

Cholelithiasis – gallstones; the presence of crystalline bodies within the gallbladder

Cirrhosis – gradual destruction of liver tissue with loss of function, and ultimately, liver failure; Figure 9-7 shows conditions associated with cirrhosis of the liver

Colorectal cancer – the presence of a malignant neoplasm in the large intestine, rectum, or appendix; also called *colon cancer*

Constipation – a decrease in the frequency of bowel movements or the passage of dry, hard stools; a common condition in elderly persons

Crohn's disease – patches of chronic digestive tract inflammation, and even ulcers, causing fever, cramps, diarrhea, weight loss, and anorexia; can affect any part of the digestive tract

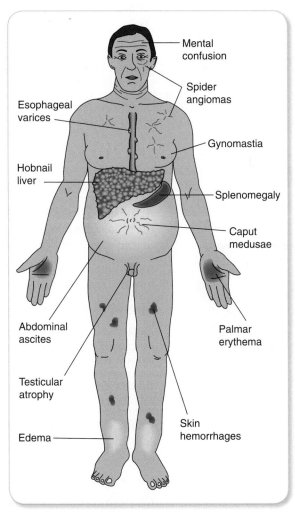

Figure 9-7 Conditions associated with cirrhosis of the liver.

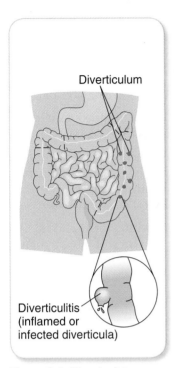

Figure 9-8 Diverticulitis.

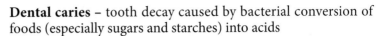

Dental caries – tooth decay caused by bacterial conversion of foods (especially sugars and starches) into acids

Diverticulitis – an inflammation of the diverticula in the wall of the digestive tract, especially in the colon

Diverticulosis – presence of one or more reticula (small pouches); commonly occurs with aging and is not harmful unless a diverticulum becomes inflamed (Figure 9-8)

Dysentery – painful intestinal inflammation often caused by the ingestion of bacteria, protozoa, parasites, or chemical irritants; produces severe diarrhea

Esophageal varices – swollen, twisted veins in the distal end of the esophagus that often cause bleeding

Fistula – an abnormal passageway between two organs, or from an organ to the body surface, such as between the rectum and anus

Flatus – gas or air in the digestive tract, particularly in the intestines

Gallstones (cholelithiasis) – formation of stones in the gallbladder, consisting of cholesterol or bilirubin, which may obstruct the biliary tract

Gastroenteritis – an inflammation of the stomach and intestine

Gastroesophageal reflux disease – a condition caused by reflux of gastric juices into the esophagus resulting in heartburn, regurgitation, inflammation, and possible damage to the esophagus; caused by weakness of the lower esophageal sphincter; commonly called *heartburn*

Heartburn – the term commonly used to describe "gastroesophageal reflux"

Hemorrhoids – a bulging blood vessel in the anus; often painful and may bleed; most appear and disappear spontaneously

Hepatitis – acute or chronic liver inflammation caused by viral infection, drugs, alcohol, parasites, or toxins; types of viral hepatitis include hepatitis A, B, C, D, E, and G

Hepatomegaly – an enlargement of the liver

Hernia – an irregular protrusion of tissue or another structure through the surrounding cavity's muscular wall

Herpetic stomatitis – inflamed lesions in (or on) the oral cavity caused by the herpes simplex virus

Hiatal hernia – a protrusion of the stomach through the opening in the diaphragm through which the esophagus passes (see Figure 9-9)

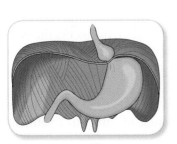

Figure 9-9 Hiatal hernia.

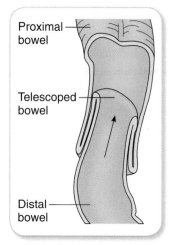

Figure 9-10 Intussusception.

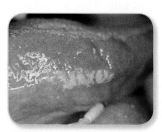

Figure 9-11 Oral leukoplakia. *Courtesy of Dr. Joseph Konzelman, School of Dentistry, Medical College of Georgia*

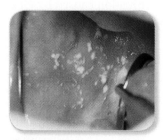

Figure 9-12 Thrush. *Courtesy of Dr. Joseph Konzelman, School of Dentistry, Medical College of Georgia*

Hirschsprung's disease (congenital megacolon) – absence of the parasympathetic nerve ganglion cells in a segment of the colon, usually in the rectosigmoid area, occurring at birth; causes colon enlargement due to obstruction

Ileus – complete or partial blockage of the small or large intestine

Intussusception – telescoping of a section of the proximal intestine into the distal intestine, causing an obstruction (Figure 9-10)

Irritable bowel syndrome (IBS) – the increased motility of the lower intestinal wall, usually precipitated by emotional stress; signs and symptoms include pain, flatulence, nausea, anorexia, constipation, diarrhea, and/or gas; also called *spastic colon*

Jaundice – yellowness of the skin, whites of the eyes, and mucous membranes caused by the presence of bile pigments, mainly **bilirubin**, in the blood; a symptom of hepatitis and other diseases of the liver and biliary system; also called **icterus**

Occult blood – blood present in the feces in such small amounts that it can be detected only microscopically or chemically; may be a sign of intestinal bleeding (*occult* means "hidden")

Oral leukoplakia – a pre-cancerous white plaque and hardening of a part of the mucous membrane in the mouth (Figure 9-11)

Pancreatitis – severe inflammation of the pancreas and surrounding tissue associated with autodigestion by pancreatic enzymes

Peptic ulcers – breaks in the mucous membrane of the stomach or proximal duodenum as a result of hyperacidity or the bacterium *Helicobacter pylori*; also known as "gastric ulcers"

Periodontal disease – infection and damage to the gingivae, bone, and ligaments around the teeth, often caused by plaque

Peritonitis – an inflammation of the peritoneum, the membrane that lines the abdominal cavity and covers the abdominal organs; may result from perforation of an ulcer, rupture of the appendix, or infection of the reproductive tract

Pyloric stenosis – a narrowing of the pyloric sphincter at the outlet of the stomach, causing an obstruction that blocks the flow of food into the small intestine; occurs as a congenital defect in newborns

Thrush – yeast infection in the mouth and throat, producing sore, white, and slightly raised patches; caused by *Candida albicans*; commonly occurs after a course of antibiotic treatment (Figure 9-12)

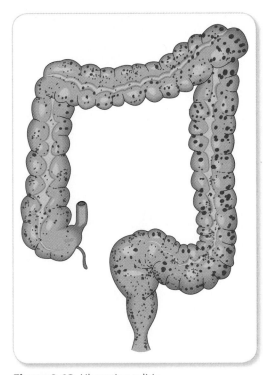

Figure 9-13 Ulcerative colitis.

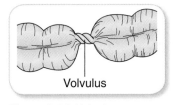

Volvulus

Figure 9-14 Volvulus.

Ulcerative colitis – a chronic inflammation and ulceration (with remissions and exacerbations) of the colon and rectum, characterized by diarrheal stools containing mucus, pus, or blood (Figure 9-13)

Volvulus – a twisting of the intestine on itself that results in an obstruction (Figure 9-14)

ABBREVIATIONS

The following abbreviations relate to terms and procedures of the digestive system.

Abbreviation	Meaning
BE	barium enema
BM	bowel movement
CBD	common bile duct
GB	gallbladder

(continues)

Abbreviation	Meaning
GERD	gastroesophageal reflux disease
GI	gastrointestinal
GI series	gastrointestinal series
HAV	hepatitis A virus
HBV	hepatitis B virus
HCl	hydrochloric acid
HCV	hepatitis C virus
HDV	hepatitis D virus
HEV	hepatitis E virus
IBD	inflammatory bowel disease
IBS	irritable bowel syndrome
LES	lower esophageal sphincter
MRI	magnetic resonance imaging
N&V	nausea and vomiting
NG	nasogastric (tube)
N/V/D	nausea, vomiting, and diarrhea
PPBS	postprandial blood sugar
SBF	small bowel follow-through
SBS	small bowel series
S&D	Stomach and duodenum
TPN	total parenteral nutrition
UGI series	upper gastrointestinal series

MEDICATIONS USED TO TREAT DIGESTIVE SYSTEM DISORDERS

The following are common medications used for digestive system conditions.

Drug Class	Generic Name	Pronunciation for Generic Name	Trade Name	Use
antacid	aluminum & magnesium hydroxide	ah-LOO-mih-num and mag-NEE-zee-um hi-DROK-side	Maalox®, Mylanta®	to neutralize stomach acid
	cimetidine	sih-MEH-tih-deen	Tagamet®	
	famotidine	fah-MAH-tih-deen	Pepcid®	
	magaldrate	MAG-al-drate	Riopan®	
	ranitidine	rah-NIH-tih-DEEN	Zantac®	

antidiarrheal	attapulgite bismuth subsalicylate loperamide	at-uh-PULL-gite BIZ-muth sub-sah-LIS-ih-late loh-PAIR-ah-mide	Kaopectate®, Diasorb® Pepto-Bismol® Imodium®	to control loose stools
antiemetic	dimenhydrinate meclizine	dy-men-HY-drih-nate MEK-lih-zeen	Dramamine® Bonine®, Antivert®	to prevent regurgitation (vomiting)
antispasmodic	dicyclomine hyoscyamine	dy-SY-klo-meen hy-oh-SY-ah-meen	Antispas®, Bentyl® Anaspaz®, Cystospaz®	to calm intestinal tract spasms
cathartic	ipecac syrup	IP-ih-kak syrup	(generic only)	to cause vomiting (after ingestion of poison)
laxative	Bisacodyl docusate psyllium senna	bis-ah-KOH-dil- DOK-yoo-sate SIL-ee-yum SEN-na	Dulcolax®, Theralax® Therevac® Metamucil® Senokot®	to relieve constipation

DRUG TERMINOLOGY

The following are common types of drugs used for digestive system conditions.

Drug Type	Pronunciation	Definition
antacids	ant-ASS-ids	agents that neutralize stomach acid; usually bases or basic salts
antidiarrheals	an-tee-dy-ah-REE-ulz	agents that control watery, loose stools; types include electrolyte solutions, bulking agents, adsorbents, and opiates
antiemetics	an-tee-eh-MET-iks	agents that prevent vomiting and nausea
antispasmodics	an-tee-spaz-MOD-iks	agents that control intestinal tract spasms by suppressing smooth muscle contraction
cathartics	ka-THAR-tiks	agents that induce vomiting; are also used for emptying the intestine by accelerating defecation
laxatives	LAK-suh-tivs	agents that induce bowels to move or loosen the stool, therefore relieving constipation; also known as "purgatives"

REVIEW EXERCISES

Multiple Choice

Select the best answer and write the letter of your choice to the left of each number.

1. Which of the following organs is not a component of the digestive tract?

   A. colon
   B. pharynx
   C. esophagus
   D. spleen

2. Which of the following is an accessory organ of digestion?

   A. stomach
   B. spleen
   C. pancreas
   D. colon

3. The portion of the small intestine that is attached to the pylorus of the stomach is the:

   A. ileum
   B. duodenum
   C. rectum
   D. jejunum

4. The middle portion of the small intestine is the:

   A. ileum
   B. jejunum
   C. duodenum
   D. pylorus

5. The portion of the small intestine that attaches to the large intestine is the:

   A. jejunum
   B. colon
   C. appendix
   D. ileum

6. Which of the following are double sheets of peritoneal membrane that hold some of the visceral organs in their proper positions?

   A. serosa
   B. flatus
   C. adventitia
   D. mesenteries

7. Which of the following terms means "telescoping of a section of the proximal intestine into the distal intestine causing an obstruction"?

    A. ileus
    B. intussusception
    C. achalasia
    D. Crohn's disease

8. A substance that increases the rates of chemical reactions is called a(n):

    A. enzyme
    B. chyme
    C. bile
    D. saliva

9. The external opening of the rectum is known as the:

    A. rugae
    B. uvula
    C. villi
    D. anus

10. Which of the following substances is stored in the gallbladder and released into the duodenum?

    A. bile
    B. pancreatic enzymes
    C. vitamin B_{12}
    D. vitamin K

11. Which of the following terms means "a twisting of the intestine on itself that results in an obstruction"?

    A. intussusception
    B. ileus
    C. volvulus
    D. rugae

12. Irregular ridges or folds in the hard palate's mucous membrane lining are referred to as:

    A. rugae
    B. uvula
    C. volvulus
    D. cecum

13. An autoimmune disorder of the small intestine causing nutrient malabsorption is known as:

    A. irritable bowel syndrome
    B. cirrhosis
    C. dysentery
    D. celiac disease

14. An inflammation of the gallbladder is referred to as:

    A. cholecystitis
    B. cirrhosis
    C. hepatitis
    D. pancreatitis

15. Patches of chronic digestive tract inflammation and/or ulcers are referred to as:

    A. fistulas
    B. ileus
    C. aphthous stomatitis
    D. Crohn's disease

Fill in the Blank

Use your knowledge of medical terminology to insert the correct terms from the list below.

villi	uvula	chyme
rectum	ileum	mastication
cecum	rugae	pyloric sphincter
hepatomegaly	defecation	jejunum
lavage	gavage	peristalsis

1. Irregular ridges or folds in the hard palate's mucous membrane lining are called _____.

2. Semi-fluid and partly digested food expelled from the stomach into the duodenum is referred to as _____.

3. Feeding via a tube passed through the nose into the esophagus is called _____.

4. The many tiny finger-like projections clustered over the entire mucous surface of the small intestine are referred to as _____.

5. An enlargement of the liver is called _____.

6. Irrigating or washing out an organ for therapeutic reasons is known as _____.

7. A cone-shaped process of connective tissue in the mouth that is suspended from the soft palate is called the _____.

8. A valvular muscle in the stomach that regulates the passage of food into the duodenum is referred to as the _____.

9. The middle part of the small intestine is known as the

_____.

10. Rippling contractions of the muscles in the digestive tract that force food through are described as a process called

_____.

Labeling – The Major Structures and Accessory Organs

Write in the terms below that correspond with each letter on the figure (left).

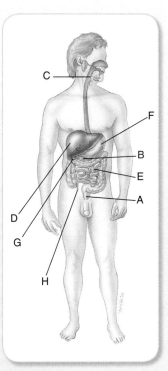

A. _____

B. _____

C. _____

D. _____

E. _____

F. _____

G. _____

H. _____

True / False

Identify each of the following statements as true or false by placing a "T" or "F" on the line beside each number.

_____ **1.** The esophagus is a collapsible tube about 25 centimeters long.

_____ **2.** The alimentary canal is a muscular tube about 8 meters long.

_____ **3.** One of the accessory organs of digestion is the spleen.

_____ **4.** The liver is located in the upper left quadrant of the abdominal cavity.

_____ **5.** Glycogen is a complex sugar formed from glucose.

_____ **6.** Waste from the digestive tract expelled through the rectum is called "feces."

_____ **7.** Deglutition means "nausea and vomiting."

_____ **8.** The palate is the roof of the mouth.

_____ **9.** The jejunum is the final section of the small intestine.

_____ **10.** The gallbladder is located in the pelvic cavity, and stores urine.

Labeling – The Structures of the Stomach

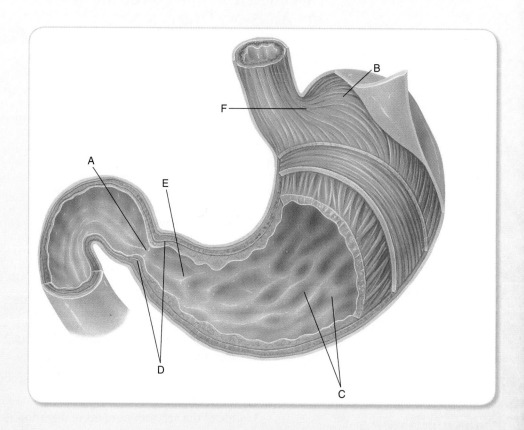

Write in the terms below that correspond with each letter on the figure above.

A. _____

B. _____

C. _____

D. _____

E. _____

F. _____

Definitions

Define each of the following words in one sentence.

1. digestion: _____

2. gingivae: _____

3. hepatocyte: _____

4. bowel: _____

5. absorption: _____

6. mastication: _____

7. saliva: _____

8. pylorus: _____

9. mesenteries: _____

10. serosa: _____

Abbreviations

Write the full meaning of each abbreviation.

Abbreviation	Meaning
1. GERD	_____
2. IBS	_____
3. HCV	_____
4. S&D	_____
5. TPN	_____
6. N&V	_____
7. BM	_____
8. NG	_____
9. IBD	_____
10. GI	_____

Matching – Terms and Definitions

Match each term with its correct definition by placing the corresponding letter on the line to its left.

_____ **1.** appendix

_____ **2.** colon

_____ **3.** rectum

A. the major organ of digestion; lies between the esophagus and the small intestine

_____ 4. small intestine

_____ 5. stomach

_____ 6. duodenum

_____ 7. pancreas

_____ 8. jejunum

_____ 9. esophagus

_____ 10. liver

B. the largest gland in the body

C. the hollow first portion of the small intestine, connecting the stomach to the jejunum

D. the middle of the small intestine; it connects with the duodenum and ileum

E. a muscular tube through which food passes from the pharynx to the stomach

F. an organ located in the abdomen that manufactures insulin

G. a storage tube for solid waste, extending from the cecum to the rectum

H. an attachment to the end of the large intestine

I. the terminal section of the digestive tract

J. the organ where most digestion occurs

Spelling

Circle the correct spelling from each pairing of terms.

1. sphancter   sphincter

2. jejenum   jejunum

3. pylorus   pilorus

4. gavage   gavaje

5. kyme   chyme

6. cecum   cekum

7. glycojen   glycogen

8. rugae   rogae

9. serosa   cerosa

10. deglotition   deglutition

Cardiovascular System

OBJECTIVES

Upon completion of this chapter, the reader should be able to:

1. Identify anatomic features of the heart.
2. Distinguish between various blood vessels.
3. Describe the major functions of the circulatory system.
4. Describe certain conditions affecting the layers of the heart.
5. Correctly define, spell, and pronounce the chapter's terms.
6. Define common abbreviations related to the cardiovascular system.
7. Identify the chambers of the heart and the pathway that blood takes through them.
8. Specify the way in which blood is supplied to the heart muscle.

Structure and Function of the Cardiovascular System

Blood circulates throughout the body in the cardiovascular system, which consists of the heart, arteries, veins, and capillaries. This system forms a continuous circuit that carries oxygen and nutrients to all cells, and removes waste products. The heart functions to pump blood that is low in oxygen to the lungs, where it is oxygenated. It then pumps oxygen-rich blood to the entire body. Each day, the heart pumps approximately 7,000 liters (1,855 gallons) of blood throughout the body.

Arteries, veins, and capillaries make up the body's blood vessels. Capillaries are the smallest of these vessels, and the sites of nutrient and gas exchange. The heart is located within the **mediastinum** of the thorax. The heart is in a tilted position, with the inferior **apex** resting on the diaphragm (Figure 10-1).

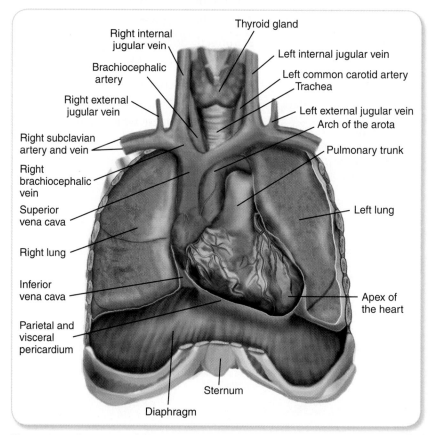

Figure 10-1 Structures of the circulatory system.

The wall of the heart consists of three layers. Moving from the innermost to outermost layers, the three layers are as follows:

1. **endocardium** – a thin membrane that lines the chambers and valves

2. **myocardium** – the thick muscle layer that makes up most of the heart wall

3. **epicardium** – a thin membrane that covers the heart

The heart's linings and layers are shown in Figure 10-2.

The **pericardium** is a serous membrane that surrounds and protects the heart, with a strengthening covering known as the **parietal pericardium**. The pericardium's inner layer is known as the **visceral pericardium**. Between these two layers is a small space called the **pericardial cavity**.

Four chambers and four valves are found within the heart. The two upper chambers are called **atria,** and the two lower chambers are known as **ventricles.** The **septum** is a wall dividing the right and left sides of the heart. The thinner atrial walls receive blood and route it to the ventricles. The ventricular walls are thicker because the ventricles pump blood through to the lungs (from the right ventricle) and throughout the entire body (from the left ventricle). Since the left ventricle must pump blood to most of the body, its muscle is thicker than those of the other chambers (Figure 10-3).

Blood that is low in oxygen and high in carbon dioxide enters the **right atrium** from the *vena cava* and from the coronary sinus.

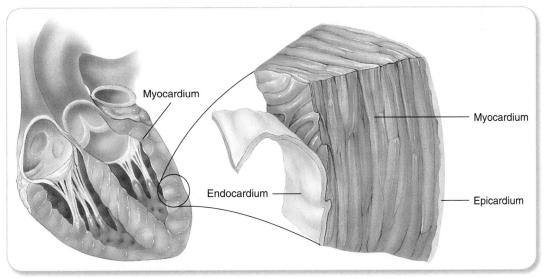

Figure 10-2 Tissues of the heart walls.

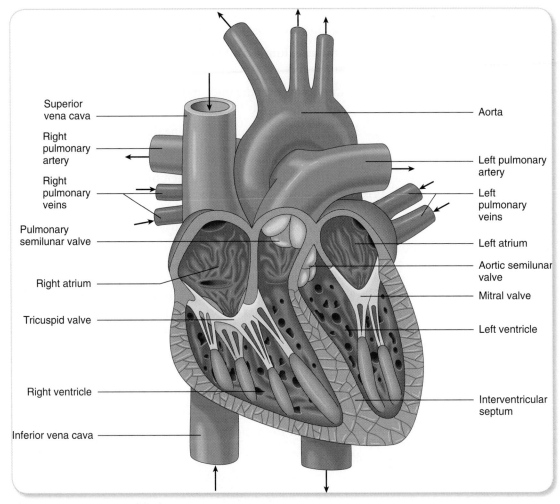

Superior vena cava

Right pulmonary artery

Right pulmonary veins

Pulmonary semilunar valve

Right atrium

Tricuspid valve

Right ventricle

Inferior vena cava

Aorta

Left pulmonary artery

Left pulmonary veins

Left atrium

Aortic semilunar valve

Mitral valve

Left ventricle

Interventricular septum

Figure 10-3 Structures of the heart.

As the right atrial wall contracts, the blood passes through the **tricuspid valve** and enters the chamber of the **right ventricle**. When the right ventricular wall contracts, the tricuspid valve closes and blood moves through the **pulmonary valve** into the trunk and its branches (*pulmonary arteries*).

From the pulmonary arteries, blood enters the capillaries associated with the alveoli of the lungs. The exchange of gases occurs between blood in the capillaries and air in the alveoli. The freshly oxygenated blood, low in carbon dioxide, returns to the heart through the pulmonary veins that lead to the left atrium.

The left atrial wall contracts, and blood moves through the mitral valve and into the chamber of the left ventricle. When the left

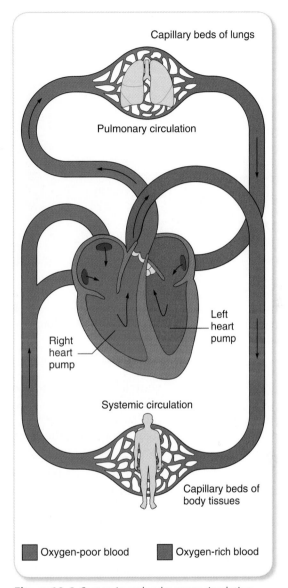

Figure 10-4 Systemic and pulmonary circulation.

ventricular wall contracts, the mitral valve closes, and blood moves through the aortic valve into the aorta and its branches (Figure 10-4).

The first two branches of the aorta, called the right and left **coronary arteries**, supply blood to the tissues of the heart. Their openings lie just beyond the aortic valve (Figure 10-5).

The cardiac conduction system coordinates and controls the contraction (**systole**) and relaxation (**diastole**) of the atria and

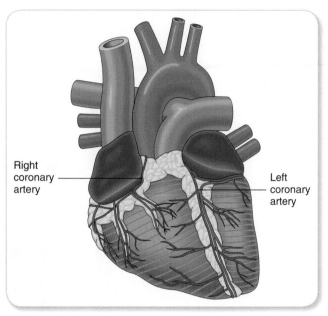

Figure 10-5 Coronary arteries.

ventricles. A key component of this conduction system is the **sinoatrial node** (or **SA node**), a small, elongated mass of specialized cardiac muscle tissue just beneath the epicardium. It is located in the right atrium near the opening of the superior vena cava and its fibers.

Impulses from the SA node travel through the myocardium to the **atrioventricular node** (or **AV node**). This node is located in the inferior portion of the septum that separates the atria just beneath the endocardium. This node coordinates the incoming impulses from the atria and relays them to the ventricles through specialized muscle fibers known as the **bundle of His**. These fibers enter the septum separating the right and left ventricles, and divide into **right** and **left bundle branches**, terminating in the **Purkinje fibers**. These fibers form the electrical impulse-conduction system of the heart and cause the ventricles to contract (Figure 10-6).

Blood vessels form a tubular network throughout the body that permits blood to flow from the heart to all living cells of the body and then back to the heart. Blood leaving the heart passes through vessels of progressively smaller diameters, referred to as *arteries*, *arterioles*, and *capillaries* (which are microscopic vessels that joint the arterial flow to the venous flow). Blood returning to the heart from the capillaries passes through vessels of progressively larger diameter, called *venules* and *veins* (Figure 10-7).

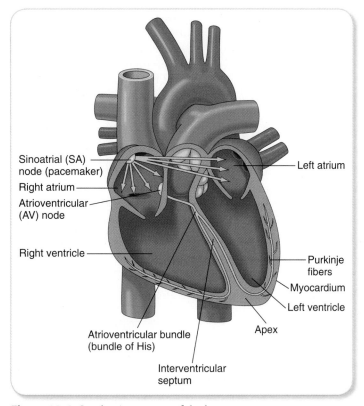

Sinoatrial (SA) node (pacemaker)

Right atrium

Atrioventricular (AV) node

Right ventricle

Left atrium

Purkinje fibers

Myocardium

Left ventricle

Apex

Atrioventricular bundle (bundle of His)

Interventricular septum

Figure 10-6 Conduction system of the heart.

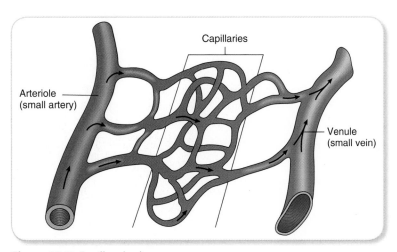

Capillaries

Arteriole (small artery)

Venule (small vein)

Figure 10-7 Capillary bed.

The thick muscle layer of the arteries (**aorta**) and its branches allows them to transport blood ejected from the heart under high pressure. The thinner muscle layer of veins allows them to distend when an increased amount of blood enters, and their one-way valves ensure that blood flows back to the heart. Capillaries facilitate the rapid exchange of materials between the blood and interstitial fluid. Figure 10-8 illustrates the anterior view of arterial circulation, and Figure 10-9 shows the anterior view of venous circulation.

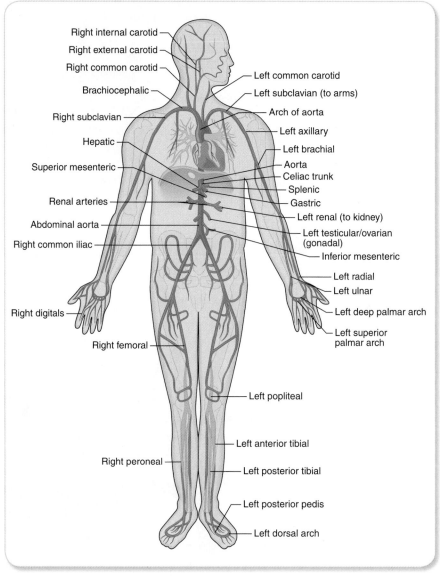

Figure 10-8 Anterior view of arterial circulation.

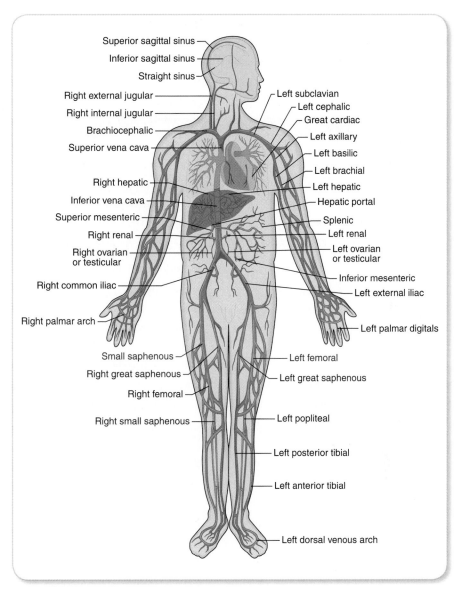

Figure 10-9 Anterior view of venous circulation.

GENERAL TERMINOLOGY RELATED TO THE CARDIOVASCULAR SYSTEM

The following are common terms that relate to the cardiovascular system.

Term	Pronunciation	Definition
anastomosis	ah-nas-toh-MOH-sis	surgical joining of two vessels to bypass an occluded area and restore normal blood flow
aorta	ay-OR-tuh	the largest blood vessel in the body; receives blood directly from the left ventricle of the heart, branches into smaller arteries, and supplies blood to the arterial side of the circulatory system
arteriole	ar-TEE-ree-ol	a small blood vessel on the arterial side of the circulatory system; arterioles are the small blood vessels that make the transition from the arteries to the capillaries
atrium	AY-tree-um	either of the two upper chambers of the heart
bicuspid valve	by-KUS-pid VALV	atrioventricular valve on the left side of the heart; also called the "mitral valve" (pronounced MY-trul VALV)
cholesterol	koh-LES-ter-ahl	fatty substance present in animal fats; circulates in the bloodstream, sometimes causing arterial plaque to form
diastole	dye-ASS-toh-lee	the period when the heart relaxes after each contraction
dysrhythmia	dis-RITH-mee-ah	any abnormal heart rhythm
endocardium	en-doh-KAR-dee-um	membranous lining of the chambers and valves of the heart; the innermost layer of heart tissue
epicardium	ep-ih-KAR-dee-um	the outer layer of heart tissue
hyperlipidemia	high-per-lip-ih-DEE-mee-ah	raised levels of fats and/or lipoproteins in the blood
left atrium	LEFT AY-tree-um	upper left heart chamber
left ventricle	LEFT VEN-trih-kul	lower left heart chamber
lumen	LOO-men	the channel formed by a hollow, tube-like anatomic structure or piece of equipment
malaise	mah-LAYZ	a general feeling of discomfort or uneasiness
mediastinum	mee-dee-ass-TYE-num	structures in the chest comprising the central thoracic cavity
myocardium	my-oh-CAR-dee-um	the muscular middle layer of the heart
occlusion	ah-KLOO-shun	blockage of vessels
pacemaker	—	the sinoatrial (SA) node, which generates electrical impulses in the heart; also, an artificial device that regulates heart rhythm
palpitation	pal-pih-TAY-shun	abnormal beating of the heart
pericardium	pair-ih-CAR-dee-um	the thin, double-walled, membranous sac that encloses the heart and the roots of the greater blood vessels

prophylactic	proh-fih-LAK-tik	used to protect against disease
pulmonary artery	PUL-moh-neh-ree artery	artery that carries blood from the heart to the lungs
pulmonary circulation	PUL-moh-neh-ree circulation	deoxygenated blood movement from the right ventricle to the lungs for oxygenation and back to the left atrium
pulmonary vein	PUL-moh-neh-ree vein	one of the vessels that carry oxygenated blood from the lungs to the left atrium
pulmonary valve	PUL-moh-neh-ree VALV	valve that controls the blood flow between the right ventricle and the pulmonary arteries
pulse	PULS	rhythmic expansion and contraction of a blood vessel, usually an artery
right atrium	RITE AY-tree-um	upper right chamber of the heart
right ventricle	RITE VEN-trih-kul	lower right chamber of the heart
sinoatrial (SA) node	sy-noh-AY-tree-al node	the pacemaker of the heart; it initiates heartbeat and helps to control its rhythm
septum	SEP-tum	the wall that divides the right and left sides of the heart
systemic circulation	sis-TEM-ik circulation	the movement of oxygenated blood away from the heart to the body, and returning of deoxygenated blood back to the heart
systole	SIS-toh-lee	the contraction phase of the heart
thrombosis	throm-BOH-sis	formation of a clot or thrombus inside a blood vessel
tricuspid valve	try-KUS-pid VALV	atrioventricular valve on the right side of the heart
valve	VALV	any of various structures that slow or prevent blood from flowing backward or forward
vasoconstriction	vaz-oh-con-STRIK-shun	narrowing of a blood vessel
vein	VAYN	any of various blood vessels carrying deoxygenated blood toward the heart (except for the pulmonary vein)
ventricle	VEN-trih-kul	either of the two lower chambers of the heart
venule	VEN-yool	a tiny vein connected to a capillary

PATHOLOGICAL CONDITIONS

The following are disorders and conditions of the cardiovascular system.

Aneurysm – a localized, abnormal dilation of a blood vessel, usually an artery, caused by weakness of the vessel wall; it may eventually burst

Angina pectoris – severe chest pain around the heart due to lack of blood and oxygen supply; also referred to as "angina"

Arrhythmia – any abnormality in the rate or rhythm of the heartbeat; also called *dysrhythmia*

Arteriosclerosis – hardening (sclerosis) of the arteries, with loss of capacity and loss of elasticity, as from fatty deposits (plaque), deposits of calcium salts, or formation of scar tissue

Ascites – accumulation of fluid in the peritoneal cavity

Atherosclerosis – the development of fatty, fibrous patches (plaques) in the lining of arteries, causing narrowing of the lumen and hardening of the vessel wall

Atrial flutter – abnormal heart rhythm in the atria; contractions occur at a rate between 250 to 400 beats per minute

Bradycardia – a slow heart rate, of less than 60 beats per minute

Bruit – an abnormal "blowing" sound or "murmur" heard while auscultating a carotid artery, organ, or gland; caused by blood flowing through a narrow or partially occluded artery

Carditis – an inflammation of the heart muscle, usually resulting from infection; in most cases, more than one layer of the heart wall is involved; chest pain, cardiac arrhythmia, circulatory failure, and damage to the structures of the heart may occur; types of carditis include endocarditis, myocarditis, and pericarditis

Claudication – cramp-like leg pains occurring in the calves, caused by poor blood circulation to the leg muscles; commonly associated with atherosclerosis

Coarctation of the aorta – abnormal narrowing of the aorta (Figure 10-10)

Congestive heart failure – any cardiac condition characterized by weakness, breathlessness, abdominal discomfort, lower body edema, and impaired pumping ability of the heart; also known as *cardiac failure*

Coronary artery disease – narrowing of the coronary arteries that prevents adequate blood supply to the myocardium, resulting in congestive heart failure

Endocarditis – inflammation of the endocardium and heart valves; characterized by lesions caused by a variety of diseases

Fibrillation – rapid, irregular, unsynchronized contractions resulting in uncoordinated twitching of the heart muscle; usually described by the part that is contracting abnormally, such as *atrial fibrillation* or *ventricular fibrillation*

Heart block – a disease that interferes with the normal electrical conduction of the heart, resulting in arrhythmia

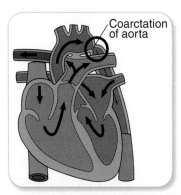

Coarctation of aorta

Figure 10-10 Coarctation of the aorta.

Heart failure – a condition caused by the inability of the heart to maintain adequate circulation of the blood; many of the symptoms associated with heart failure are caused by the dysfunction of organs other than the heart, especially the lungs, kidneys, and liver

Hypertension – a common disorder that is a known cardiovascular disease risk factor; characterized by elevated blood pressure over the normal values of 120/80 mm Hg in an adult over 18 years of age; this elevation is characterized by persistent readings of more than 140/90 mm Hg

Hypotension – an abnormal condition in which the blood pressure is not adequate for normal perfusion and oxygenation of the tissues; an expanded intravascular space, hypovolemia, or diminished cardiac output may be the cause

Infarct – an area of localized necrosis in a tissue resulting from anoxia; caused by a blockage or a narrowing of the artery that supplies the area

Intermittent claudication – a form of cramp-like pains in the leg muscles that is manifested only at certain times, usually after walking, and is relieved by rest

Ischemia – a decreased supply of oxygenated blood to a body part; often marked by pain and organ dysfunction, as in ischemic heart disease; some causes of ischemia are arterial embolism, atherosclerosis, thrombosis, and vasoconstriction

Mitral valve prolapse – a drooping of the mitral valve into the left atrium during ventricular systole, resulting in incomplete closure and mitral insufficiency

Murmur – an abnormal heart sound resulting from turbulent blood flow

Myocardial infarction – a heart attack; a life-threatening condition caused by occlusion of coronary arteries resulting from inadequate blood supply

Myocarditis – inflammation of the myocardium that is usually caused by viral, bacterial, or fungal infection, rheumatic fever, or chemical agents

Occlusion – a blockage in a canal, vessel, or passage of the body

Patent ductus arteriosus – a congenital defect involving an abnormal opening in the heart caused by failure of the fetal ductus arteriosus to close after birth (Figure 10-11)

Pericarditis – inflammation of the pericardium associated with trauma, malignant neoplastic disease, infection, uremia, and myocardial infarction

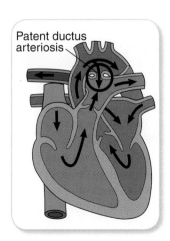

Patent ductus arteriosis

Figure 10-11 Patent ductus arteriosus.

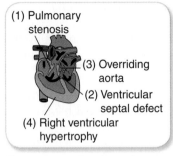

(1) Pulmonary stenosis

(3) Overriding aorta

(2) Ventricular septal defect

(4) Right ventricular hypertrophy

Figure 10-12 Tetralogy of Fallot.

Raynaud's phenomenon – intermittent attacks of ischemia of the extremities of the body, especially the fingers, toes, ears, and nose; caused by exposure to cold, or by emotional stimuli; attacks are characterized by severe blanching of the extremities, followed by cyanosis, then redness, usually accompanied by numbness, tingling, burning, and often pain

Rheumatic fever – a systemic inflammatory disease that may develop as a delayed reaction to an inadequately treated infection of the upper respiratory tract by group A beta-hemolytic streptococci; usually occurs in school-age children and may affect the heart, joints, skin, and brain

Tetralogy of Fallot – a set of congenital cardiac defects including ventricular septal defect, pulmonary valve stenosis, dextroposition of the aorta, and hypertrophy of the right ventricle (Figure 10-12)

Thrombophlebitis – vein inflammation due to the formation of a clot (thrombus); occurs most commonly as the result of trauma to the vessel wall, and is also called *phlebitis*

Transposition of the great vessels – a congenital cardiac anomaly in which the pulmonary artery arises from the left ventricle and the aorta from the right ventricle; there is no communication between the systemic and pulmonary circulations

Varicose veins – enlarged, superficial veins with incompetent valves that have become twisted and dilated; may be caused by thrombophlebitis, pregnancy, and obesity; common, especially in women, and usually painless

ABBREVIATIONS

The following abbreviations are related to terms and procedures of the cardiovascular system.

Abbreviation	Meaning
AF	atrial fibrillation
AMI	acute myocardial infarction
AS	aortic stenosis
ASCVD	arteriosclerotic cardiovascular disease
ASD	atrial septal defect
ASHD	arteriosclerotic heart disease
AV	atrioventricular
BBB	bundle branch block

BP	blood pressure
CABG	coronary artery bypass graft
CAD	coronary artery disease
cath	catheterization
CCU	coronary care unit
CHD	coronary heart disease
CHF	congestive heart failure
CPK	creatine phosphokinase
CPR	cardiopulmonary resuscitation
CVA	cerebrovascular accident
CVD	cardiovascular disease
DVT	deep vein thrombosis
ECG	electrocardiogram
ECHO	echocardiogram
GOT	glutamic oxaloacetic transaminase
HDL	high-density lipoprotein
LDH	lactate dehydrogenase
LDL	low-density lipoprotein
LV	left ventricle
LVH	left ventricular hypertrophy
MI	myocardial infarction
MR	mitral regurgitation
MRI	magnetic resonance imaging
MS	mitral stenosis
MVP	mitral valve prolapse
PACs	premature atrial contractions
PAT	paroxysmal atrial tachycardia
PDA	patent ductus arteriosus
PET	positron emission tomography
PTCA	percutaneous transluminal coronary angioplasty
PVC	premature ventricular contraction
SA	sinoatrial
SV	stroke volume
VLDL	very low-density lipoprotein
VSD	ventricular septal defect
VT	ventricular tachycardia

MEDICATIONS USED TO TREAT CARDIOVASCULAR SYSTEM DISORDERS

Various medications are used for the treatment of cardiovascular system disorders and conditions. Sometimes, surgical procedures are also required. The following are common medications used for cardiovascular system conditions.

Drug Class	Generic Name	Pronunciation for Generic Name	Trade Name	Use
ACE inhibitors	benazepril	beh-NAH-zeh-pril	Lotensin®	to ease heart-pumping and lower blood pressure by dilating arteries
	captopril	KAP-toh-pril	Capoten®	
	enalapril	eh-NAL-ah-pril	Vasotec®	
	lisinopril	lih-SIH-no-pril	Zestril®, Prinivil®	
	quinapril	QWIH-nah-pril	Accupril®	
	ramipril	RAH-mih-pril	Altace®	
angiotensin II receptor blockers	irbesartan	ir-beh-SAR-tan	Avapro®	to block the action of angiotensin II (which narrows and dilates blood vessels, lowering blood pressure)
	losartan	loh-SAR-tan	Cozaar®	
	valsartan	val-SAR-tan	Diovan®	
Antiarrhythmics	amiodarone	ah-mee-oh-dah-ROAN	Cordarone®	to alter the electrical flow through the heart's conduction system and regulate fast or irregular heartbeats
	disopyramide	dy-soh-PEER-ah-myed	Norpace®, Norpace CR®	
	flecainide	fleh-KAY-nyed	Tambocor®	
	mexiletine	MEK-sih-leh-teen	Mexitil®	
	moricizine	mor-IH-sih-zeen	Ethmozine®	
	procainamide	pro-KAY-nah-myed	Procan SR®, Pronestyl®	
	propafenone	pro-PAF-en-oan	Rythmol®	
	quinidine	QUIN-ih-dyen	Cardioquin®, Quinaglute Dura-Tabs®	
	sotalol	SOH-tah-lol	Betapace®	
	tocainide	toh-KAY-nyed	Tonocard®	
anticoagulants, anti-clotting agents	dicumarol	dy-CYOO-mah-rol	—	to reduce proteins involved in blood clotting so clots cannot form as easily
	enoxaparin	ee-NOK-sah-prin	Lovenox®	
	heparin	HEH-prin	—	
	warfarin	WAR-fah-rin	Coumadin®	

antiplatelet medications	aspirin	AS-pih-rin	(many names)	to reduce ability of blood platelets to clot
	clopidogrel	kloh-pih-DOH-grel	Plavix®	
	dipyridamole	dy-peer-ID-ah-moal	Persantine®	
beta blockers	atenolol	ah-TEH-no-lol	Tenormin®	to reduce contraction strength of heart muscle, lower blood pressure, and slow heartbeat
	bisoprolol	by-SOH-pro-lol	Zebeta®	
	carvedilol	kar-VEH-dih-lol	Coreg®	
	labetalol	la-BEH-tah-lol	Normodyne®, Trandate®	
	metoprolol	meh-TAH-pro-lol	Lopressor®	
	nadolol	NAY-doh-lol	Corgard®	
	pindolol	PIN-doh-lol	Visken®	
	propranolol	pro-PRAH-noh-lol	Inderal®	
	timolol	TIM-oh-lol	Blocadren®, Timoptic®	
bile acid sequestrants	cholestyramine	koh-leh-STEER-ah-meen	Prevalite®, Questran®	lipid-lowering medications that require more body cholesterol to create other bile acids; more cholesterol is used up and lowered
	colesevelam	koh-leh-SEH-veh-lam	Welchol®	
	colestipol	koh-LEH-stih-pol	Colestid®	
calcium channel blockers	amlodipine	am-LOD-ih-peen	Norvasc®	to inhibit calcium ions from entering the heart and blood vessel muscle cells; used to reduce heart rate, lower strength of heart contraction, lower blood pressure, dilate coronary arteries, and normalize certain fast or irregular heartbeats
	bepridil	BEH-prih-dil	Vascor®	
	diltiazem	dil-TY-ah-zem	Cardizem®, Dilacor XR®	
	felodipine	feh-LOD-ih-peen	Plendil®	
	nicardipine	nih-KAR-dih-peen	Cardene®	
	nifedipine	ny-FED-ih-peen	Procardia®, Adalat®	
	verapamil	veh-RAP-ah-mil	Calan®, Isoptin®	
centrally acting hypertensive agents	clonidine	KLON-ih-deen	Catapres®	to decrease blood pressure by affecting brain control centers
	guanabenz	GWAH-nah-benz	Wytensin®	
	guanfacine	GWAN-fah-seen	Tenex®	
	methyldopa	meh-thil-DOH-pa	Aldomet®	
coronary vasodilators	isosorbide dinitrate	eye-soh-SOR-byed dy-NY-trayt	Isordil®, Sorbitrate®	to dilate blood vessels; used to treat angina, myocardial infarction, and congestive heart failure
	isosorbide mononitrate	eye-soh-SOR-byed maw-noh-NY-trayt	Monoket®, IMDUR®	
	nitroglycerin	ny-troh-GLIS-er-in	Nitrodisc®, Nitro-Dur®	
	pentaerythritol tetranitrate	pen-tah-eh-RITH-rih-tol teh-tra-NY-trayt	Peritrate SA®	

(continues)

Drug Class	Generic Name	Pronunciation for Generic Name	Trade Name	Use
direct-acting vasodilators	hydralazine	hy-DRAH-lah-zeen	Apresoline®	to lower blood pressure by relaxing blood vessel walls
	minoxidil	mih-NOK-sih-dil	Loniten®	
diuretics	amiloride	ah-MIL-oh-ryed	Midamor®	to remove water via the kidneys to lower blood pressure and relieve edema
	bumetanide	byoo-MEH-tah-nyed	Bumex®	
	furosemide	fyoo-ROS-eh-myed	Lasix®	
	hydrochlorothiazide	hy-droh-klor-oh-THY-ah-zyed	Esidrix®, HydroDIURIL®	
	spironolactone	spih-ron-oh-LAK-toan	Aldactone®	
	triamterene	try-AM-ter-een	Dyrenium®	
diuretics (combination)	hydrochlorothiazide plus amiloride	hy-droh-klor-oh-THY-ah-zyed plus ah-MIL-oh-ryed	Moduretic®	same as the diuretics
	hydrochlorothiazide plus spironolactone	hy-droh-klor-oh-THY-ah-zyed plus spih-ron-oh-LAK-toan	Aldactazide®	
	hydrochlorothiazide plus triamterene	hy-droh-klor-oh-THY-ah-zyed plus try-AM-ter-een	Maxzide®	
hemorrheologic agents	pentoxifylline	pen-tok-SIF-ih-lin	Pentoxil®, Trental®	to decrease blood viscosity; used to treat claudication
inotropic agents	digitalis	dih-jih-TAH-lis	—	to increase the amount of blood the heart can pump by increasing the heart muscle's strength
	digitoxin	dih-jih-TOK-sin	Crystodigin®	
	digoxin	dih-JOK-sin	Lanoxin®, Lanoxicaps®	
	dobutamine	doh-BYOO-tah-meen	Dobutrex®	
	dopamine	DOH-pah-meen	Intropin®	
	molindone	MOH-lin-doan	Moban®	
lipid-lowering medications	atorvastatin	ah-TOR-vah-stah-tin	Lipitor®	to reduce triglycerides and cholesterol
	clofibrate	klo-FY-brayt	Atromid-S®	
	fluvastatin	FLOO-vah-stah-tin	Lescol®	
	gemfibrozil	jem-FY-broh-zil	Lopid®	
	lovastatin	LOH-vah-stah-tin	Mevacor®	
	niacin	NY-ah-sin	Nicobid®	
	pravastatin	PRAH-vah-stah-tin	Pravachol®	
	simvastatin	SIM-vah-stah-tin	Zocor®	

peripherally acting hypertensive agents	doxazosin	dok-SAH-zoh-sin	Cardura®	to lower blood pressure by affecting nerves involved in blood pressure regulation
	guanadrel	GWAH-nah-drel	Hylorel®	
	guanethidine	GWAH-neh-thih-deen	Ismelin®	
	mecamylamine	mek-ah-MY-lah-meen	Inversine®	
	prazosin	PRAH-zoh-sin	Minipress®	
Thrombolytics	anistreplase	ah-NIS-treh-plays	Eminase®	to dissolve blood clots
	reteplase	REH-teh-plays	Retavase®	
	streptokinase	strep-TOH-kih-nays	Streptase®	
	tissue-type plasminogen activator (tPA, TPA)	plaz-MIN-oh-jen	Activase®	
	urokinase	yoo-ROK-ih-nays	Abbokinase®	

DRUG TERMINOLOGY

The following are common types of drugs used for cardiovascular system conditions.

Drug Type	Pronunciation	Definition
angiotensin-converting enzyme (ACE) inhibitors	an-jee-oh-TEN-sin	used for heart failure and other cardiovascular problems; they dilate arteries to lower blood pressure and help the heart to pump easier
antianginals	an-tee-AN-jih-nals	used to relieve or prevent attacks of angina
antiarrhythmics	an-tee-ah-RITH-mics	used to help regulate cardiac rhythm
anti-clotting agents	—	same as anticoagulants below
anticoagulants	an-tee-coh-AG-yoo-lents	prevent the formation of dangerous clots
antihypertensives	an-tee-hy-per-TEN-sivs	help to control high blood pressure
beta blockers	BAY-tah blockers	to lower blood pressure by reducing contraction strength of heart muscle and slowing heartbeat
calcium channel blockers	—	to reduce calcium ions entering heart and blood vessel muscle cells; to lower blood pressure and normalize certain arrhythmias
cardiotonics	kar-dee-oh-TON-iks	increase the force of contractions of the myocardium; used for congestive heart failure
diuretics	dy-yoo-RET-iks	promote the excretion of urine

(continues)

Drug Type	Pronunciation	Definition
heparin	HEP-ah-rin	naturally found in the body; the synthetic version is administered to prevent clotting
lipid-lowering agents	LIH-pid lowering agents	aid in lowering cholesterol levels
nitrates	NY-trayts	dilate veins, arteries, or coronary arteries; used to control angina
Statins	STAH-tinz	the most frequently used class of lipid-lowering agents
thrombolytics	throm-boh-LIT-iks	dissolve thrombi
tissue-type plasminogen activators (tPA, TPA)	plaz-MIH-no-jen	prevent thrombi from forming
vasoconstrictors	vay-soh-kon-STRIK-tors	narrow blood vessels
Vasodilators	vay-soh-dy-LAY-tors	dilate or widen blood vessels

REVIEW EXERCISES

Multiple Choice

Select the best answer and write the letter of your choice to the left of each number.

1. Hardening of the arteries caused by a fatty substance is referred to as:

   A. arteriorrhagia
   B. arteriosclerosis
   C. atherosclerosis
   D. arterioliposclerosis

2. Blood that is low in oxygen and high in carbon dioxide enters which of the following chambers of the heart?

   A. right ventricle
   B. left ventricle
   C. right atrium
   D. left atrium

3. The key of the conduction system is the:

   A. SA node
   B. AV node
   C. bundle of His
   D. Purkinje fibers

4. Cramp-like leg pains caused by blood circulation is called:

   A. edema
   B. angina pectoris
   C. aneurysm
   D. claudication

5. Formation of a clot inside a blood vessel is referred to as:

   A. occlusion
   B. thrombosis
   C. ischemia
   D. vasoconstriction

6. Which of the following is an inflammatory disease that may develop after a streptococcal infection of the upper respiratory tract?

   A. Lyme disease
   B. thrombophlebitis
   C. arteriosclerosis
   D. rheumatic fever

7. A small red or purple spot caused by a minor capillary hemorrhage is referred to as:

    A. thrombosis
    B. aneurysm
    C. petechiae
    D. ischemia

8. Which of the following chambers contracts and pumps deoxygenated blood through the pulmonary valve into the pulmonary trunk?

    A. left atrium
    B. right atrium
    C. vena cava
    D. right ventricle

9. Which of the following are the smallest vessels?

    A. veins
    B. arterioles
    C. arteries
    D. capillaries

10. Accumulation of fluid in the peritoneal cavity is referred to as:

    A. edema of the legs
    B. occlusion
    C. ascites
    D. asthenia

11. The heart lies in the thoracic cavity between the lungs, in an area called the:

    A. vena cava
    B. ventricle
    C. mediastinum
    D. sternum

12. Which of the following is the purpose of the four valves in the heart?

    A. preventing infection
    B. gateway to the heart
    C. blood receives oxygen
    D. blood flows in only one direction

13. Which of the following are commonly used for lipid lowering?

    A. statins
    B. nitrates

    C. vasoconstrictors
    D. beta blockers

14. Which of the following blood vessels carries blood from the heart to the lungs?

    A. coronary artery
    B. pulmonary vein
    C. pulmonary artery
    D. superior vena cava

15. A localized and abnormal dilation of a blood vessel, usually an artery, is called:

    A. coarctation of the aorta
    B. atherosclerosis
    C. arteriosclerosis
    D. aneurysm

Fill in the Blank

Use your knowledge of medical terminology to insert the correct term from the list below.

Tetralogy of Fallot	arteriosclerosis	endocarditis
myocarditis	bruit	diastole
murmur	hepatomegaly	malaise
fibrillation	epicardium	lumen
ischemia	systole	atherosclerosis

1. A(n) _____ is an abnormal heart sound resulting from turbulent blood flow.

2. The condition of having an enlarged liver is called _____.

3. A hardening of the arteries, with loss of capacity and loss of elasticity, is known as _____.

4. An unusual sound made by blood rushing past an obstruction is referred to as a(n) _____.

5. A local deficiency of blood supply caused by an obstruction of the blood circulation is known as _____.

6. An inflammation of the heart muscle that is usually caused by viral or bacterial infections is called _____.

7. An inflammation of the inner layer of the heart is referred to as _____.

8. A general feeling of discomfort or uneasiness is known as _____.

9. The contraction phase of the heart is called _____.

10. A congenital heart condition consisting of pulmonary valve stenosis, ventricular septal defect, dextroposition of the aorta, and hypertrophy of the right ventricle is known as _____.

Labeling – The Anterior External View of the Heart

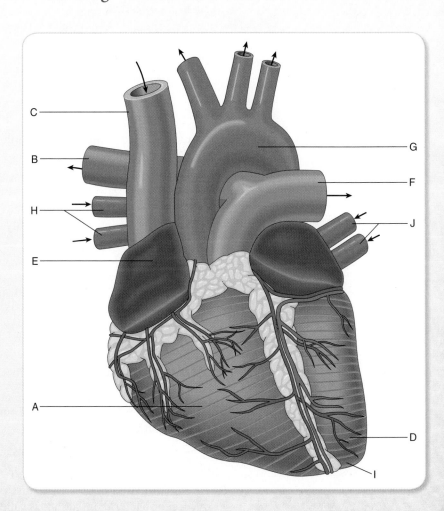

Write in the terms below that correspond with each letter on the figure above.

A. _____

B. _____

C. _____

D. _____

E. _____

F. _____

G. _____

H. _____

I. _____

J. _____

True / False

Identify each of the following statements as true or false by placing a "T" or "F" on the line beside each number.

_____ 1. Pericarditis is an inflammation of the heart muscle.

_____ 2. Mitral valve prolapse is a drooping of the mitral valve into the left atrium during ventricular systole.

_____ 3. A varicose vein is an enlargement of a superficial vein.

_____ 4. A condition of the two major heart arteries being reversed is called *Tetralogy of Fallot*.

_____ 5. A closing off of a vessel is known as an *occlusion*.

_____ 6. Any abnormality of the rhythm of the heartbeat is referred to as a *murmur*.

_____ 7. Bradycardia is a heart rate of more than 100 beats per minute.

_____ 8. Vasodilator agents widen blood vessels.

_____ 9. Inflammation of the heart is called *anastomosis*.

_____10. A palpitation is an abnormal beating of the heart.

Labeling – The Anterior Cross-Section View of the Heart

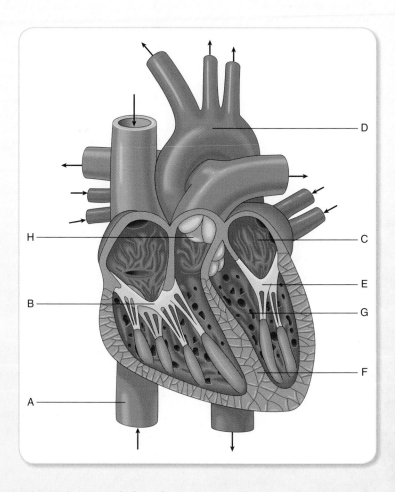

Write in the terms below that correspond with each letter on the figure above.

A. _____

B. _____

C. _____

D. _____

E. _____

F. _____

G. _____

H. _____

Definitions

Define each of the following words in one sentence.

1. arrhythmia: _____
2. bicuspid valve: _____
3. diastole: _____
4. endocardium: _____
5. bruit: _____
6. epicardium: _____
7. infarction: _____
8. pacemaker: _____
9. petechiae: _____
10. ischemia: _____

Abbreviations

Write the full meaning of each abbreviation:

Abbreviation	Meaning
1. AF	_____
2. CAD	_____
3. BP	_____
4. CVD	_____
5. LDL	_____
6. MS	_____
7. CPR	_____
8. LDH	_____
9. LV	_____
10. MI	_____

Matching – Terms and Definitions

Match each term with its correct definition by placing the corresponding letter on the line to its left.

_____ 1. heart block

_____ 2. vein

_____ 3. hypertension

_____ 4. flutter

A. the condition of having an enlarged liver

B. prevents blood from flowing backward or forward

_____ **5.** thrombosis

_____ **6.** hepatomegaly

_____ **7.** aneurysm

_____ **8.** valve

_____ **9.** pulse

_____**10.** patent ductus arteriosus

C. blood vessels carry generally deoxygenated blood toward the heart

D. rhythmic expansion and contraction of a blood vessel, usually an artery

E. a localized, abnormal dilation of a blood vessel

F. a congenital defect of the heart

G. a condition of higher-than-normal blood pressure

H. an abnormal heart rhythm occurring at a rate between 250 and 400 beats per minute

I. formation of a clot within a blood vessel

J. interferes with normal electrical conduction of the heart

Spelling

Circle the correctly spelled term in each pairing.

1. dysrrythmia   dysrhythmia

2. aneurysm   anorysm

3. malayse   malaise

4. thrombusis   thrombosis

5. ischemia   iskemia

6. varikose   varicose

7. prophylactic   propfylactic

8. aortae   aorta

9. palpitation   palpitasion

10. fibrilation   fibrillation

CHAPTER

Blood

11

OUTLINE

OBJECTIVES

Upon completion of this chapter, the reader should be able to:

1. Describe the composition of blood plasma.
2. Explain the functions of the blood.
3. Differentiate types of white blood cells.
4. Describe plasma and its functions.
5. Interpret abbreviations used for components of the blood.
6. List and describe 10 disorders of the blood.
7. Correctly define, spell, and pronounce this chapter's terms.
8. List and define four common types of drugs used for blood conditions.

STRUCTURE AND FUNCTION OF BLOOD

Blood is the fluid that circulates in the cardiovascular system. It is a type of connective tissue, with cells suspended in a liquid extracellular matrix. It is vital in transporting substances between body cells and the external environment. This activity promotes homeostasis. The total adult blood volume is about 5 liters. Blood circulates through the vessels, bringing oxygen and nourishment to all cells, and carrying away carbon dioxide and other waste products. It also distributes body heat and carries special substances such as antibodies and hormones.

Whole blood is slightly heavier and three to four times thicker than water. Its cells, which form mostly in the red bone marrow, include red blood cells that transport gases. They also include white blood cells that fight disease. Blood also contains cellular fragments called *platelets* that help to control blood loss. Together, the cells and platelets are termed "formed elements" of the blood, in contrast to the liquid portion, which is called **plasma**. It is identical in composition to interstitial fluid, except for the presence of plasma proteins.

Plasma is the fluid portion of the blood within which cellular elements are suspended. Water is the main component of plasma, accounting for about 92 percent of its weight. Proteins account for about 7 percent. The remaining 1 percent consists of dissolved organic molecules—amino acids, glucose, lipids, nitrogenous wastes, ions, trace elements, vitamins, dissolved oxygen (O_2) and carbon dioxide (CO_2).

Plasma proteins include albumins, globulins, and fibrinogen. They are primarily manufactured by the liver.

- **albumins** – These are the most prevalent type of protein in the plasma (making up about 60 percent of the total). Albumins help to maintain normal blood volume and the **osmotic** pressure of the plasma.

- **globulins** – Making up about 36 percent of the plasma proteins, these can be subdivided into alpha, beta, and gamma globulins. Globulins have a variety of functions, including transport of lipids and fat-soluble vitamins. Lymphatic tissues produce the gamma globulins, which are a type of antibody.

- **fibrinogen** – Constituting only about 4 percent of the plasma proteins, fibrinogen is the largest plasma protein (in size), and is essential for blood-clotting (coagulation). Fibrin is derived from fibrinogen for use in the clotting process.

A blood sample contains about 45 percent red blood cells by volume. This percentage is called the **hematocrit**. The white blood cells and platelets account for less than 1 percent of the blood. The remaining 55 percent of the blood is made up of plasma (a clear, straw-colored liquid). Plasma is a complex mixture of water, amino acids, proteins, carbohydrates, lipids, vitamins, hormones, electrolytes, and cellular waste.

In the blood, the solid components (cells and fragments of cells) are known as the *formed elements*, which are suspended in the plasma. **Hemopoiesis** is the process of the production of these formed elements in the blood. After birth, most of the production of blood cells occurs in the red bone marrow of the skull, sternum, ribs, vertebrae, and pelvis. Figure 11-1 shows the various formed elements found in the blood.

Red blood cells are also known as **erythrocytes**. They are tiny bi-concaved discs that are thinner in the center than they

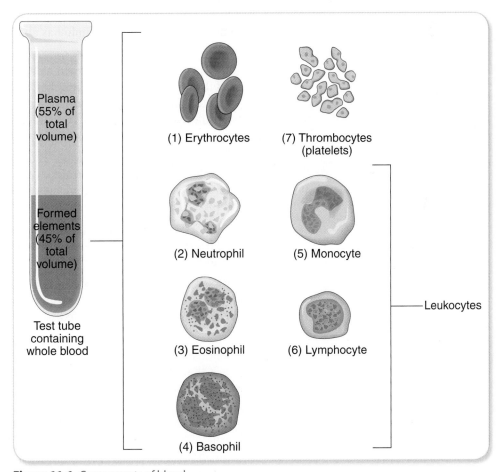

Figure 11-1 Components of blood.

are at the edges. They have a life span of only about 120 days. A mature red blood cell lacks a nucleus. They mostly consist of **hemoglobin**, which is made up of iron (**heme**) and protein (**globin**). Oxygen is transported in combination with hemoglobin (**oxyhemoglobin**). Carbon dioxide is transported from the tissue cells to the lungs for excretion in combination with hemoglobin (**carboxyhemoglobin**).

Many components of hemoglobin are recycled. The *heme* groups are converted by cells of the spleen and liver to a colored pigment called bilirubin. This pigment is carried by plasma albumin to the liver, where it is metabolized and incorporated into a secretion called **bile**. It is secreted into the digestive tract, and the bilirubin metabolites are filtered from the blood in the kidneys, where they contribute to the yellow color of urine.

Red blood cells (RBCs) transport oxygen to the body's cells, and are the most numerous of the formed elements found in the blood. A healthy adult male has about 4.5 to 6 million RBCs per cubic millimeter of blood. A healthy adult female has about 4.8 million per cubic millimeter of blood.

White blood cells (WBCs) are also known as **leukocytes**. They are larger than erythrocytes, but fewer in number. In contrast with erythrocytes, a mature leukocyte has a nucleus. Leukocytes are grouped into two different types: granulocytes and agranulocytes.

- **granulocytes** – The three types of leukocytes include neutrophils, eosinophils, and basophils. They have granules in their cytoplasm that absorb certain dyes that are used when preparing a slide for microscope viewing (such as in a "Wright's stain").

- **neutrophils** – These cells are **phagocytic** (engulfing and destroying bacteria). They make up about 60 to 70 percent of all WBCs, and have multi-lobed nuclei.

- **eosinophils** – These cells proliferate in response to allergic reactions. They constitute about 2 to 4 percent of all white blood cells, and their nuclei are bi-lobed.

- **basophils** – These cells secrete histamine (released during allergic reactions) and **heparin** (a natural anticoagulant). They constitute less than 1 percent of all white blood cells, and also have bi-lobed nuclei. Tissue basophils are called **mast cells**.

- **agranulocytes** – These are cells made up of monocytes and lymphocytes that do not have granules in their cytoplasm, and do not stain a dark color. They have large nuclei that are not multi-lobed.

- **monocytes** – These cells are phagocytic, and constitute about 3 to 8 percent of all WBCs. They are the largest of the white blood cells in size, and have kidney bean-shaped, bi-lobed nuclei. Monocytes that leave circulation and enter the tissues develop into **macrophages**.

- **lymphocytes** – These cells play an important role in immunity. Some of them are phagocytic, while others produce antibodies that destroy bacteria. They constitute about 20 to 25 percent of all WBCs and have large, spherical nuclei. Lymphocytes are the smallest white blood cells. Lymphocytes are sometimes called **immunocytes** because they are responsible for specific immune responses directed against invaders.

Platelets (also known as **thrombocytes**), are small, disc-shaped fragments of very large cells called **megakaryocytes**. Platelets are essential for normal coagulation (blood-clotting) and contain no hemoglobin. There are about 250,000 to 500,000 platelets in each cubic millimeter of blood. The typical life span of a platelet is about 10 days. Platelets are always present in the blood, but they are not active unless damage has occurred to the walls of the circulatory system.

GENERAL TERMINOLOGY RELATED TO THE BLOOD

The following are common terms that relate to the blood.

Term	Pronunciation	Definition
agglutinin	ah-GLOO-tin-in	substance in blood plasma that causes clumping when it interacts with a specific antigen
agglutinogen	ah-GLOO-tih-no-jen	protein substance on the red blood cell membrane that reacts to agglutinins
agglutination	ah-gloo-tih-NAY-shun	the clumping of cells and other particles due to agglutinins
albumin	al-BEW-min	the major protein in blood plasma; some drugs bind themselves to albumin, and the drug molecules that are bound to albumin are pharmacologically inactive until they detach themselves from the protein
anisocytosis	an-ih-soh-sigh-TOH-sis	unequal size of the red blood cells, as found in anemia and other blood conditions
antibody	AN-tih-baw-dee	a substance developed within the immune system and designed to identify and destroy foreign substances
antigen	AN-tih-jen	a substance that stimulates formation of antibodies

(continues)

Term	Pronunciation	Definition
basophil	BAY-soh-fill	a granulocytic white blood cell that normally comprises less than 1% of the total number of white blood cells; granules contain heparin and histamine
bilirubin	bill-ih-ROO-bin	a pigment released into blood after the destruction of old or damaged red blood cells; the liver recycles bilirubin into new hemoglobin
blood pH	—	a measure of the blood's acidity; the hydrogen ion concentration in the blood
coagulation	koh-ag-yoo-LAY-shun	the complex process of blood-clotting
deoxyhemoglobin	dee-ok-see-HEE-moh-gloh-bin	the form of hemoglobin without oxygen
eosinophil	ee-oh-SIN-oh-fill	a granulocytic bi-lobed leukocyte; eosinophils constitute 1% to 3% of the white blood cells of the body, increase in number with allergies and some parasitic conditions, and decrease with steroid administration
erythroblast	eh-RITH-roh-blast	an immature form of a red blood cell; normally found only in bone marrow; contains hemoglobin
erythrocyte	eh-RITH-roh-sight	a mature red blood cell that is the major cellular element of the circulating blood, and transports oxygen as its principal function
erythropoiesis	eh-rith-roh-poy-EE-sis	the process of erythrocyte production in the bone marrow, involving the maturation of a nucleated precursor into a hemoglobin-filled, nucleus-free erythrocyte that is regulated by erythropoietin, a hormone produced by the kidney
fibrin	FIH-brin	a protein formed from fibrinogen that forms a net-like structure that allows a blood clot to organize and anchor itself to a blood vessel wall
fibrinogen	fih-BRIN-oh-jen	a blood-clotting factor responsible for forming fibrin; without fibrinogen and fibrin, blood would not be able to form the clots necessary to stop blood flow
globulin	GLOB-yew-lin	a class of proteins that circulate in blood; many of the globulins are essential components of the immune system
granulocyte	GRAN-yew-loh-sight	a white blood cell that has granules in its cytoplasm
hematology	hee-mah-TALL-oh-jee	the scientific study of blood and the tissue that forms blood
heme	HEEM	the pigmented iron-containing non-protein part of the hemoglobin molecule
hemoglobin	hee-moh-GLOH-bin	a complex protein-iron compound in the blood that carries oxygen to the cells from the lungs, and carbon dioxide away from the cells to the lungs

hemolysis	hee-MALL-ih-sis	the breakdown of red blood cells and the release of hemoglobin that occurs normally at the end of the life span of a red blood cell
hemostasis	hee-moh-STAY-sis	the termination of bleeding by mechanical or chemical means, or by the complex coagulation process of the body
heparin	HEP-er-in	a naturally occurring anti-clotting agent
leukocyte	LOO-koh-syt	a white blood cell; five types of white blood cells circulate in human blood: neutrophils, basophils, eosinophils, lymphocytes, and monocytes
lipoprotein	lih-poh-PROH-teen	a protein combined with a lipid
macrophage	MAK-roh-fayj	phagocytic cell derived from a monocyte
mast cells	MAST SELLS	mastocytes; the cells containing granules that are rich in histamine and heparin; they play a major role in allergy and anaphylaxis
megakaryocyte	meg-ah-KAIR-ee-oh-sight	a very large bone marrow cell, which serves as a precursor cell for platelets
monocyte	MON-oh-sight	the largest of the white blood cells, which normally represents 3% to 7% of the circulating white blood cells
myeloid	MY-eh-loyd	relating to the bone marrow or spinal cord
neutrophil	NOO-troh-fill	a white blood cell that is capable of ingesting bacteria and foreign materials in the blood; neutrophils normally account for 55% to 65% of white blood cells in the blood
oxyhemoglobin	ok-see-HEE-moh-gloh-bin	the oxygen-loaded form of hemoglobin
pancytopenia	pan-sigh-toh-PEE-nee-ah	a large reduction in RBCs, WBCs, and platelets
plasma	PLAZ-muh	the fluid portion of blood that remains after all blood cells have been removed; plasma consists of water, dissolved proteins, amino acids, glucose, fats, fatty acids, electrolytes, gases, and metabolic wastes
plasma protein	PLAZ-muh PRO-teen	any of the proteins in blood plasma
platelet	PLAYT-let	a blood cell formed in bone marrow that initiates blood-clotting; platelets are essential for controlling bleeding episodes, but they can also trigger inappropriate blood clots inside veins, leading to myocardial infarctions, strokes, or pulmonary emboli
prothrombin	proh-THROM-bin	a precursor of thrombin synthesized in the liver when adequate vitamin K is present

(continues)

Term	Pronunciation	Definition
reticulocyte	reh-TIK-yoo-loh-sight	a newly formed red blood cell; reticulocytes normally account for only 1% of circulating red blood cells
serology	see-RALL-oh-jee	the scientific study of blood serum for infection
serum	SEE-rum	the clear, sticky fluid portion of the blood that remains after removal of all cells and clots; serum differs from plasma in that plasma still contains clotting factors
stem cell	—	a type of cell in bone marrow that generates all other blood cells; stem cells give rise to cells that eventually differentiate themselves into red and white blood cells and platelets
thrombin	THROM-bin	an enzyme in blood that converts fibrinogen to fibrin; necessary for the blood to clot normally
thromboplastin	throm-boh-PLAST-in	a substance that starts the clotting process by converting prothrombin into thrombin when calcium ions are present
thrombus	THROM-bus	a blood clot that forms in the cardiovascular system; thrombi may form in a blood vessel or in a chamber of the heart; a thrombus that breaks away from its site of formation and floats through the bloodstream is called an *embolus*

PATHOLOGICAL CONDITIONS

The following are disorders and conditions of the blood.

Allergy – a reaction to a food, drug, environmental condition, or substance triggered by the body's immune system; while all allergies to drugs are considered side effects, not all side effects are allergies—the immune system must be involved in order for a drug reaction to be considered an allergy

Anaphylactic shock – a life-threatening allergic reaction; characterized by a drop in blood pressure, and often associated with difficulty breathing; usually fatal unless appropriate emergency treatment is given

Anaphylaxis – an immediate and serious allergic reaction following exposure to a drug or other chemical

Anemia – a pathologic condition caused by a decreased red blood cell count and deficient hemoglobin

Aplastic anemia – a condition caused by production failure in bone marrow

Disseminated intravascular coagulation – a disorder of the clotting cascade characterized by simultaneous hemorrhage and thrombosis

Dyscrasia – a general term applied to any blood disease where the number or physical structure of one or more of the cellular components of the blood cells is abnormal; blood dyscrasias may occur naturally or as the result of exposure to drugs, toxins, or radiation

Granulocytosis – an abnormally high number of granulocytes in the circulating blood

Edema – the accumulation of fluid in the interstitial space

Hematoma – blood loss into a tissue, organ, or other confined space; may compress nearby organs, causing pain and impairing their function; hematomas are most common after trauma, or as a side effect of anticoagulant medications; in many cases, must be surgically drained

Hemochromatosis – a disorder caused by deposition of hemosiderin (a protein that promotes storage of iron) in the tissues of the body; can cause cirrhosis of the liver, destruction of the pancreas, and heart failure

Hemolytic anemia – a condition characterized by extreme reduction and destruction of red blood cells

Hemophilia – hereditarily linked inability of the body to control blood-clotting

Hemorrhage – a loss of a large amount of blood in a short time period, either externally or internally; may be arterial, venous, or capillary

Hyperalbuminemia – an increased level of albumin in the blood

Hyperlipemia – an excessive level of triglycerides in the blood; may be due to dietary factors, or metabolic disease, such as diabetes mellitus

Hyperlipidemia – a general term indicating excessive levels of any specific fat or fats in the blood; includes excess cholesterol, triglycerides, or low-density lipoprotein (LDL)

Leukemia – cancer of the blood or bone marrow signified by proliferation of leukocytes; the increased white blood cell production interferes with normal clotting

Leukocytosis – an abnormally high number of white blood cells in the blood

Leukopenia – any condition in which the number of leukocytes in the circulating blood is lower than normal

Multiple myeloma – a cancer of the bone marrow that rapidly spreads through the marrow and invades the surrounding bone, including the skull; eventually, the tumors destroy bone and lead to multiple bone fractures and pain

Myeloma – a tumor that develops in the blood cell-forming tissue of the bone marrow

Neutrophilia – a condition of increased neutrophils in the blood

Nutritional anemia – a type of anemia caused by nutritional deficiencies

Pernicious anemia – a condition resulting from deficiency of mature RBCs and the formation and circulation of megaloblasts (large, immature, nucleated RBCs) with variations of RBC sizes and shapes

Polycythemia vera – an abnormal increase in production of red blood cells; a serious condition that can be controlled by removing blood and by chemotherapy that reduces the activity of bone marrow cells; characterized by bone marrow overproduction, leading to erythrocytosis

Sickle cell anemia – a genetically based disease of the red blood cells characterized by abnormal hemoglobin and the tendency of the cells to form into a sickle shape; the red blood cells in sickle cell anemia are diminished in number, and fragile; because of their abnormal shape, sickled cells can obstruct capillaries and cause extreme pain

Splenomegaly – enlargement of the spleen; causes include cirrhosis of the liver, hemolytic anemia, certain infections, and leukemia

Thalassemia – any of a group of inherited disorders of hemoglobin metabolism in which there is impaired formation of one or more of the protein chains of globin

Thrombocytopenia – a deficiency of platelets in circulating blood; severe thrombocytopenia can allow spontaneous hemorrhaging; the most common cause of thrombocytopenia is cancer chemotherapy

ABBREVIATIONS

The following abbreviations are related to terms and procedures concerning the blood.

Abbreviation	Meaning
Ab	antibody
Ag	antigen
ALL	acute lymphatic leukemia
AML	acute myelogenous leukemia
B-cell	B-lymphocyte
BMT	bone marrow transplantation
CBC	complete blood (cell) count
chol	cholesterol
DIC	disseminated intravascular coagulation
EPO	erythropoietin
Fe	iron
Hb (or Hbg)	hemoglobin
HbO_2	oxyhemoglobin
HCT	hematocrit
HDL	high-density lipoprotein
LDL	low-density lipoprotein
lymph	lymphocyte
MCH	mean corpuscular hemoglobin
MCHC	mean corpuscular hemoglobin concentration
MCV	mean corpuscular volume
O_2	oxygen
PA	pernicious anemia
PCV	packed cell volume
PRBCs	packed red blood cells
PSA	prostate-specific antigen
PT	prothrombin time
PTA	prothrombin tissue activator
PTT	partial thromboplastin time
RBC	red blood cell
T-cell	T-lymphocyte
TPA	tissue plasminogen activator
VLDL	very-low-density lipoprotein
WBC	white blood cell

MEDICATIONS USED TO TREAT BLOOD DISORDERS

The following are common medications used for blood disorders.

Drug Class	Generic Name	Pronunciation for Generic Name	Trade Name	Use
Anticoagulants	dipyridamole	dy-per-ID-ah-mol	Persantine®	to dissolve blood clots
	enoxaparin	eh-NOK-sah-pah-rin	Lovenox®	
	heparin	HEP-ah-rin	various	
	warfarin	WAR-fah-rin	Coumadin®	
clotting agent; coagulant	phytonadione, vitamin K	fy-toh-nah-DY-own	Mephyton®	aids in clotting blood
Hemostatics	aminocaproic acid	ah-mee-noh-cah-PRO-ik acid	Amicar®	to stop bleeding
	recombinant factor VIIa	—	NovoSeven®	
Thrombolytics	alteplace	AL-teh-plays	Activase®	to dissolve blood clots
	streptokinase	strep-TOK-in-ays	Streptase®	
	urokinase	yoo-ROK-in-ays	Abbokinase®	

DRUG TERMINOLOGY

The following are common types of drugs used for blood conditions.

Drug Type	Pronunciation	Definition
Anticoagulants	an-tee-koh-AG-yoo-lents	agents that prevent blood clot formation
Coagulants	koh-AG-yoo-lents	agents that promote clotting
Hemostatics	hee-moh-STAT-iks	agents that stop bleeding
Thrombolytics	throm-boh-LIT-iks	agents that dissolve blood clots

REVIEW EXERCISES

Multiple Choice

Select the best answer and write the letter of your choice to the left of each number.

1. Which of the following medical terms means "the stoppage of bleeding"?

    A. embolism
    B. coagustasis
    C. hemostasis
    D. erythropoiesis

2. Which of the following defines "hematoma"?

    A. pain within the blood system
    B. an abnormally low erythrocyte count
    C. an alternate term for "erythrocytes"
    D. an extravascular mass of clotted blood

3. Which of the following is the fluid portion of blood?

    A. serum
    B. plasma
    C. fibrin
    D. thrombin

4. Which of the following cells may assist in clot formation?

    A. erythrocytes
    B. monocytes
    C. leukocytes
    D. thrombocytes

5. Which of the following agents are able to dissolve blood clots?

    A. thrombolytics
    B. hemostatics
    C. anticoagulants
    D. coagulants

6. Which of the following blood cells are agranular?

    A. monocytes
    B. erythrocytes
    C. eosinophils
    D. neutrophils

7. Which of the following blood cells is described as an "immature erythrocyte"?

   A. a leukocyte
   B. a reticulocyte
   C. a lymphocyte
   D. a basophil

8. Which of the following is a bone marrow cancer that may lead to many bone fractures?

   A. hemophilia
   B. hemochromatosis
   C. thalassemia
   D. multiple myeloma

9. A disorder of the clotting cascade characterized by simultaneous hemorrhage and thrombosis is referred to as:

   A. hematoma
   B. thrombocytopenia
   C. polycythemia vera
   D. disseminated intravascular coagulation

10. How many types of leukocytes are qualified as granulocytes?

   A. two
   B. three
   C. four
   D. five

11. Heparin is classified as an:

   A. antihistamine
   B. antidepressant
   C. anticoagulant
   D. antibody

12. The smallest white blood cell is called a(n):

   A. eosinophil
   B. neutrophil
   C. monocyte
   D. lymphocyte

13. Plasma minus fibrinogen is referred to as:

   A. plasmin
   B. serum
   C. antibody
   D. hemoglobin

14. Which of the following is the largest white blood cell?

    A. monocyte
    B. lymphocyte
    C. erythrocyte
    D. thrombocyte

15. Which of the following is a condition caused by production failure in bone marrow?

    A. hematoma
    B. aplastic anemia
    C. hemophilia
    D. leukemia

Fill in the Blank

Use your knowledge of medical terminology to insert the correct term from the list below into the appropriate statement.

anemia	leukemia	myeloma
thalassemia	granulocytosis	erythropoiesis
neutrophilia	pernicious anemia	hemolysis
thrombocytopenia	erythropoiesis	polycythemia vera
purpura	hemostasis	erythremia

1. A cancer of the blood or bone marrow signified by proliferation of leukocytes is known as _____.

2. An abnormal increase in the number of red blood cells is called _____.

3. The breakdown of red blood cells and the release of hemoglobin is called _____.

4. A _____ is a white blood cell that has granules in its cytoplasm.

5. A hereditary type of hemolytic anemia that causes hemoglobin production to be deficient is referred to as _____.

6. The termination of bleeding by the complex coagulation process of the body is known as _____.

7. A _____ is a tumor that develops in the blood cell-forming tissue of the bone marrow.

8. Pinpointed red or purple skin hemorrhages signify a condition called _____.

9. A deficiency of platelets in circulating blood is referred to as _____.

10. The process of red blood cell production in the bone marrow involving the maturation of a nucleated precursor into a hemoglobin-filled cell is called _____.

True / False

Identify each of the following statements as true or false by placing a "T" or "F" on the line beside each number.

_____ 1. A pigment released into blood after the destruction of old or damaged red blood cells is an antibody.

_____ 2. The major protein in the blood plasma is immunoglobulin.

_____ 3. Basophils contain heparin and histamine.

_____ 4. An immediate and serious allergic reaction following exposure to a drug is anaphylaxis.

_____ 5. An excessive level of blood triglycerides in the blood is called *hypolipemia*.

_____ 6. The white blood cells consist of three types of leukocytes.

_____ 7. A complex protein-iron compound in the blood that carries oxygen to the cells is known as *hemoglobin*.

_____ 8. Sickle cell anemia is a chronic and hereditary type of hemolytic anemia.

_____ 9. Fibrinogen is a blood-clotting factor responsible for forming fibrin.

_____ 10. Eosinophil is a type of leukocyte which lacks granules.

Definitions

Define each of the following words in one sentence.

1. hemostasis: _____

2. erythropoiesis: _____

3. antigen: _____

4. heparin: _____

5. hemolysis: _____

6. leukemia: _____

7. purpura: _____

8. hemochromatosis: _____

9. stem cell: _____

10. myeloma: _____

Abbreviations

Write the full meaning of each abbreviation.

Abbreviation	Meaning
1. B-cell	_____
2. PCV	_____
3. PTA	_____
4. LDL	_____
5. CBC	_____
6. PA	_____
7. PSA	_____
8. Hb	_____
9. Ab	_____
10. chol	_____

Matching – Terms and Definitions

Match each term with its correct definition by placing the corresponding letter on the line to its left.

_____ 1. monocyte

_____ 2. globulin

_____ 3. fibrinogen

_____ 4. basophil

_____ 5. neutrophil

_____ 6. megakaryocyte

_____ 7. lymphocyte

_____ 8. platelet

_____ 9. erythrocyte

_____ 10. anisocytosis

A. unequal size of red blood cells

B. a phagocytic white blood cell that has a multi-lobed nucleus

C. a very large bone marrow cell that serves as a precursor cell for platelets

D. the smallest white blood cell; it plays an important role in immunity

E. a blood cell that is essential for controlling bleeding episodes

F. a blood-clotting factor

G. a mature red blood cell

H. the largest of the white blood cells; it normally represents 3 to 7 percent of these cells in the blood circulation

I. a granulocytic white blood cell that contains histamine

J. a class of proteins in the blood; this class consists of essential components of the immune system

Spelling

Circle the correctly spelled term in each pairing of words.

1. oxyhemoglubin   oxyhemoglobin

2. fibrinogen   fibrinogan

3. anaphylaxis   anaphilaxis

4. anizocytosis   anisocytosis

5. billirubin   bilirubin

6. agglutination   aglutination

7. hemorrage   hemorrhage

8. lipoprotein   lypoprotein

9. spllenomegaly   splenomegaly

10. hemophillia   hemophilia

Lymphatic and Immune Systems

OBJECTIVES

Upon completion of this chapter, the reader should be able to:

1. Identify the structure of the lymphatic and immune systems.

2. Describe the functions of the immune system.

3. Discuss the locations and functions of the thymus and spleen.

4. Distinguish between innate (non-specific) and adaptive (specific) defenses.

5. Interpret the meaning of the abbreviations presented in this chapter.

6. Define, pronounce, and spell the diseases and disorders discussed in this chapter.

7. Discuss the origins and actions of the five different types of immunoglobulins.

8. Explain how allergic reactions arise from immune mechanisms.

STRUCTURE AND FUNCTION OF THE IMMUNE SYSTEM

The **lymphatic system** consists of vessels that transport fluids, and is made up of many different cells and biochemicals, as well as the organs and glands that produce them. The lymphatic vessels transport excess fluid away from tissues, returning it to the bloodstream.

The lymphatic system has a second major function, which allows humans to exist along with many different types of organisms that may exist in or on their bodies, potentially causing infectious diseases. Cells and biochemicals of the lymphatic system attack "foreign" particles, allowing the body to destroy infectious microorganisms and viruses. This immunity against disease also provides protection against toxins and cancer. When the body's immune response is abnormal, the result may be autoimmune disorders, allergies, persistent infections, and even cancer. The following organs make up the lymphatic system, and are involved with immunity:

- **lymphatic vessels** – Beginning as lymphatic capillaries, these tiny tubes merge to form larger lymphatic vessels. These lead to larger vessels that unite with veins in the chest (Figure 12-1). The walls of the lymphatic vessels are similar to veins, but thinner, with flap-like valves that help prevent the backflow of lymph. The larger lymphatic vessels lead to specialized organs called *lymph nodes*.

- **lymph nodes (lymph glands)** – Located along the lymphatic pathways, these structures contain large numbers of *lymphocytes* and *macrophages*, which fight invading microorganisms. Lymph nodes occur in groups or chains in the larger lymphatic vessels, but do not exist in the central nervous system. Lymph nodes have two primary functions:

  - to filter particles from the lymph fluid that may be potentially harmful before returning the fluid to the bloodstream

  - to monitor body fluids with the lymphocytes and macrophages in a process known as **immune surveillance**

  The lymph nodes, along with the red bone marrow, produce lymphocytes, which attack invading viruses, bacteria, and other parasitic cells that the lymphatic vessels bring to the nodes. Macrophages inside the nodes engulf and then destroy **cellular debris**, foreign substances, and damaged cells.

- **thymus** – This gland is a soft, bi-lobed structure enclosed in a connective tissue capsule. It is located posterior to the upper part of the sternum. The thymus is larger during infancy and early childhood, but shrinks after puberty, becoming very small in adults. When an adult becomes elderly, the lymphatic tissue in the thymus is replaced by adipose and connective

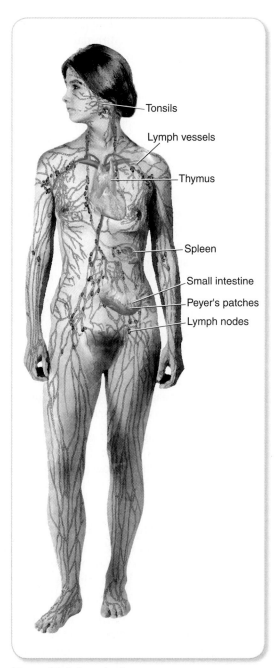

Figure 12-1 Lymphatic system.

tissues. Epithelial cells inside the thymus secrete *thymosins* (hormones that stimulate maturation of **T-lymphocytes** after they migrate to other lymphatic tissues).

- **spleen** – Located in the upper left portion of the abdomen, just below the diaphragm, the spleen is the largest lymphatic organ in the body. It resembles a large lymph node and is subdivided into lobules. The venous sinuses (spaces) of the spleen are filled with blood instead of lymph. The spleen is also a major site of production of immunoglobulin by B-lymphocytes that have differentiated into antibody-producing plasma cells.

There are two types of tissue within the splenic lobules. White pulp is distributed throughout the spleen in tiny groups, and is composed of splenic nodules, containing many lymphocytes. The red pulp fills the remaining lobule spaces and surrounds the venous sinuses. It contains many red blood cells, lymphocytes, and macrophages.

When a **pathogen** (a disease-causing microorganism) multiplies, an **infection** may be the result. Pathogens include bacteria, fungi, viruses, and protozoans. The human body has a variety of defenses against disease, including mechanical, chemical, and other defenses. When pathogens try to enter the body, they are often stopped by the skin, the cilia of the lower nasal cavity, and the mucous membranes. All of these structures act as barriers to pathogen intrusion.

If pathogens get past the mechanical defenses, they may be killed by chemical barriers, including the gastric juices in the stomach. Pathogens in the bloodstream may be destroyed by **phagocytosis** (the ingestion of foreign substances by the specialized cells known as macrophages). Humans are resistant to some diseases that affect other animals, and may be harmed by some diseases that do not affect other animals. This natural resistance occurs because a pathogen may not be able to survive in a human's internal body environment. Substances called **antigens** in the bloodstream may cause an immune response to a specific disease to occur.

There are three major types of **immunity**, which are defenses of the immune system that resist particular pathogens. **Natural immunity** is the body's natural resistance to diseases, and varies between individuals based on unique body chemistry and genetics. **Acquired active immunity** occurs either by producing natural antibodies to a disease, or by vaccination against the disease. **Vaccination** or **immunization** is the injection of an antigen from another organism, causing active immunity due to antibody production. A **vaccine** is the substance that is injected.

Acquired active immunity is of two types: **humoral immunity** (provided by **plasma cells** that produce **immunoglobulins**, which are a type of antibody), and **cell-mediated immunity** (provided by the action of T cells, which respond to antigens by producing **interferons** and **interleukins**). These substances may be antiviral or affect how body cells act. T cells are of four types:

- **cytotoxic cells** – help to destroy infected cells
- **helper cells** – stimulate the immune response
- **suppressor cells** – suppress B cells and other immune cells
- **natural killer cells** – kill cells by releasing proteins that cause cell death

Acquired passive immunity is provided as antibodies or antitoxins that have developed in another person or species. It is used to treat snakebite, tetanus, and other conditions when immediate immunity is required. An **antitoxin** is an antibody with action directed against specific toxins. This type of immunity is used to reduce the chance of catching a disease such as the flu (influenza). **Gamma globulin** consists of collected antibodies that may be given to prevent or treat hepatitis A, rabies, and varicella.

GENERAL TERMINOLOGY RELATED TO THE IMMUNE SYSTEM

The following are common terms that relate to the immune system.

Term	Pronunciation	Definition
acquired immunity	ah-KWY-erd ih-MYOO-nih-tee	resistance to a communicable disease, either by being exposed to the infectious agent, or by having been vaccinated against it; also called *active immunity*
allergen	AH-ler-jen	an environmental substance that can produce a hypersensitive allergic reaction in the body, but may not be intrinsically harmful
allergy	AH-ler-jee	a hypersensitive reaction to common, often intrinsically harmless substances, most of which are environmental
anaphylaxis	ah-nuh-fih-LAK-sis	an exaggerated, life-threatening hypersensitivity reaction to a previously encountered antigen
antibody	AN-tih-baw-dee	a substance developed within the immune system and designed to identify and destroy foreign substances
antigen	AN-tih-jen	a substance that stimulates formation of antibodies

(continues)

Term	Pronunciation	Definition
antitoxin	AN-tih-tok-sin	a substance containing antibodies directed against a particular disease or poison
autoimmune	aw-toh-ih-MYOON	pertaining to an immune response to a person's own tissue
B cell	BEE SEL	a lymphocyte that matures in lymphoid tissue, and is active in producing antibodies
candidiasis	kan-dih-DY-ah-sis	a fungal infection of the *Candida* species; commonly known as a *yeast infection* or *thrush*
cell-mediated immunity	SEL MEE-dee-ay-ted ih-MYOO-nih-tee	the mechanism of acquired immunity characterized by the dominant role of T cell lymphocytes
cytotoxic	sy-toh-TOK-sik	capable of destroying infected cells throughout the body
Epstein-Barr virus	EP-steen-BAR VY-rus	human herpesvirus; a virus of the herpes family that is one of the most common viruses in humans; commonly causes infectious mononucleosis (glandular fever)
gamma globulin	GAH-muh GLAW-byoo-lin	the protein in blood plasma that contains antibodies; given for passive transfer of immunity
globulin	GLAW-byoo-lin	a class of proteins that circulate in blood; many globulins are essential components of the immune system
humoral immunity	HYOO-moh-rul ih-MYOO-nih-tee	resistance to infectious disease provided by plasma cells and antibody production
hypersensitivity	hy-per-sen-sih-TIH-vih-tee	an overreaction to a foreign material within the body; hypersensitivity reactions are produced by an inappropriate immune system response to a material that the body senses as a threat
hypersplenism	hy-per-SPLEH-nih-zum	overactivity of the spleen, causing it to rapidly and prematurely destroy blood cells
immune	ih-MYOON	pertaining to the state of being resistant to an infectious disease due to the presence of antibodies against that disease
immune surveillance	ih-MYOON ser-VAY-lens	the constant monitoring by the immune system of microorganisms, foreign tissue, and diseases caused by altered cells, especially cancer
immunity	ih-MYOO-nih-tee	the state or condition of being resistant to invading microorganisms
immunization	ih-myoo-nih-ZAY-shun	a process by which resistance to an infectious disease is induced
immunoglobulin	ih-myoo-no-GLAW-byoo-lin	an antibody; immunoglobulins are classified into five categories, each abbreviated with a capital letter: IgG, IgM, IgA, IgD, and IgE
immunology	ih-myoo-NAW-loh-jee	the study of the reaction of tissues of the immune system to antigenic stimulation
immunosuppressed	ih-myoo-no-suh-PREST	a condition in which the immune response is inadequate

immunotherapy	ih-myoo-noh-THEH-ruh-pee	treatment of disease involving inducing, enhancing, or suppressing an immune response
interferon	in-ter-FEE-ron	a natural glycoprotein formed by cells exposed to a virus or another foreign particle of nucleic acid
interleukin	in-ter-LOO-kin	one of a large group of proteins produced mainly by T cells that are important in the inflammatory response
lymph	LIMF	a clear fluid of slightly yellowish color that is produced by many organs of the body; it enters into the lymphatic vessels
lymph node	LIMF NOHD	a specialized organ that filters harmful substances from the tissues, and assists in the immune response
lymphocyte	LIM-foh-syt	an agranular leukocyte active in immunity (T cells and B cells); found in both the blood and in lymphoid tissue
macrophage	MAH-kroh-fayj	a phagocytic cell derived from a monocyte; usually located within the tissues; macrophages process antigens for T cells
monocyte	MAW-noh-syt	an agranular phagocytic leukocyte
natural immunity	NAH-trul ih-MYOO-nih-tee	a usually inherent, non-specific form of immunity to a specific disease; also called *genetic immunity* or *innate immunity*
natural killer cell	NAH-trul KIH-ler SEL	a lymphocyte that is capable of binding to and killing virus-infected cells, and some tumor cells, by releasing cytotoxins
passive immunity	PAH-siv ih-MYOO-nih-tee	a form of acquired immunity resulting from antibodies that are transmitted naturally through the placenta to a fetus or infant, or artificially by injection of antiserum for treatment or prophylaxis; passive immunity is not permanent and does not last as long as active immunity
pathogen	PAH-tho-jen	a disease-causing agent
phagocytosis	fah-go-sih-TOH-sis	the engulfing of foreign material by white blood cells
plasma cells	PLAHZ-muh SELS	mature forms of B cells that produce antibodies
suppressor cell	suh-PREH-sor SEL	a T cell that suppresses B cells and other immune cells
T cell	TEE SEL	a lymphocyte that matures in the thymus gland, and attacks foreign cells directly; this type of cell is responsible for cellular immunity
T helper cells	TEE HEL-per sels	lymphocytes that improve the immune system's effectiveness by helping other cells to engulf and kill infected cells
thymosin	THY-moh-sin	a hormone secreted by the thymus gland that aids in distribution of thymocytes and lymphocytes
tonsils	TAWN-sils	tissues located in the throat (pharynx) that filter inhaled or swallowed materials, and aid in immunity early in life
vaccination	vak-sih-NAY-shun	the act of giving a vaccine, usually by injection
vaccine	vak-SEEN	a preparation of material derived from microorganisms administered to confer immunity to one or more infectious diseases; vaccines may be prepared from bacteria, viruses, or rickettsiae

PATHOLOGICAL CONDITIONS

The following are pathological conditions of the lymphatic and immune systems.

Acquired immunodeficiency syndrome – a progressive impairment of the immune system caused by the human immunodeficiency virus (HIV); gradually destroys the immune system, affecting many organ systems, with ultimately fatal consequences; HIV attacks helper T lymphocytes, which normally guard the body against tumors, viruses, and parasites

Autoimmune hemolytic anemia – an autoimmune condition in which red blood cells are destroyed by antibodies; because of failure of immune response, B cell–produced antibodies cannot identify RBCs as part of the body, resulting in an attack on, and destruction of, the red blood cells

Cytomegalovirus – a virus of the herpes family that is opportunistic, usually infecting **immunosuppressed** patients; can affect the bone marrow, retinas of the eyes, and salivary glands

Idiopathic thrombocytopenic purpura – an acquired disorder that results from an isolated deficiency of platelets with unknown cause; symptoms are related to an inability of the blood to clot and include spontaneous bleeding in the internal organs, mucous membranes, or skin

Infectious mononucleosis – an acute herpesvirus infection caused by the **Epstein-Barr virus**, characterized by atypical lymphocytes, abnormal liver function, bruising, enlargement of the spleen and liver, fever, sore throat, and swollen lymph glands; usually transmitted by droplet infection, but not highly contagious; young people are most often affected, and in childhood, the disease is mild and usually not noticed—the older the patient, the more severe the symptoms are likely to be; infection confers permanent immunity

Kaposi's sarcoma – a skin cancer that most commonly appears in people with a damaged immune system, particularly those with AIDS; Kaposi's sarcoma may also occur in elderly men, diabetics, and persons with other types of cancer; lesions appear as purple or blue patches or nodules that grow in size, appearing on various body parts, and may eventually metastasize to the lymph nodes and internal organs (Figure 12-2)

Lymphadenitis – an inflammatory condition of the lymph nodes, usually the result of systemic neoplastic disease, bacterial infection, or other inflammatory condition; nodes may be enlarged, hard, smooth or irregular, and may feel hot to the

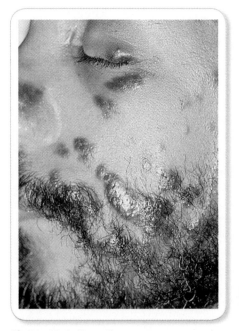

Figure 12-2 Kaposi's sarcoma. *Courtesy of Robert A. Silverman, M.D., Clinical Associate Professor, Department of Pediatrics, Georgetown University*

touch; location of the affected node is indicative of the site or origin of disease

Lymphangitis – an inflammation of one or more lymphatic vessels, usually resulting from an acute streptococcal infection of one of the extremities

Lymphedema – a primary or secondary condition characterized by the accumulation of lymph in soft tissue, and the resultant swelling caused by inflammation, obstruction, or removal of lymph channels

Lymphoma – a malignant cancer of the lymphatic system that normally appears as a single, painless, enlarged lymph node, usually in the neck; later signs and symptoms include anemia, fever, weakness, and weight loss; this disease may spread to the bones, gastrointestinal tract, liver, and spleen; lymphomas are usually categorized as *Hodgkin's* or *non-Hodgkin's* lymphomas

Myasthenia gravis – a chronic, progressive neuromuscular disease that is thought to be an autoimmune disorder, causing skeletal muscle weakness and fatigue; symptoms usually start in the face and throat, spreading to the rest of the body; mainly affects women between the ages of 20 and 40, and men over the age of 60

Rheumatoid arthritis – a chronic, painful inflammation of the joints that most commonly affects the hands and feet, but can affect multiple joints throughout the body; initiated when the body's immune system attacks connective tissue in the joints, causing swelling of affected joints, often with permanent disfigurement; mostly affects women during middle age

Sarcoidosis – a chronic disorder of unknown origin that causes nodules to form in the eyes, liver, lungs, lymph nodes, skin, spleen, and small bones of the hands and feet; nodules usually disappear over time, but leave scar tissue on the affected areas

Scleroderma – a chronic, progressive immune system disorder characterized by sclerosis (hardening) of the skin and scarring of certain internal organs; may progress to affect the digestive tract, heart, kidneys, and lungs

Severe combined immunodeficiency (SCID) – a group of disorders resulting from a disturbance in T cell and B cell development and function leading to an absence of both cell-mediated (T cell) and antibody-mediated (B cell) immunity; manifests as severe, recurrent infections with bacteria, fungi, protozoa, and viruses; occurs by age 3 to 6 months, when the natural material placental immunity begins to deplete; most commonly seen infections are *Pneumocystis* pneumonia and mucoutaneous **candidiasis**; the infant fails to thrive and experiences chronic otitis media and diarrhea

Systemic lupus erythematosus – a chronic, inflammatory autoimmune disease affecting connective tissue in nearly every organ of the body; may cause anemia, fatigue, hair loss, inflammation of heart tissue, kidney failure, nerve damage, skin rash, and weakness

Thymic hypoplasia or aplasia – a congenital immunodeficiency condition resulting from a small or absent thymus that affects young children; thymus and parathyroid glands are absent or underdeveloped; affected infant exhibits signs of *tetani* due to hypocalcemia caused by hypoparathyroidism; T cells are very low in number or absent, while B cells are present but produce lower-than-normal amounts of antibodies

X-linked agammaglobulinemia – a condition of severe B cell deficiency only seen in male infants; causes severe, recurrent infections such as bacterial otitis media, bronchitis, meningitis, and pneumonia, usually occurring after 4 to 6 months of age; all five immunoglobulin classes are usually absent, as are circulating B cells, but there are still normal numbers of circulating T cells

ABBREVIATIONS

The following abbreviations are related to common terminology of the immune system.

Abbreviation	Meaning
Ab	antibody
Ag	antigen
AIDS	acquired immunodeficiency syndrome
ARC	AIDS-related complex
AZT	azathioprine
CMV	cytomegalovirus
EBV	Epstein-Barr virus
HD	Hodgkin's disease
HIV	human immunodeficiency virus
IFN	interferon
Ig	immunoglobulins
IgA	immunoglobulin A
IgD	immunoglobulin D
IgE	immunoglobulin E
IgG	immunoglobulin G
IgM	immunoglobulin M
Ks	Kaposi's sarcoma
NHL	non-Hodgkin's lymphoma
NK cell	natural killer cell
RT	reverse transcriptase
SCID	severe combined immunodeficiency
SLE	systemic lupus erythematosus
T_C cell	cytotoxic T cell
T_H cell	helper T cell
T_S cell	suppressor T cell

MEDICATIONS USED TO TREAT IMMUNE SYSTEM DISORDERS

The following medications are commonly used for lymphatic and immune system disorders.

Drug Class	Generic Name	Pronunciation for Generic Name	Trade Name	Use
immunosuppressants	antithymocyte globulin	an-tih-THY-moh-syt GLAW-byoo-lin	Atgam®	to suppress organ rejection for various organ and bone marrow transplants
	azathioprine	ah-zuh-THY-oh-preen	AZT®	to treat autoimmune diseases, in organ transplantation, for inflammatory bowel diseases, and for multiple sclerosis
	basiliximab	bay-sih-LIK-sih-mab	Simulect®	a monoclonal antibody used to suppress organ rejection for various organ transplants and prolong life of transplanted organs
	cyclosporine	sy-kloh-SPOH-rin	Restasis®	to suppress cell destruction and improve survival rates for individuals with organ transplants
	daclizumab	dah-KLIH-zuh-mab	Zenapax®	a monoclonal antibody used to suppress organ rejection for various organ transplants and prolong life of transplanted organs
	intravenous γ-immunoglobulin (IVIg)	in-trah-VEE-nus IH-myoo-no-glaw-byoo-lin	Vigam®	a biological response modifier used to treat a variety of infections as well as chronic lymphatic leukemia
	muromonab-CD3	myoo-RAW-moh-nab-CD3	Orthoclone® OKT3®	a monoclonal antibody used to suppress organ rejection for various organ transplants and prolong life of transplanted organs
	mycophenolate mofetil	my-koh-PHEH-no-layt MOH-feh-til	CellCept®	to suppress organ rejection for various organ transplants

Rh$_0$ [D] immune globulin	R H zero D ih-MYOON GLAW-byoo-lin	RhoGAM®	given to Rh negative pregnant women who have been exposed to Rh positive blood, in order to prevent erythroblastosis fetalis in the fetus
	sirolimus	sih-ROH-lih-mus	Rapamune®	a macrolide used to suppress organ rejection in patients receiving kidney transplants
	tacrolimus	tah-KROH-lih-mus	Prograf®	a macrolide used orally or by injection to suppress organ rejection in liver or kidney transplants; used topically for severe atopic dermatitis

DRUG TERMINOLOGY

The following are common types of drugs used for lymphatic and immune system conditions.

Drug Type	Pronunciation	Definition
antianaphylaxis agents	an-tih-ah-nuh-fih-LAK-sis AY-jents	medications that make a patient insensitive to an antigen by desensitization
antibiotic	an-tih-by-AW-tik	a drug used against a bacterial infection
antihistamine	an-tih-HIS-tuh-meen	a drug that works against histamine
antilymphocyte globulin	an-tih-LIM-foh-syt GLAW-byoo-lin	a substance that interferes with cellular immunity by depleting T cell numbers
antiviral (for AIDS)	an-tih-VY-rul	a drug that stops the development of a virus
attentuated vaccine	ah-TEN-yoo-ay-ted vak-SEEN	a vaccine in which the antigen's ability to produce disease has been lessened or eliminated
corticosteroids	kor-tih-koh-STEH-royds	anti-inflammatory, immunosuppressant drugs
cytotoxic agents	sy-toh-TOK-sik AY-jents	chemical drugs that kill cells
inactivated vaccine	in-AK-tih-vay-ted vak-SEEN	a vaccine in which only the viral coat or bacterial cell wall are present
radiation therapy	ray-dee-AY-shun THEH-ruh-pee	a method of treatment involving the use of targeted x-rays
vaccines	vak-SEENS	drugs administered to induce an immune response

REVIEW EXERCISES

Multiple Choice

Select the best answer and write the letter of your choice to the left of each number.

1. Which of the following T lymphocytes stimulate the immune response?

   A. natural killer cells
   B. cytotoxic cells
   C. helper cells
   D. suppressor cells

2. Administration of gamma globulin may produce:

   A. passive immunity
   B. active immunity
   C. both active and passive immunity
   D. neither active nor passive immunity

3. A substance that stimulates formation of antibodies is called a(n):

   A. gamma globulin
   B. thymosin
   C. antitoxin
   D. antigen

4. Which of the following microorganisms may cause infectious mononucleosis?

   A. viruses
   B. fungi
   C. bacteria
   D. protozoans

5. Kaposi's sarcoma commonly appears in patients with damaged immune systems, particularly those with AIDS, as a cancer of the:

   A. brain
   B. bones
   C. skin
   D. inner ear

6. A chronic, progressive immune system disorder characterized by hardening of the skin and scarring of certain internal organs is referred to as:

   A. sarcoidosis
   B. scleroderma
   C. severe combined immunodeficiency
   D. systemic lupus erythematosus

7. A hypertensive reaction to a substance is called a(n):

   A. immunity
   B. toxicity
   C. allergy
   D. interferon

8. Glandular fever is also known as:

   A. Kaposi's sarcoma
   B. infectious mononucleosis
   C. autoimmune hemolytic anemia
   D. myasthenia gravis

9. Which of the following systems in the human body lacks lymph nodes?

   A. the respiratory system
   B. the central nervous system
   C. the urinary system
   D. the circulatory system

10. One of the primary functions of the lymph nodes is to monitor body fluids with lymphocytes and macrophages in a process known as:

   A. immunization
   B. humoral immunity
   C. passive immunity
   D. immune surveillance

11. Vaccines may be prepared from:

   A. bacteria or viruses
   B. protozoans or fungi
   C. fungi or rickettsiae
   D. viruses, bacteria, or rickettsiae

12. Which of the following white blood cells produce antibodies?

   A. monocytes
   B. T lymphocytes
   C. B lymphocytes
   D. macrophages

13. An exaggerated, life-threatening hypersensitivity reaction to a previously encountered antigen is called:

   A. humoral immunity
   B. anaphylaxis
   C. autoimmune
   D. phagocytosis

14. Which of the following blood cells may be stimulated or matured by the hormone known as *thymosin*?

    A. T-lymphocytes
    B. macrophages
    C. B-lymphocytes
    D. none of the above

15. Which of the following organs in the body is a major site of production of immunoglobulin by plasma cells?

    A. the thymus
    B. the lungs
    C. the heart
    D. the spleen

Fill in the Blank

Use your knowledge of medical terminology to insert the correct term from the list below.

humoral immunity	cytotoxic cells	cell-mediated immunity
natural killer cells	antigen	macrophages
interleukins	pathogen	interferons
immunoglobulin	monocyte	T-helper cells
lymphocyte	suppressor cells	allergen

1. An agranular phagocytic leukocyte is called a(n) _____.

2. T lymphocytes help to destroy infected cells, and are referred to as _____.

3. Resistance to infectious disease provided by plasma cells and antibody production is called _____.

4. Lymphocytes that improve the immune system's effectiveness by helping other cells to engulf and kill infected cells are known as _____.

5. An agranular leukocyte active in immunity is called a(n) _____.

6. A disease-causing agent is referred to as a(n) _____.

7. A T lymphocyte that abolishes B cells and other immune cells is called a(n) _____.

8. A phagocytic cell derived from a monocyte is known as a(n) _____.

9. An immune response to a person's own tissue is known as a(n) _____ response.

10. Any antibody is also known as a(n) _____.

True / False

Identify each of the following statements as true or false by placing a "T" or "F" on the line beside each number.

_____ 1. The walls of lymphatic vessels are similar to those of the arteries.

_____ 2. Macrophages are able to destroy cellular debris.

_____ 3. The thymus shrinks in early infancy and early childhood.

_____ 4. The spleen is located in the upper right portion of the abdomen.

_____ 5. An antitoxin is an antibody with action directed against specific viruses.

_____ 6. Gamma globulin may be given to prevent or treat rabies and varicella.

_____ 7. Acquired immunity is also called *active immunity*.

_____ 8. Candidiasis is known as a yeast infection or thrush.

_____ 9. Epstein-Barr virus commonly causes pericarditis.

_____ 10. Natural immunity is also called *genetic immunity*.

Definitions

Define each of the following words in one sentence.

1. thymosin: _____

2. phagocytosis: _____

3. vaccine: _____

4. immunity: _____

5. antigen: _____

6. interferon: _____

7. antitoxin: _____

8. gamma globulin: _____

9. allergen: _____

10. lymph: _____

Abbreviations

Write the full meaning of each abbreviation.

Abbreviation	Meaning
1. IgM	_____
2. SLE	_____
3. Ks	_____
4. AIDS	_____
5. Ag	_____
6. HIV	_____
7. EBV	_____
8. ARC	_____
9. Ab	_____
10. SCID	_____

Matching

Match each term with its correct definition by placing the corresponding letter on the line to its left.

_____ 1. plasma cell

_____ 2. passive immunity

_____ 3. T helper cell

_____ 4. natural immunity

_____ 5. suppressor cell

_____ 6. candidiasis

_____ 7. lymphangitis

_____ 8. thymic aplasia

_____ 9. lymphadenitis

_____ 10. sarcoidosis

A. of unknown origin, it causes nodules to form in the eyes, liver, and lungs

B. an inflammation of the lymphatic vessels

C. a fungal infection

D. an inflammatory condition of the lymph nodes

E. a congenital immunodeficiency condition resulting from an absent or small thymus

F. a usually inherent, non-specific form of immunity to a specific disease

G. a T cell that suppresses B cells

H. a form of acquired immunity resulting in the formation of antibodies

I. mature forms of B cells that produce antibodies

J. lymphocytes that improve the immune system's effectiveness by assisting other cells

Spelling

Circle the correct spelling from each pairing of words.

1. immunosupressed   immunosuppressed
2. humural immunity   humoral immunity
3. phagocytosis   phagosytosis
4. macrophage   microphage
5. surveillance   surveilance
6. thymozin   thymosin
7. immunoglobulin   immunoglabulin
8. interferon   interfiron
9. anafylaxis   anaphylaxis
10. globulin   glubulin

Respiratory System

OBJECTIVES

Upon completion of this chapter, the reader should be able to:

1. List the structures of the upper respiratory tract.
2. Describe the anatomy of the lungs.
3. Identify the functions of the respiratory system.
4. Describe certain conditions affecting the lungs that are related to specific types of work.
5. Identify the structures of the chest cavity.
6. Classify the common types of drugs used for respiratory conditions.
7. Define, pronounce, and spell 10 diseases and disorders from this chapter.
8. Define the terms *hemothorax*, *hypercapnia*, *hyperoxia*, and *hypoxemia*.

OUTLINE

STRUCTURE AND FUNCTION OF THE RESPIRATORY SYSTEM

Obtaining oxygen and removing carbon dioxide are the primary functions of the respiratory system, which includes tubes that remove particles from (filter) incoming air and transport air into and out of the lungs. The entire process of gas exchange between the atmosphere and cells is called **respiration**. The organs of the respiratory system can be divided into two groups. The upper respiratory tract includes the nose, nasal cavity, paranasal sinuses, and pharynx. The lower respiratory tract includes the larynx, trachea, bronchial tree, and lungs (Figure 13-1).

The nasal cavity is a hollow space behind the nose. The **nasal septum**, composed of bone and cartilage, divides the nasal cavity into right and left portions. Bones and processes that curve out from the nasal cavity walls, dividing the cavity into passages, are called

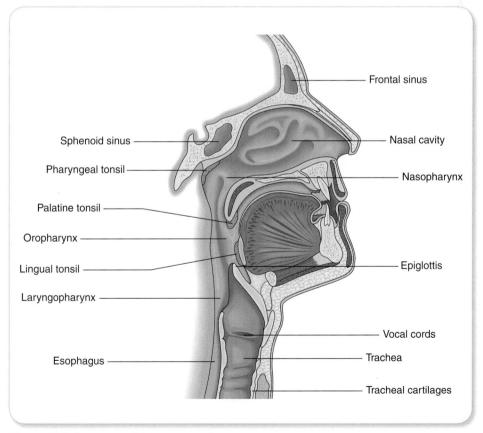

Figure 13-1 Structures of the upper respiratory tract.

nasal conchae. The **paranasal sinuses** are air-filled spaces within the maxillary, frontal, and ethmoid bones of the skull opening into the nasal cavity. Mucous membranes line the sinuses and are continuous with the lining of the nasal cavity. The paranasal sinuses lighten the skull and help to enhance the sound of the voice.

The **pharynx**, or throat, is behind the oral cavity, the nasal cavity, and the larynx. The pharynx is divided into the **nasopharynx**, the **oropharynx**, and the **laryngopharynx**. The larynx contains the vocal cords, which are the structures that make vocal sounds possible. The vocal cords are two folds of tissue that stretch across the larynx and vibrate as air passes through the space between them, producing sound. During normal breathing, the vocal cords are relaxed.

The opening between the vocal cords is called the **glottis**. The epiglottic cartilage supports a flap-like structure called the **epiglottis**. This structure usually stands upright and allows air to enter the larynx. During swallowing, however, the larynx rises, and the epiglottis presses downward to partially cover the opening into the larynx. This helps to prevent foods and liquids from entering the air passages.

The **trachea**, or *windpipe*, is a flexible, cylindrical tube about 2.5 centimeters in diameter and 12.5 centimeters in length. It extends downward anterior to the esophagus and into the thoracic cavity, where it splits into right and left bronchi (Figure 13-2).

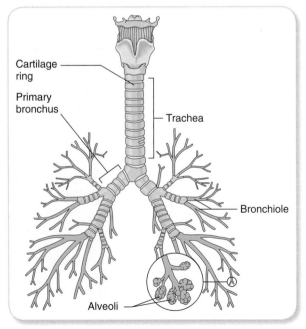

Figure 13-2 The trachea, bronchial tree, and alveoli.

The two bronchi lead to the lungs and subdivide into smaller tubes called **bronchioles**. The bronchi make up the **bronchial tree**, which begins with right and left **primary bronchi**. As the bronchial tree branches out into smaller and smaller tubes, it leads to thin **alveolar ducts** that lead to outpouchings called **alveolar sacs**, ending at the microscopic **alveoli** (air sacs, or *pulmonary parenchyma*), which have very thin walls that allow for gas exchange between the lungs and the blood.

The **lungs** are soft, spongy, cone-shaped organs in the thoracic cavity. The mediastinum separates the right and left lungs medially, and the diaphragm and thoracic cage enclose them (Figure 13-3).

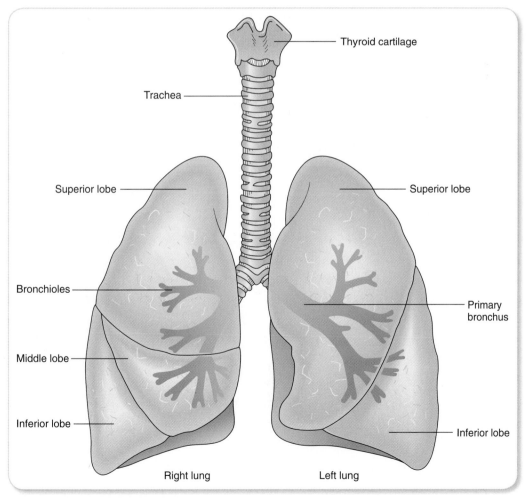

Figure 13-3 Structures of the lungs.

Each lung consists of smaller divisions called *lobes*. Two lobes exist in the left lung, which must also accommodate the heart in the chest cavity, while three lobes exist in the right lung. They are surrounded by **pleura**, which are double-folded membranes divided into the **parietal pleura** (the outer layer), and **visceral pleura** (the inner layer). The pleura are separated by a potential space known as the **pleural cavity** (Figure 13-4).

The process of breathing occurs because of muscular control that changes the air capacity of the thoracic cavity. When a person inhales, the thoracic cavity expands, and the lungs fill with air. When exhalation occurs, the cavity reduces in size and the lungs expel air outward. The diaphragm (which lies below the lungs) and **intercostal muscles** (which lie between the ribs) handle the majority of the contractions that control breathing. When the diaphragm contracts, it lowers to allow more air space in the thoracic cavity. When the intercostal muscles contract, they pull the ribs up and out, also allowing more air space.

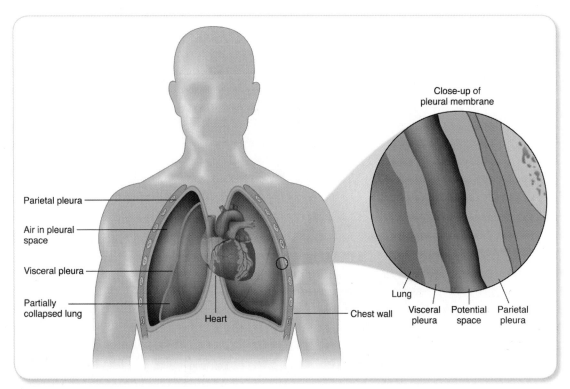

Figure 13-4 The pleura.

GENERAL TERMINOLOGY RELATED TO THE RESPIRATORY SYSTEM

The following are common terms that relate to the respiratory system.

Term	Pronunciation	Definition
adenoids	ADD-eh-noydz	collections of lymphoid tissue in the nasopharynx; also called **pharyngeal tonsils**
alveolus	al-VEE-oh-lus	air sacs at the end of each bronchiole
apex	AY-peks	the uppermost section of the lung
aphonia	ah-FOH-nee-ah	loss of voice
bradypnea	bray-DIP-nee-ah	abnormally slow breathing
bronchus	BRONG-kus	one of the two airways from the trachea to the lungs
bronchiole	BRONG-key-ohl	a small branch of a bronchus within the lung
bronchospasm	BRONG-koh-spaz-um	a sudden contraction in the bronchi that causes coughing
cilia	SIL-ee-ah	hair-like extensions of a cell's surface that usually provide some protection by sweeping foreign particles away
cyanosis	sy-ah-NO-sis	blue discoloration of the skin, lips, and nail beds due to low levels of oxygen in the blood
diaphragm	DYE-ah-fram	a dome-shaped musculofibrous partition that separates the thoracic and abdominal cavities
dyspnea	DISP-nee-ah	difficulty breathing
epiglottis	ep-ih-GLOT-iss	a thin, leaf-shaped cartilaginous structure that overhangs the larynx like a lid and prevents food from entering the larynx and trachea while swallowing
epistaxis	ep-ih-STAK-sis	bleeding from the septum of the nose
eupnea	YOOP-nee-ah	normal breathing
expiration	ek-spih-RAY-shun	expulsion of air from the lungs; breathing out; **exhalation**
glottis	GLOT-iss	part of the larynx, consisting of the vocal folds of mucous membrane and muscle
hilum	HIGH-lum	the midsection of the lung, where the vessels and nerves enter and exit
inspiration	in-spih-RAY-shun	taking air into the lungs; breathing in; **inhalation**
intubation	in-too-BAY-shun	insertion of a tube into the trachea
laryngopharynx	lah-ring-go-FAIR-inks	the lowest region of the pharynx, situated near the larynx
larynx	LAIR-inks	the organ of voice production in the respiratory tract, between the pharynx and trachea; also called the **voice box**

(continues)

Term	Pronunciation	Definition
mediastinum	mee-dee-ass-TYE-num	a part of the thoracic cavity in the middle of the thorax, between the pleural sacs containing the two lungs; extends from the sternum to the vertebral column and contains all the thoracic viscera except the lungs
nares	NAIRZ	the external nostrils (openings at the base of the nose)
nasopharynx	nay-zoh-FAIR-inks	the portion of the throat above the soft palate
oropharynx	or-oh-FAIR-inks	the back portion of the mouth
orthopnea	or-THOP-nee-ah	shortness of breath caused by lying flat
paranasal sinuses	pair-ah-NAY-zul SIGN-nuss-ez	the area of the nasal cavity where external air is warmed by blood in the mucous membrane lining
parietal pleura	pah-RYE-eh-tal PLOO-rah	the portion of the pleura closest to the ribs
pharynx	FAIR-inks	the passageway at the back of the mouth for air and food; the **throat**
pleura	PLOO-rah	the double layer of membrane making up the outside of the lungs
pleural cavity	PLOO-ral KAV-ih-tee	the space between the two pleura
septum	SEP-tum	a cartilaginous division, as in the nose
snore	SNOR	noise produced by vibrations in the structures of the nasopharynx
surface tension	SER-fus TEN-shun	a force created by the attraction of water molecules that makes it hard for the alveoli to inflate, and may cause their collapse
surfactant	serf-AK-tent	a mixture of lipids and proteins synthesized by alveolar cells that is continuously secreted into alveolar air spaces; reduces the tendency of the alveoli to collapse, especially during low lung volume
thorax	THOH-raks	the chest cavity
trachea	TRAY-kee-ah	the airway from the larynx into the bronchi; the **windpipe**
visceral pleura	VISS-er-al PLOO-rah	the portion of the pleura that is closest to the internal organs
wheezes	WEE-zez	whistling sounds heard on inspiration in certain breathing disorders, especially asthma

PATHOLOGICAL CONDITIONS

The following are pathological conditions of the respiratory system.

Anoxia – an abnormal condition characterized by a local or systemic lack of oxygen in body tissues; may result from an inadequate supply of oxygen to the respiratory system, or an inability of the blood to carry oxygen to the tissues

Anthracosis – a chronic lung disease characterized by the deposit of coal dust in the lungs, and by the formation of black nodules on the bronchioles, resulting in focal emphysema; occurs in coal miners and is aggravated by cigarette smoking

Apnea – absence or severe reduction in breathing

Asbestosis – a chronic lung disease caused by the inhalation of asbestos fibers that results in the development of alveolar and pleural fibrosis; asbestos miners and workers have been most frequently affected, but the disease sometimes occurs in other people who have been exposed to asbestos building materials

Asphyxia – severe hypoxia leading to hypoxemia and hypercapnia, loss of consciousness, and, if not corrected, death

Aspiration – removal by suction of fluid or gas from a body cavity

Asthma – a respiratory condition characterized by difficulty exhaling and by wheezing; caused by smooth muscle spasms in the airways, especially the bronchi, that reduce airflow and cause inflammation and accumulation of mucus in the air passages; more common in children than in adults

Atelectasis – an abnormal condition characterized by the collapse of alveoli, preventing the respiratory exchange of carbon dioxide and oxygen in a part of the lungs

Bradypnea – an abnormally low rate of breathing

Bronchiectasis – an abnormal condition of the bronchial tree characterized by irreversible dilation and destruction of the bronchial walls

Bronchiolectasis – chronic dilation of the bronchioles

Bronchitis – an inflammation, usually due to infection of the mucous membranes lining the bronchi

Bronchogenic carcinoma – the most common malignant lung tumors that originate in bronchi

Byssinosis – an occupational respiratory disease characterized by shortness of breath, coughing, and wheezing; an allergic reaction to dust or fungi in cotton, flax, and hemp fibers

Chronic obstructive pulmonary disease (COPD) – a group of disorders, almost always a result of smoking, that obstruct bronchial flow; one or more of the following is present in varying degrees: emphysema, chronic bronchitis, bronchospasm, and bronchitis

Cor pulmonale – serious cardiac disease associated with chronic lung disorders such as emphysema

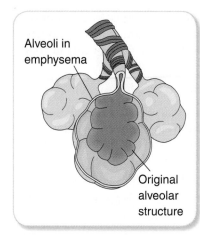

Alveoli in emphysema

Original alveolar structure

Figure 13-5 Emphysema.

Croup – an inflammation of the airway that produces a hoarse cough and wheezing; a childhood disorder that is usually caused by a viral infection

Cystic fibrosis – hereditary disorder of the exocrine glands characterized by excess mucus production in the respiratory tract, pancreatic deficiency, and other symptoms

Emphysema – a lung condition characterized by the destruction of alveoli and bronchioles (Figure 13-5) in which the loss of large numbers of alveoli reduces air exchange with the blood; as the condition progresses, patients experience increasing shortness of breath following minimal exertion; inhaling smoke from tobacco products is the most common cause; the resulting lung damage is usually irreversible, but stopping smoking usually ceases or slows the progression of the disease

Empyema – pus in a body space, usually due to an infection

Hemothorax – an accumulation of blood and fluid in the pleural cavity, usually the result of trauma

Hypercapnia – excessive carbon dioxide in the blood

Hyperoxia – abnormally high oxygen tension in the blood

Hyperpnea – an exaggerated, deep, rapid, or labored respiration; occurs normally with exercise and abnormally with aspirin overdose, pain, fever, or any condition in which the supply of oxygen is inadequate, such as cardiac disease and respiratory disease

Hyperventilation – deep, prolonged, and rapid breathing

Hypoxemia – an abnormal deficiency in the concentration of oxygen in arterial blood

Hypoxia – inadequate oxygen tension at the cellular level, characterized by tachycardia, hypertension, peripheral vasoconstriction, dizziness, and mental confusion

Laryngitis – inflammation of the mucous membranes in and around the larynx; primary symptom is hoarseness or total loss of voice; most often due to either voice strain or a viral infection

Mesothelioma – a rare malignant tumor of the mesothelium of the pleura, associated with exposure to asbestos

Nasal polyps – masses of tissue in the nasal cavity that bulge outward from the normal surface level

Pertussis – an acute, highly contagious respiratory disease, also known as *whooping cough,* that is characterized by paroxysmal coughing ending in a loud, "whooping" inspiration; occurs primarily in infants and children less than four years of age who have not been immunized

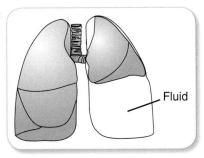

Figure 13-6 Pleural effusion.

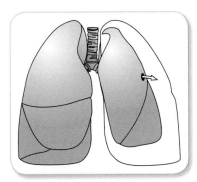

Figure 13-7 Pneumothorax.

Pharyngitis – inflammation or infection of the mucous membranes that line the throat; also called *sore throat;* some causes are diphtheria, herpes simplex virus, infectious mononucleosis, and streptococcal infection

Pleural effusion – an abnormal accumulation of fluid in the pleural space of the lungs; characterized by chest pain, dyspnea, and non-productive cough (Figure 13-6)

Pleuritis (pleurisy) – an inflammation of the pleural lining of the lungs; causes intense pain during breathing

Pneumoconiosis – any lung disease caused by chronically breathing dust or other particles; *black lung disease,* found in coal miners, is one form

Pneumonia – inflammation of the lungs characterized by fluid filling the alveoli and bronchioles; may be caused by inhaling irritating chemicals or by infection with bacteria, viruses, fungi, or protozoa; a condition known as **lobar pneumonia** affects an entire lobe of a lung

Pneumothorax – the presence of air or gas in the pleural space, causing a lung to collapse; may be the result of an open chest wound that permits the entrance of air (Figure 13-7)

Pulmonary edema – the accumulation of extravascular fluid in lung tissues and alveoli, caused most commonly by congestive heart failure

Pulmonary embolism – the blockage of a pulmonary artery by fat, air, tumor tissue, or thrombus that usually arises from a peripheral vein (most frequently one of the deep veins of the legs)

Rhinitis – inflammation of the mucous membranes in the nose; signs and symptoms include itching, sneezing, congestion, and production of excess mucus; allergic rhinitis (hay fever) is a common example

Sarcoidosis – granulomatous lesions of unknown cause of lungs and other organs

Silicosis – a lung disorder caused by continued long-term inhalation of the dust of an inorganic compound, silicon dioxide, which is found in sands, quartzes, and many other stones; incidence is highest among industrial workers exposed to silica powder in manufacturing processes

Sinusitis – an inflammation, usually due to infection, of the mucous membranes lining the paranasal sinuses; can cause fever, congestion, and severe pain

Tachypnea – abnormally rapid breathing; often develops during fever and with respiratory disease

Tonsillitis – inflammation of the tonsils, usually due to infection

Tracheotomy – an incision made into the trachea, through the neck below the larynx, performed to gain access to the airway below a blockage with a foreign body, tumor, or edema of the glottis

Tuberculosis – an infection caused by *Mycobacterium tuberculosis;* most commonly affects the lungs, but can also invade any part of the body, including bone, the gastrointestinal tract, and the kidneys; tuberculosis lesions are characterized by death of affected tissue with sloughing (shedding) of tissue and formation of cavities

ABBREVIATIONS

The following abbreviations are related to terms and procedures concerning the respiratory system.

Abbreviation	Meaning
AFB	acid-fast bacilli
AIDS	acquired immunodeficiency syndrome
AP	anteroposterior
ARD	acute respiratory disease
ARDS	adult respiratory distress syndrome
ARF	acute respiratory failure
BS	breath sounds
CF	cystic fibrosis
COLD	chronic obstructive lung disease
COPD	chronic obstructive pulmonary disease
CPR	cardiopulmonary resuscitation
CXR	chest X-ray
DOE	dyspnea on exertion
DPT	diphtheria, pertussis, and tetanus (combined vaccination)
HDM	hyaline membrane disease
IMV	intermittent mandatory ventilation
IPPB	intermittent positive pressure breathing
IRDS	infant respiratory distress syndrome
LLL	left lower lobe (of the lungs)
LUL	left upper lobe (of the lungs)
PA	posteroanterior
PE	pulmonary embolism

Abbreviation	Meaning
PFT	pulmonary function test
R	respiration
RD	respiratory disease
RDS	respiratory distress syndrome
RLL	right lower lobe (of the lungs)
RUL	right upper lobe (of the lungs)
SIDS	sudden infant death syndrome
SOB	shortness of breath
TB	tuberculosis
TPR	temperature, pulse, and respiration
URI	upper respiratory infection

MEDICATIONS USED TO TREAT RESPIRATORY SYSTEM DISORDERS

The following are common medications used for respiratory disorders.

Generic Name	Trade Name	Drug Class	Use
codeine	(generic only)	antitussives	to relieve coughing
dextromethorphan	Benylin®, Pertussin®		
diphenhydramine	Allermax®, Benadryl		
albuterol	Ventolin®, Proventil®	bronchodilators	to dilate bronchial walls and prevent spasms
ephedrine	Bronkaid®, Primatene®		
epinephrine	Bronkaid Mist®, Primatene Mist®		
omalizumab	Xolair®		
terbutaline	Brethaire®, Brethine®		
theophylline	Theo-Dur®, Slo-Bid®		
pseudoephedrine	Drixoral®, Sudafed®	decongestants	to lower and prevent buildup of mucus
xylometazoline	Otrivin®		
guiafenesin	Humibid®, Robitussin®	expectorants	to promote coughing and mucus expulsion

DRUG TERMINOLOGY

The following are common types of drugs used for respiratory conditions.

Drug Type	Pronunciation	Definition
antitussive	an-tee-TUS-siv	an agent that controls coughing
bronchodilator	brong-koh-dy-LAY-tor	an agent that dilates the bronchial walls
decongestant	dee-kon-JEST-ant	an agent that relieves mucus congestion of the upper respiratory tract
expectorant	ek-SPEK-toh-rant	an agent that promotes coughing and expulsion of mucus
nebulizer	NEB-yoo-ly-zer	a device that delivers medication through the nose or mouth, in a fine spray, to the respiratory tract
ventilator	VEN-tih-lay-tor	a mechanical breathing device

REVIEW EXERCISES

Multiple Choice

Select the best answer and write the letter of your choice to the left of each number.

1. Which of the following is part of the lower respiratory tract?

   A. paranasal sinuses
   B. pharynx
   C. larynx
   D. nasal cavity

2. The pharynx is also called the:

   A. septum
   B. conchae
   C. voice box
   D. throat

3. A small branch of a bronchus within the lung is referred to as a(n):

   A. bronchiole
   B. alveolus
   C. hilum
   D. septum

4. A mixture of lipids and proteins formed by alveolar cells is known as a:

   A. mucoid
   B. globulin
   C. sebum
   D. surfactant

5. The lowest part of the pharynx is referred to as the:

   A. laryngopharynx
   B. nasopharynx
   C. epiglottis
   D. trachea

6. A chronic lung disease caused by coal dust is called:

   A. byssinosis
   B. anthracosis
   C. asbestosis
   D. bronchiectasis

7. Which of the following disorders is usually caused by a viral infection?

    A. empyema
    B. emphysema
    C. byssinosis
    D. croup

8. Which of the following terms means "low concentration of oxygen in a tissue"?

    A. eupnea
    B. hypercapnia
    C. hypothermia
    D. hypoxemia

9. An acute, highly contagious respiratory disease characterized by paroxysmal coughing that occurs primarily in infants or children is referred to as:

    A. pneumonia
    B. pleuritis
    C. pertussis
    D. pulmonary edema

10. Rhinitis is also called:

    A. nose bleed
    B. hay fever
    C. sore throat
    D. asthma

11. Severe hypoxia leading to hypoxemia and hypercapnia, with loss of consciousness, is referred to as:

    A. croup
    B. apnea
    C. anoxia
    D. eupnea

12. What is the total number of lobes in both lungs?

    A. 2
    B. 3
    C. 4
    D. 5

13. Which of the following is the medical term for the nostrils?

    A. polyps
    B. tonsils
    C. adenoids
    D. nares

14. The medical term for "nose bleed" is:

    A. pus
    B. coryza
    C. epistaxis
    D. sputum

15. An abnormal condition characterized by the collapse of alveoli is referred to as:

    A. bronchiectasis
    B. emphysema
    C. asthma
    D. atelectasis

Fill in the Blank

Use your knowledge of medical terminology to insert the correct term from the list below into the appropriate statement.

pleural cavity	aphonia	apnea
oropharynx	dyspnea	aspiration
intubation	septum	snore
hilum	trachea	hyperoxia
apex	anoxia	hemothorax

1. A _____ is an accumulation of blood in the pleural cavity.

2. The back portion of the mouth is called the _____.

3. The condition of "losing your voice" is referred to as _____.

4. The _____ is the midsection of the lung where the vessels and nerves enter or exit.

5. The uppermost section of the lung is called the _____.

6. A noise produced by vibration in the structures of the nasopharynx is called a(n) _____.

7. Insertion of a tube into the trachea is called _____.

8. _____ is the removal by suction of fluid or gas from a body cavity.

9. An abnormal condition characterized by a local or systemic lack of oxygen in body tissues is referred to as _____.

10. Difficulty in breathing is called _____.

Labeling – The Structures of the Upper Respiratory Tract

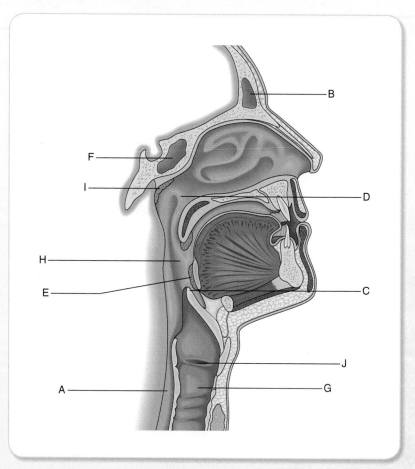

Write in the term below that corresponds with each letter on the figure above.

A. _____

B. _____

C. _____

D. _____

E. _____

F. _____

G. _____

H. _____

I. _____

J. _____

True / False

Identify each of the following statements as true or false by placing a "T" or "F" on the line beside each number.

_____ 1. The throat is a passageway for air only.

_____ 2. The pleura are moist layers of membrane surrounding the lungs.

_____ 3. The hilum is the lowest portion of the lung.

_____ 4. Only the left lung has a middle lobe.

_____ 5. The pharynx contains the vocal cords.

_____ 6. The paranasal sinuses include the maxillary and frontal openings into the nasal cavity.

_____ 7. During normal breathing, the vocal cords are relaxed.

_____ 8. The lungs are soft, spongy, and cone-shaped organs.

_____ 9. The visceral pleura is located in the inner layer.

_____ 10. The diaphragm is the membranous wall that separates the lungs.

Labeling – The External View of the Lungs

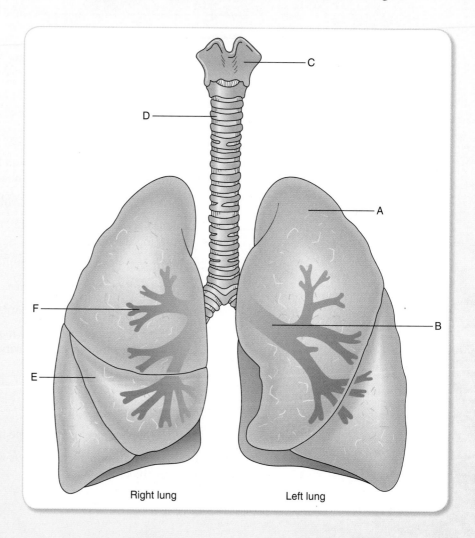

Right lung   Left lung

Write in the term below that corresponds with each letter on the figure above.

A. _____

B. _____

C. _____

D. _____

E. _____

F. _____

Definitions

Define each of the following words in one sentence.

1. pleurisy: _____

2. rhinitis: _____

3. apnea: _____

4. anthracosis: _____

5. hypoxia: _____

6. hemothorax: _____

7. eupnea: _____

8. dysphonia: _____

9. atelectasis: _____

10. wheezes: _____

Abbreviations

Write the full meaning of each abbreviation.

Abbreviation	Meaning
1. AP	_____
2. COLD	_____
3. ARF	_____
4. DOE	_____
5. RDS	_____
6. LUL	_____
7. IRDS	_____
8. RD	_____
9. TB	_____
10. SOB	_____

Matching – Terms and Definitions

Match each term with its correct definition by placing the corresponding letter on the line to its left.

_____ 1. expiration

_____ 2. cyanosis

_____ 3. thorax

_____ 4. snore

A. fibrotic lung disease from inhaling particles

B. cancer arising from the cells lining the pleura

_____ **5.** bradypnea

_____ **6.** crackles

_____ **7.** mesothelioma

_____ **8.** pneumonia

_____ **9.** pulmonary embolism

_____ **10.** silicosis

C. popping sounds heard in lung collapse

D. the blockage of a pulmonary artery by fat or air that usually arises from a peripheral vein

E. inflammation of the lungs

F. blue discoloration of the lips

G. the chest cavity

H. noise produced by vibrations in the structures of the nasopharynx

I. expulsion of air from the lungs

J. abnormally slow breathing

Spelling

Circle the correct spelling from each pairing of words.

1. alveoli	alvioli
2. medyastinum	mediastinum
3. epiglotis	epiglottis
4. tonsills	tonsils
5. epistaxis	epistacksis
6. trachai	trachea
7. pharynx	pharinx
8. snor	snore
9. wheezes	wheizes
10. asphysia	asphyxia

Urinary System

OBJECTIVES

Upon completion of this chapter, the reader should be able to:

1. Describe the anatomy of the kidneys.
2. Identify the function of the urinary system.
3. List and define the major pathological conditions of the urinary system.
4. Identify the organs of the urinary system.
5. Describe the process of the production of urine.
6. Define, pronounce, and spell urinary terminology.
7. Classify the common types of drugs used for urinary system conditions.
8. Define abbreviations related to the urinary system.

Structure and Function of the Urinary System

The urinary system includes a pair of kidneys, which remove substances from the blood, form urine, and help regulate certain metabolic processes. It also includes a pair of tubular ureters, which transport urine from the kidneys to the urinary bladder. The urinary bladder stores urine. A tubular urethra then conveys urine outside of the body (Figure 14-1).

A **kidney** is a bean-shaped organ with a smooth surface. It is enclosed in a tough, fibrous capsule. The kidneys are positioned **retroperitoneally**, which means they are behind the peritoneum (the membrane that lines the abdominal and pelvic cavities). The lateral surface of each kidney is convex (bulging outward), but its medial (middle) side is deeply concave (curving inward). The

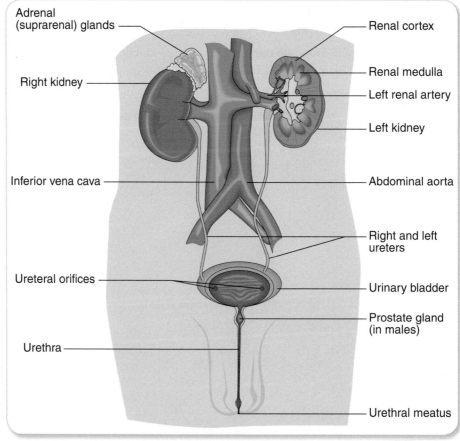

Figure 14-1   The urinary system.

resulting medial depression leads into a hollow chamber called the **renal sinus**. The entrance of this sinus is called the *hilum*, through which blood vessels, nerves, lymphatic vessels, and the ureter pass.

The upper end of the ureter expands to form a funnel-shaped sac called the **renal pelvis** inside the renal sinus. The pelvis is subdivided into two or three tubes, called *major calyces*. These are further subdivided into several *minor calyces* (Figure 14-2).

A series of small elevations called *renal papillae* project into the renal sinus from its wall. Tiny openings that lead into a minor calyx pierce each projection. Each kidney has two distinct regions: an outer cortex and an inner medulla. The **renal medulla** is composed of conical masses of tissue called *renal pyramids* and appears striated. The **renal cortex** forms a shell around the medulla and dips into the medulla between renal pyramids, forming *renal columns*. The kidney's functional units, called **nephrons**, are mainly located in the cortex (Figure 14-3).

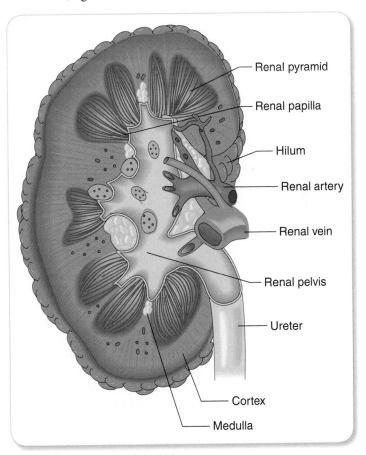

Renal pyramid

Renal papilla

Hilum

Renal artery

Renal vein

Renal pelvis

Ureter

Cortex

Medulla

Figure 14-2 Structures of the kidney.

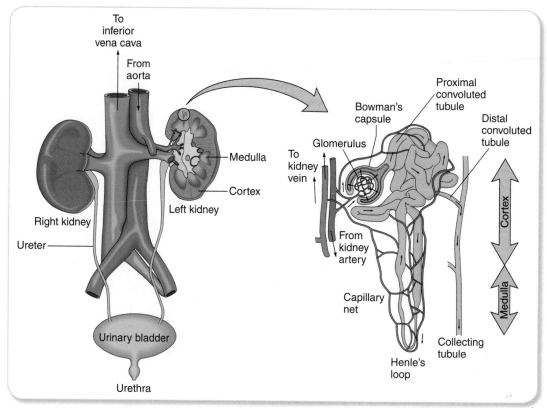

Figure 14-3 The nephron.

Each kidney contains more than a million nephrons. A nephron consists of small tubes or **tubules**, and associated small blood vessels. Fluid formed by capillary filtration enters the tubules and is subsequently modified by transport processes. The resulting fluid that leaves the tubules is urine.

Arterial blood enters the kidney through the renal artery, which divides into interlobar arteries. The **afferent arterioles** move blood into the **glomeruli**, which are capillary networks that produce a blood filtrate that enters the urinary tubules. The blood remaining in a glomerulus leaves through an **efferent arteriole**, which delivers the blood into another capillary network—the **peritubular capillaries** surrounding the renal tubules. The tubular portion of a nephron consists of a *glomerular capsule*, a *proximal convoluted tubule*, a *descending limb of the loop of Henle*, an *ascending limb of the loop of Henle*, and a *distal convoluted tubule*.

The primary function of the kidneys is the regulation of the volume of blood plasma, the concentration of waste products in the blood, the concentration of electrolytes, and the pH of plasma. Each of the nephrons receives a blood filtrate from a capillary bed called the **glomerulus**. The filtrate is similar to plasma, but it is modified as it passes through different regions of the nephron and is thereby changed into urine. Each **ureter** is a tube about 25 centimeters long that begins from the renal pelvis. The ureters descend behind the peritoneum and join the urinary bladder.

The **urinary bladder** is a hollow, distensible, muscular organ that stores urine and forces it into the urethra. It lies in the pelvic cavity, behind the symphysis pubis (the middle joint of the pubic bones). The internal floor of the bladder includes a triangular area called the **trigone**, which has an opening at each of its three angles.

The **urethra** is a tube that conveys urine from the urinary bladder to the outside of the body. Its wall is lined with mucous membranes and has a thick layer of smooth muscle tissue. The urethral wall also has numerous mucous glands, called *urethral glands*, which secrete mucus into the urethral canal.

In females, the urethra is about 4 centimeters long. Its opening, the external urethral orifice (urinary meatus) is anterior to the vaginal opening and posterior to the clitoris. In males, the urethra functions as part of both the urinary system and the reproductive system, and extends from the bladder to the tip of the penis (Figure 14-4).

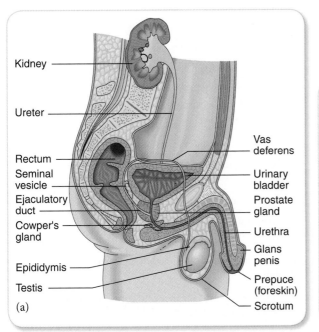
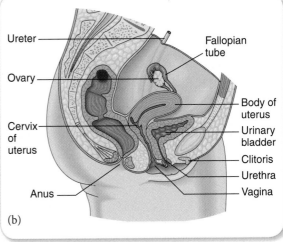

Figure 14-4 The urinary bladder (a) male (b) female.

GENERAL TERMINOLOGY RELATED TO THE URINARY SYSTEM

The following are common terms that relate to the urinary system.

Term	Pronunciation	Definition
bladder	BLAD-der	storage site for urine before it is excreted from the body
Bowman's capsule	BOW-manz CAP-sool	spherical structure that surrounds the glomerulus and collects filtrate
calyx	KAY-liks	one of the cup-shaped structures in the renal pelvis for the collection of urine
cortex	KOR-teks	tissue layer of the kidney just beneath the renal capsule
creatine	KREE-ah-tin	a substance found in urine; elevated levels of creatine may indicate muscular dystrophy
creatinine	kree-AT-in-in	a component of creatine
filtration	fil-TRAY-shun	the process of separating solids from a liquid by passing it through a porous substance
glomerulus	glom-AIR-yoo-lus	a group of capillaries in a nephron
hilum	HIGH-lum	a portion of the kidney where blood vessels and nerves enter and exit
meatus	mee-AY-tus	the external opening of a canal, such as the urethra
medulla	meh-DULL-ah	the central portion of the kidney
micturition	mik-chuh-RISH-un	the act of eliminating urine from the bladder; also called *voiding* or *urination*
nephrolith	NEF-roh-lith	a renal calculus; also known as a *kidney stone*
nephron	NEF-ron	the functional unit of the kidney
nephropathy	neh-FRAW-pah-thee	any disease of the kidneys
nocturia	nok-TOO-ree-ah	increased frequency and urgency of urination during the night
oliguria	ol-ih-GYOO-ree-ah	decreased production of urine associated with kidney failure
polyuria	paw-lee-YOO-ree-ah	excessive production of urine associated with diabetes mellitus and diabetes insipidus
prostate	PRAW-stayt	the gland surrounding the urethra in the male; active in the ejaculation of semen
pyuria	py-YOO-ree-ah	the presence of pus in the urine; may be caused by kidney disease or a urinary tract infection
renal pelvis	REE-nuhl PELL-viss	the collecting area for urine in the center of the kidney

renin	REH-nin	an enzyme produced in the kidneys to regulate the filtration rate of blood by increasing blood pressure as necessary
residual urine	rih-ZID-yoo-al YOO-rin	urine remaining in the bladder after urination
retroperitoneal	reh-tro-per-ih-toh-NEE-al	posterior to the peritoneum
trigone	TRY-gon	triangular area at the base of the bladder through which the ureters enter and the urethra exits the bladder
urea	yoo-REE-ah	a waste product of nitrogen metabolism excreted in normal adult urine
ureter	YOO-reh-ter	the tube that transports urine from the kidney to the bladder
urethra	yoo-REE-thrah	the tube through which urine is transported from the bladder to the exterior of the body
uric acid	YOO-rik AS-sid	a nitrogenous waste excreted in the urine
urination	YOO-rih-NAY-shun	the act of eliminating urine from the body; also called *micturition* or *voiding*
urine	YOO-rin	the fluid released by the kidneys for elimination through the urethra; normally clear, straw-colored, and slightly acidic
voiding	VOY-ding	the act of eliminating urine from the body; also called *micturition* or *urination*

PATHOLOGICAL CONDITIONS

The following are pathological conditions of the urinary system.

Cystitis – urinary bladder inflammation; commonly caused by a bacterial infection of the bladder, particularly in women, because of the short length of the urethra

Glomerulonephritis – inflammation of the glomerulus (of the kidneys)

Hematuria – blood in the urine; may be caused by a kidney stone, bladder cancer, or cystitis

Hydronephrosis – enlargement of the kidney due to constant pressure from backed-up urine in the ureter due to an obstructing stone or structure (Figure 14-5)

Nephrolithiasis – kidney stone or calculus formation in the urinary system

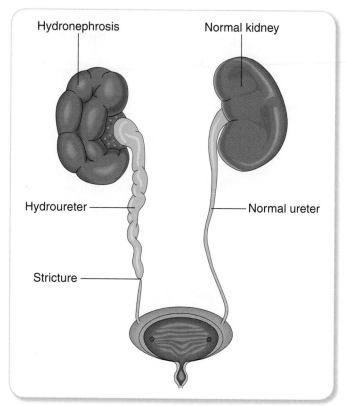

Figure 14-5 Hydronephrosis.

Nephrotic syndrome – also called *nephrosis*; occurs as a result of another existing kidney disorder and is characterized by proteinuria, hypoproteinemia, generalized edema, and hyperlipidemia; the basement membrane of renal glomeruli is primarily affected; may become evident after glomerulonephritis, kidney transplants, allergic reactions, diabetes mellitus, pregnancy, infections, or exposure to toxins

Neurogenic bladder – a condition of urinary retention due to lack of innervation of the nerves of the bladder; caused by a spinal cord injury, multiple sclerosis, Parkinson's disease, or spina bifida

Polycystic kidney disease – a hereditary kidney disorder involving grape-like sacs or cysts filled with fluid that replace normal kidney tissue (Figure 14-6)

Pyelitis – an inflammation of the renal pelvis

Pyelonephritis – a bacterial infection in the renal pelvis with abscesses

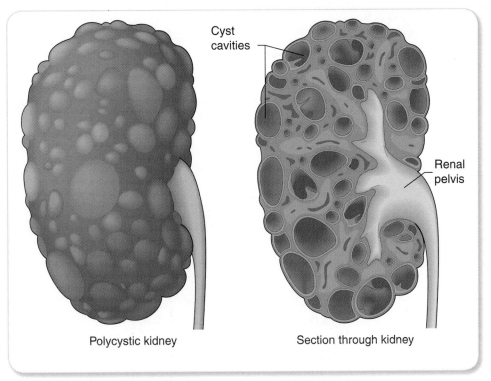

Figure 14-6 Polycystic kidney disease.

Renal calculi – stone formations occurring in the kidney

Renal cell carcinoma – a malignant kidney tumor that occurs in adulthood

Renal failure – the loss of kidney function; may result from other conditions, such as diabetes mellitus

Uremia – the presence of high levels of the waste product urea and/or ammonia in the blood, resulting in renal failure; the kidneys are unable to remove urea

Urethritis – an inflammation of the urethra; painful, especially when passing urine, and most commonly caused by infection

Vesicoureteral reflux – an abnormal reflux (backflow) of urine from the bladder to the ureter

Wilm's tumor – a malignant kidney tumor occurring in children that arises from residual embryonic or fetal tissue; also known as a **nephroblastoma**

ABBREVIATIONS

The following abbreviations are related to terms and procedures concerning the urinary system.

Abbreviation	Meaning
ADH	antidiuretic hormone
AGN	acute glomerular nephritis
ARF	acute renal failure
BUN	blood urea nitrogen
CAPD	continuous ambulatory peritoneal dialysis
CCPD	continuous cycling peritoneal dialysis
CRF	chronic renal failure
C&S	culture and sensitivity
cysto	cystoscopy
EPO	erythropoietin
ESRD	end-stage renal disease
GFR	glomerular filtration rate
HD	hemodialysis
I&O	intake and output
IVP	intravenous pyelogram
K	potassium
KUB	kidneys, ureters, bladder
pH	potential hydrogen; the abbreviation for the degree of acidity or alkalinity of a solution
RP	retrograde pyelogram
UA	urinalysis
UTI	urinary tract infection
VCUG	voiding cystourethrogram

MEDICATIONS USED TO TREAT URINARY SYSTEM CONDITIONS

The following are common medications used for urinary conditions.

Generic Name	Trade Name	Drug Class	Use
phenazopyridine	Pyridium®, Urogesic®	analgesic	to relieve pain
amoxicillin	Amoxil®, Wymox®	antibiotics	to treat infections (especially urinary tract infections), including those with fungal causes
ciprofloxacin	Cipro®		
levofloxacin	Levaquin®		
tetracycline	Sumycin®		
trimethoprim	Trimpex®		
vasopressin	Pitressin®	antidiuretic	to control urine secretion
oxybutynin	Ditropan®	antispasmodics	to relax muscles, relieve pain, and decrease the urgency to urinate
tolterodine	Detrol®		
bethanecol	Duvoid®, Urecholine®	diuretics	to increase urination

DRUG TERMINOLOGY

The following are common types of drugs used for urinary conditions.

Drug Type	Pronunciation	Definition
antispasmodics	an-tee-spaz-MOD-iks	pharmacological agents that relieve spasms and decrease frequency of urination
diuretics	die-yoo-RET-iks	pharmacological agents that increase urination

REVIEW EXERCISES

Multiple Choice

Select the best answer and write the letter of your choice to the left of each number.

1. The upper end of the ureter expands to form a funnel-shaped sac called:

   A. the hilum
   B. the renal sinus
   C. the renal pelvis
   D. the major calyces

2. The kidney's functional units are referred to as:

   A. the renal sinuses
   B. the renal calyces
   C. the glomeruli
   D. the nephrons

3. Which of the following is not part of the primary function of the kidneys?

   A. regulation of plasma pH
   B. regulation of waste products in the blood
   C. regulation of the blood volume
   D. regulation of the blood protein levels

4. The spherical structure that surrounds the glomerulus is known as the:

   A. calyx
   B. cortex
   C. renal pelvis
   D. Bowman's capsule

5. Urine remaining in the bladder after urination is called:

   A. residual urine
   B. voiding
   C. micturition
   D. oliguria

6. The triangular area at the base of the bladder is referred to as the:

   A. meatus
   B. hilum
   C. trigone
   D. calyx

7. Which of the following is a hereditary kidney disorder involving grape-like sacs that replace normal kidney tissue?

   A. nephrotic syndrome
   B. polycystic kidney disease
   C. pyelonephritis
   D. Wilm's tumor

8. The presence of high levels of ammonia in the blood, resulting in renal failure, signifies a condition called:

   A. uremia
   B. uropathy
   C. hemoglobinopathy
   D. hemochromatosis

9. Which of the following disorders or conditions may be caused by a kidney stone, bladder cancer, or cystitis?

   A. hydronephrosis
   B. nephrolithiasis
   C. nephrotic syndrome
   D. hematuria

10. Urine is carried to the urinary bladder by:

    A. blood vessels
    B. lymphatics
    C. the ureters
    D. the urethra

11. The outermost layer of kidney tissue is the:

    A. renal cortex
    B. renal medulla
    C. major calyx
    D. minor calyx

12. Urine is produced by the:

    A. gall bladder
    B. urinary bladder
    C. ureter
    D. kidney

13. An abnormally low position of a kidney is called:

    A. nephrolithiasis
    B. nephroptosis
    C. hydronephrosis
    D. polycystic kidney disease

14. Nitrogenous waste excreted in the urine is referred to as:

   A. uric acid
   B. renin
   C. bile acid
   D. histamine

15. Which of the following substances is produced in the kidneys to regulate the filtration rate of blood by increasing blood pressure as necessary?

   A. urea
   B. uric acid
   C. renin
   D. creatinine

Fill in the Blank

Use your knowledge of medical terminology to insert the correct term from the list below.

glomerulus	renal sinus	hilum
calyx	trigone	bladder
urethra	renal medulla	medulla
meatus	prostate	cortex
renal pelvis	ureter	capsule

1. The storage site for urine before it is excreted from the body is called the _____.

2. A _____ is a tube that transports urine from the kidney to the bladder.

3. The _____ is a gland surrounding the urethra in the male.

4. A cup-shaped structure in the renal pelvis for the collection of urine is referred to as the _____.

5. A group of capillaries in a nephron is called a _____.

6. The portion of the kidney where blood vessels enter or exit is known as the _____.

7. A triangular area at the floor of the urinary bladder is called the _____.

8. A collecting area for urine in the center of the kidney is called the _____.

9. The external opening of the canal of the urethra is referred to as the _____.

10. The region of the kidney just beneath the renal capsule is known as the _____.

Labeling – The Urinary System

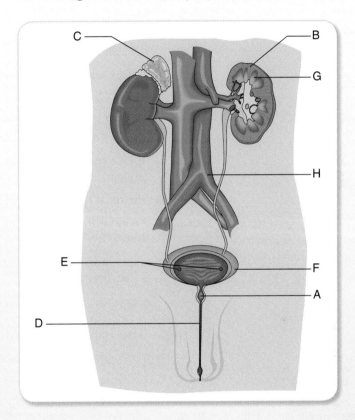

Write in the term below that corresponds with each letter on the figure above.

A. _____

B. _____

C. _____

D. _____

E. _____

F. _____

G. _____

H. _____

True / False

Identify each of the following statements as true or false by placing a "T" or "F" on the line beside each number.

_____ **1.** The act of eliminating urine from the body is referred to as "filtration."

_____ **2.** The collecting area for urine in the center of the kidneys is called the "nephron."

_____ **3.** The renal calculi are stone formations occurring in the kidney.

_____ **4.** Wilm's tumor is also known as a "nephroblastoma."

_____ **5.** Grape-like cysts filled with fluid that replace normal kidney tissues are signs of polycystic kidney disease.

_____ **6.** Kidneys are located inside the peritoneum.

_____ **7.** The ureter is a tube about 4 centimeters long in females.

_____ **8.** The renal papillae project into the nephrons.

_____ **9.** An elevation of creatinine may indicate muscular dystrophy.

_____ **10.** Urine remaining in the bladder after urination is called "hydronephrosis."

Labeling – The Internal Anatomy of the Kidney

Write in the term below that corresponds with each letter on the figure left.

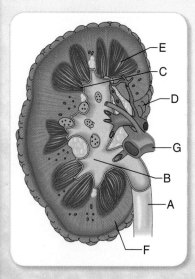

A. _____

B. _____

C. _____

D. _____

E. _____

F. _____

G. _____

Definitions

Define each of the following words in one sentence.

1. renal calculi: _____

2. cystitis: _____

3. oliguria: _____

4. pyuria: _____

5. renin: _____

6. urea: _____

7. nocturia: _____

8. renal cell carcinoma: _____

9. hydronephrosis: _____

10. polyuria: _____

Abbreviations

Write the full meaning of each abbreviation.

Abbreviation	Meaning
1. C&S	_____
2. ADH	_____
3. CRF	_____
4. EPO	_____
5. IVP	_____
6. UA	_____
7. K	_____
8. BUN	_____
9. ARF	_____
10. HD	_____

Matching – Terms and Definitions

Match each term with its correct definition by placing the corresponding letter on the line to its left.

_____ 1. pyuria

_____ 2. urea

_____ 3. urethra

_____ 4. ureter

A. the central portion of the kidney

B. the functional unit of the kidney

_____ 5. creatine

_____ 6. calyx

_____ 7. medulla

_____ 8. cortex

_____ 9. meatus

_____ 10. nephron

C. the tissue layer of the kidney just beneath the renal capsule

D. a cup-shaped structure in the renal pelvis

E. a waste product of nitrogen metabolism

F. the external opening of a canal

G. a tube through which urine is transported from the bladder to the exterior of the body

H. a tube that transports urine from the kidney to the bladder

I. a substance found in urine that may indicate muscular dystrophy

J. the presence of pus in the urine

Spelling

Circle the correct spelling from each pairing of words.

1. trigone   trigane

2. peritonum   peritoneum

3. glumerulus   glomerulus

4. papillae   papilae

5. hillum   hilum

6. nocturia   nochuria

7. calyx   kalyx

8. filltration   filtration

9. nephrolithiasis   nephrolitiasis

10. michurition   micturition

Male Reproductive System

OBJECTIVES

Upon completion of this chapter, the reader should be able to:

1. Describe the structures and functions of the male reproductive system.
2. Define the contents and functions of semen.
3. Label a diagram of the male reproductive system.
4. List and define the major pathological conditions of the male reproductive system.
5. Define, pronounce, and spell male reproductive system terminology.
6. Interpret abbreviations related to the male reproductive system.
7. Classify the common types of drugs used for male reproductive conditions.
8. Describe the hormone released from the testes and its functions.

STRUCTURE AND FUNCTION OF THE MALE REPRODUCTIVE SYSTEM

The male reproductive system consists of the testes, the internal genitalia (accessory glands and ducts), and the external genitalia. The external genitalia consists of the **penis** and the **scrotum**, a sac-like structure that contains the testes (testicles). The urethra serves as a common passageway for sperm and urine, although not simultaneously. It runs through the anterior shaft of the penis and is surrounded by a spongy column of tissue known as the **corpus spongiosum**. The corpus spongiosum and two columns of tissue called the **corpora cavernosa** constitute the erectile tissue of the penis.

The tip of the penis is enlarged into a region called the **glans** that, at birth, is covered by a layer of skin called the **foreskin** or **prepuce**. In some cultures, the foreskin is removed surgically in a procedure called a *circumcision*. The scrotum is an external sac into which the testes migrate during fetal development. This location outside the abdominal cavity is necessary because normal sperm development requires a temperature that is 2 to 3 degrees (Fahrenheit) lower than the core body temperature.

The failure of one or both testes to descend is known as **cryptorchidism**. Those that remain in the abdomen through puberty become sterile and are unable to produce sperm. The male accessory glands and ducts include the **prostate gland**, the **seminal vesicles**, and the **bulbourethral (Cowper's) glands**. The bulbourethral glands and seminal vesicles empty their secretions into the urethra through ducts (Figure 15-1).

The prostate gland is the best known of the three accessory glands because of its medical significance. Cancer of the prostate is the second most common form of cancer in men (next to lung cancer), and *benign prostatic hypertrophy* (enlargement) creates problems for many men after age 50.

The human testes are paired ovoid structures. The testes have a tough outer fibrous capsule that encloses masses of coiled **seminiferous tubules**. Between these tubules is interstitial tissue consisting primarily of blood vessels and the testosterone-secreting Leydig cells.

The seminiferous tubules leave each testis and join the **epididymis**, a single duct that forms a tightly coiled cord on the surface of the testicular capsule. Sperm are released into the lumen of the seminiferous tubule, along with secreted fluid. **Sertoli cells** of the

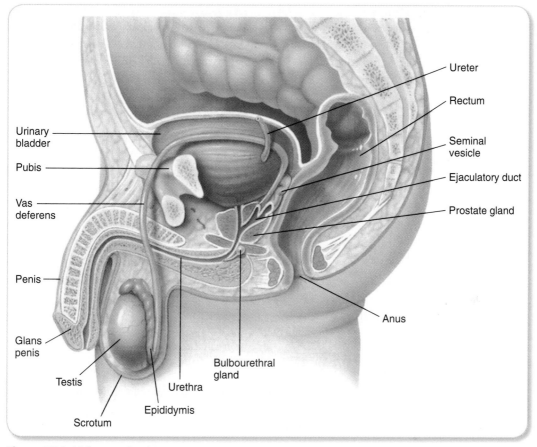

Figure 15-1 Male reproductive system.

seminiferous tubules regulate sperm development. These cells provide nourishment for the developing sperm.

Accessory glands of the male reproductive tract include the bulbourethral gland, seminal vesicles, and prostate. The prostate's primary function is to secrete various fluid mixtures. When sperm leave the vas deferens during ejaculation, they are joined by these secretions, resulting in a sperm–fluid mixture known as *semen*.

GENERAL TERMINOLOGY RELATED TO THE MALE REPRODUCTIVE SYSTEM

The following are common terms that relate to the male reproductive system.

Term	Pronunciation	Definition
bulbourethral glands	buhl-boh-yoo-REE-thral glands	two small glands located on each side of the prostate, draining to the wall of the urethra; secrete a fluid component of the seminal fluid; also called *Cowper's glands*
circumcision	sir-kum-SIH-zhun	the surgical procedure that removes the foreskin of the penis; widely performed on newborns
corpus cavernosum	KOR-pus kah-ver-NO-sum	a type of spongy erectile tissue within the penis; becomes engorged with blood during sexual excitement
corpus spongiosum	KOR-pus spun-jee-OH-sum	one of the cylinders of spongy tissue, with the corpora cavernosa, on the dorsum of the penis
ductus deferens	DUK-tus DEH-feh-renz	the extension of the epididymis of the testis that ascends from the scrotum into the abdominal cavity and joins the seminal vesicle to form the ejaculatory duct
dysuria	dis-YOO-ree-ah	pain or difficulty when passing urine
ejaculation	ee-jack-yoo-LAY-shun	the sudden emission of semen from the male urethra, usually during copulation, masturbation, or as a nocturnal emission
ejaculatory duct	ee-JACK-yoo-lah-toh-ree DUKT	one of two ducts which begin at the vas deferens and pass through the prostate gland to empty into the urethra
epididymis	ep-ih-DID-ih-mis	one of a pair of long, tightly coiled ducts that carry sperm from the seminiferous tubules of the testes to the vas deferens
foreskin	FOR-skin	a loose fold of skin that covers the end of the penis; also called the "prepuce"
glans penis	GLANZ PEE-nis	the conical tip of the penis that covers the end of the corpora cavernosa and corpus spongiosum like a cap; the urethral orifice is normally located at the distal tip of the glans penis
gonads	GOH-nadz	the primary organs of the male reproductive system; the testes (singular: *testicle* or *testis*); the male sex glands
orchidopexy	OR-kid-oh-peck-see	an operation to mobilize an undescended testis, bring it into the scrotum, and attach it so that it will not retract
perineum	pair-ih-NEE-um	the region surrounding the penis and the anus
prostate	PROSS-tayt	a gland in males that surrounds the neck of the bladder and the deepest part of the urethra, and produces a fluid that becomes part of semen; a firm structure, about the size of a chestnut, located in the pelvic cavity
prostatectomy	pross-tah-TEK-toh-mee	surgical removal of a part of the prostate gland, or the total excision of the gland
rete testis	REE-TEE TES-tis	a structure composed of a fibrous network or mesh in the center of the testis
scrotum	SKROH-tum	the pouch of skin containing the testes and parts of the spermatic cords
semen	SEE-men	a combination of spermatozoans, seminal fluid, prostaglandins, and enzymes

seminal vesicles	SEM-in-uhl VESS-ih-kuls	the tubular gland that produces a secretion that contains a thick and yellowish fluid
seminiferous tubules	SEM-in-IF-er-us TOO-byoolz	long, thread-like tubes packed in areolar tissue in the lobes of the testes
spermatozoan	sper-mat-oh-ZOH-ahn	a mature male germ cell that develops in the seminiferous tubules of the testes; resembles a tadpole, and has a head with a nucleus, a neck, and a tail that provides propulsion; term is sometimes spelled "spermatozoon"; plural form is "spermatozoa"
testicles	TESS-tih-kuls	the male gonads that produce sperm and testosterone; adult testes are suspended in the scrotum by the spermatic cords
testosterone	tess-TOSS-ter-own	a male hormone secreted by the testes that is responsible for promoting the functional maturation of sperm; also determines secondary sex characteristics, stimulates overall metabolism, and stimulates sexual behaviors and the sex drive
urethra	yoo-REE-thrah	a small, tubular structure that drains urine from the bladder; in males, it is about 20 centimeters long and begins at the bladder, passing through the center of the prostate gland, where it joins the ejaculatory duct and serves as a passageway for semen during ejaculation
vas deferens	VAS DEF-er-enz	the extension of the epididymis of the testis that ascends from the scrotum into the abdominal cavity and joins the seminal vesicle to form the ejaculatory duct; also called the **spermatic duct**, **testicular duct**, and the *ductus deferens*
vasectomy	vah-SEK-toh-mee	a surgical procedure in males to prevent their ability to impregnate a female; it is accomplished via a small incision at the base of the scrotum

PATHOLOGICAL CONDITIONS

The following are disorders and conditions of the male reproductive system.

Acquired immunodeficiency syndrome – a deadly virus that may be sexually transmitted involving destruction of the body's immune system by invading T cells

Anorchism – the congenital absence of one or both testes; also called "anorchia"

Balanitis – an inflammation of the glans penis and the mucous membrane beneath it

Benign prostatic hyperplasia – a non-malignant, non-inflammatory enlargement of the prostate gland that is most common among men over 50 years of age; usually progressive and may lead to urethral obstruction, interference with urine flow, increased urinary frequency, nocturia, dysuria, and urinary tract infections

Chancre – a skin lesion, usually of primary syphilis, that begins at the infection site as a papule and develops into a red, bloodless, painless ulcer with a scooped-out appearance; heals without treatment and leaves no scar; two or more chancres may develop at the same time, usually in the genital area, but sometimes on the hands, face, or other body surface

Chlamydia – a microorganism capable of causing urinary tract infections; one of the most common sexually transmitted organisms in North America, and a frequent cause of sterility

Cryptorchidism – a developmental defect in which one or both testicles fail to descend into the scrotum and are retained in the abdomen or inguinal canal (Figure 15-2a)

Epididymitis – an inflammation of the epididymis; may result from venereal disease, a urinary tract infection, prostatitis, or prolonged use of catheters (Figure 15-2b)

Epispadias – a congenital defect in which the urethra opens on the dorsum of the penis at any point below the internal sphincter (Figure 15-3)

Genital herpes – a chronic infection caused by type 2 herpes simplex virus; usually transmitted by sexual contact; causes painful vesicular eruptions on the skin and mucous membranes of the genitalia of males and females (Figure 15-4); *also discussed in the chapter on the female reproductive system*

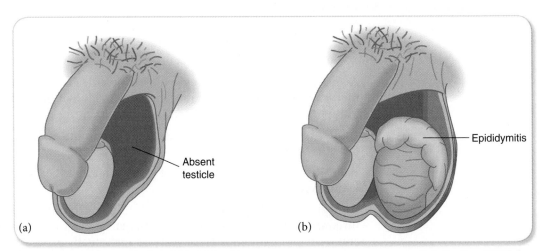

Figure 15-2 (a) Cryptorchidism (b) Epididymitis.

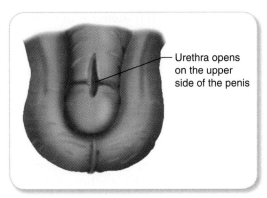

Figure 15-3 Epispadias.

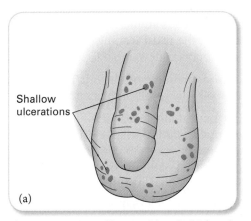

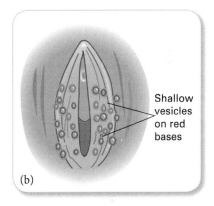

Figure 15-4 Genital herpes (a) male (b) female.

Genital warts – small, soft, moist, pink or red swelling of the genitals that becomes pedunculated (stalk-like), and may be painless; may be solitary, or in a cauliflower-like group present in a certain area of the genitalia; caused by a sexually transmitted disease (human papillomavirus)

Gonorrhea – a common sexually transmitted disease that usually affects the genitourinary tract, and occasionally the pharynx or rectum; results from contact with an infected person or with secretions containing the causative organism *Neisseria gonorrhoeae*

Hydrocele – an accumulation of fluid around the testicles; caused by inflammation of the epididymis or testis

Hypospadias – a developmental anomaly in males in which the urethra opens on the central portion of the penis or on the perineum (Figure 15-5)

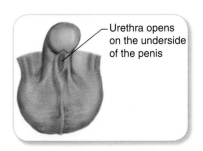

Figure 15-5 Hypospadias.

Impotence – the inability of the adult male to achieve penile erection or, less commonly, to ejaculate after achieving an erection

Orchitis – inflammation of one or both of the testes, characterized by swelling and pain; often caused by mumps, syphilis, or tuberculosis

Phimosis – a tightness of the foreskin of the penis that prevents retraction of the foreskin over the glans; usually congenital, but may be the result of infection

Priapism – an abnormal condition of prolonged or constant penile erection, often painful, and seldom associated with sexual arousal; may result from localized infection, a lesion in the penis or central nervous system, or the use of certain drugs

Prostate cancer – a slowly progressive adenocarcinoma of the prostate that affects an increasing proportion of American males after age 50; the third leading cause of cancer deaths; cause is unknown, but is believed to be hormone-related

Prostatitis – an acute or chronic inflammation of the prostate gland, usually the result of infection

Syphilis – a sexually transmitted disease caused by a spirochete (*Treponemal pallidum*), characterized by distinct stages of effects over a period of years; any organ system may become involved; the spirochete is able to pass through the human placenta, producing congenital syphilis

Testicular cancer – a malignant neoplastic disease of the testis occurring most frequently in men between 20 and 35 years of age; an undescended testicle is often involved

Testicular torsion – rotation of the spermatic cord that causes an interruption in the blood supply to the tissue

Varicocele – a dilation of the pampiniform venous complex of the spermatic cord; forms a soft, elastic swelling that can cause pain; most common in men between 15 and 25 years of age (Figure 15-6)

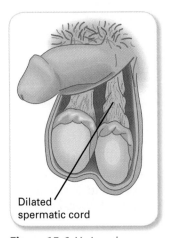

Dilated
spermatic cord

Figure 15-6 Varicocele.

ABBREVIATIONS

The following abbreviations are related to terms and procedures concerning the male reproductive system.

Abbreviation	Meaning
AIDS	acquired immunodeficiency syndrome
BPH	benign prostatic hyperplasia

DRE	digital rectal examination
ED	erectile dysfunction
FTA-ABS	fluorescent treponemal antibody-absorption test; a serological test used to detect syphilis
GC	gonococcus (*Neisseria gonorrhoeae*)
GU	genitourinary
HPV	human papillomavirus
HSV	herpes simplex virus
NGU	nongonococcal urethritis
PAP	prostatic acid phosphatase
PED	penile erectile dysfunction
PSA	prostate-specific antigen
STD	sexually transmitted disease
STS	serological test for syphilis
TRUS	transrectal ultrasound
TSE	testicular self-examination
TURP	transurethral resection of the prostate
VD	venereal disease
VDRL	venereal disease research laboratory

MEDICATIONS USED TO TREAT MALE REPRODUCTIVE SYSTEM DISORDERS

The following are common medications used for male reproductive system disorders.

Drug Class	Generic Name	Pronunciation for Generic Name	Trade Name	Use
treatments for benign prostatic hypertrophy	alfuzosin	al-FYOO-zoh-sin	Uroxatral®	to relieve or cure enlargement of the prostate
	doxazosin	dok-ZAY-zoh-sin	Cardura®	
	dutasteride	doo-TAS-teh-ride	Avodart®	
	finasteride	fih-NAS-teh-ride	Proscar®	
	tamsulosin	tam-SOO-loh-sin	Flomax®	
	terazosin	teh-RAZ-oh-sin	Hytrin®	
treatments for erectile dysfunction	sildenafil	sil-DEN-ah-fil	Viagra®	to achieve or lengthen the duration of erections
	tadalafil	tah-DAH-lah-fil	Cialis®	
	vardenafil	var-DEN-ah-fil	Levitra®	

DRUG TERMINOLOGY

The following are common types of drugs used for male reproductive system conditions.

Drug Type	Pronunciation	Indication
alpha blockers	AL-fah BLOK-ers	used along with finasteride or dutasteride to treat prostate enlargement
antibiotics	an-tee-by-OT-iks	used along with antimicrobials to treat genital tract inflammation
chemotherapeutics	kee-moh-thair-ah-PYOO-tiks	used to treat prostate cancer; commonly include Adriamycin,® docetaxel, estramustine, mitoxantrone, paclitaxel, and prednisone
dopamine agonists	DOH-pa-meen AG-oh-nists	used to treat gonadotropin deficiency or suppression, and hyperprolactinemia
glucocorticoids	gloo-koh-KOR-tih-koidz	used to treat sperm autoimmunity that can cause infertility
vasodilators	vay-zoh-dy-LAY-tors	used along with cholinergic antihistamines to treat coital disorders; commonly include sildenafil

REVIEW EXERCISES

Multiple Choice

Select the best answer and write the letter of your choice to the left of each number.

1. The fold of skin that covers the tip of the penis is the:

   A. penile urethra
   B. glans penis
   C. prepuce
   D. corpus spongiosum

2. The tubular gland that produces a secretion containing a thick and yellowish fluid is called the:

   A. preputial gland
   B. seminal vesicle
   C. prostate gland
   D. corpus cavernosum

3. The erectile tissue that surrounds the urethra is the:

   A. corpus spongiosum
   B. corpus cavernosum
   C. membranous urethra
   D. glans penis

4. Which of the following describes the condition known as "cryptorchidism"?

   A. The foreskin has been surgically removed
   B. Sperm cells are not produced
   C. The prostate gland is enlarged
   D. The testes fail to descend into the scrotum

5. The gland that surrounds the urethra and produces an alkaline secretion is the:

   A. Bartholin's gland
   B. prostate gland
   C. preputial gland
   D. bulbourethral gland

6. Which of the following is the site of sperm production?

   A. the rete testis
   B. the seminal vesicles
   C. the seminiferous tubules
   D. the ductus deferens

7. Which of the following structures carries sperm from the epididymis to the urethra?

   A. ductus deferens
   B. seminal vesicle
   C. ejaculatory duct
   D. corpus cavernosum

8. Which of the following is also called the "Cowper's gland"?

   A. prostate gland
   B. pineal gland
   C. bulbourethral gland
   D. seminal vesicle

9. The erectile tissue that surrounds the urethra is referred to as the:

   A. corpus spongiosum
   B. corpus cavernosum
   C. ejaculatory duct
   D. ductus deferens

10. Which of the following disorders causes painful vesicular eruptions on the skin of the male genitalia?

    A. genital herpes
    B. genital warts
    C. epispadias
    D. syphilis

11. Which of the following medical terms means "a tightness of the foreskin of the penis"?

    A. epispadias
    B. priapism
    C. impotence
    D. phimosis

12. Non-malignant and non-inflammatory enlargement of the prostate is called:

    A. cryptorchidism
    B. epispadias
    C. benign prostatic hyperplasia
    D. carcinoma of the prostate

13. Which of the following malignant tumors occurs most frequently in men between 20 and 35 years of age?

    A. prostate cancer
    B. testicular cancer
    C. testicular torsion
    D. genital warts

14. Which of the following structures of the male reproductive system is also called the "spermatic duct"?

    A. rete testis
    B. seminal vesicle
    C. bulbourethral gland
    D. vas deferens

15. A structure composed of a fibrous network in the testis is called the:

    A. testicular duct
    B. spermatic duct
    C. rete testis
    D. epididymis

Fill in the Blank

Use your knowledge of medical terminology to insert the correct term from the list below.

ductus deferens	chancre	genital warts
circumcision	epispadias	testicular torsion
orchidopexy	chlamydia	prostate cancer
perineum	testicular cancer	priapism
epididymis	varicocele	genital herpes

1. A dilation of the pampiniform venous complex of the spermatic cord is called a _____.

2. A rotation of the spermatic cord that causes an interruption in the blood supply to the tissue is known as _____.

3. Moist red swellings of the genitals that become pedunculated are known as _____.

4. The _____ is the region surrounding the urogenital and anal openings.

5. An operation to mobilize an undescended testis is called an _____.

6. A congenital defect in which the urethra opens on the dorsum of the penis is known as _____.

7. A skin lesion of primary syphilis is called a _____.

8. An abnormal condition of prolonged penile erection is known as _____.

9. A _____ is a surgical procedure that removes the foreskin.

10. The _____ is the structure that carries sperm from the epididymis to the urethra.

Labeling – The Organs and Ducts of the Male Reproductive System

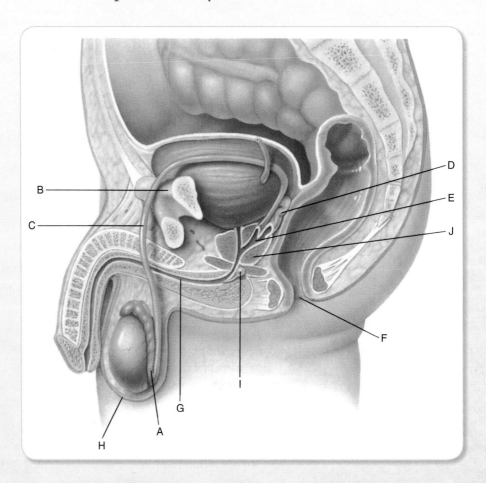

Write in the term that corresponds with each letter on the figure above.

A. _____

B. _____

C. _____

D. _____

E. _____

F. _____

G. _____

H. _____

I. _____

J. _____

True / False

Identify each of the following statements as true or false by placing a "T" or "F" on the line beside each number.

_____ **1.** The ductus deferens is the structure that carries sperm from the prostate to the epididymis.

_____ **2.** The primary organs of the male reproductive system are known as "gonads."

_____ **3.** Difficulty passing urine is called "purulence."

_____ **4.** A male hormone secreted by the testes is referred to as "progesterone."

_____ **5.** An inflammation of the glans penis and the mucous membrane beneath it is called "balanitis."

_____ **6.** "Purulent" means "producing or containing pus."

_____ **7.** Syphilis is a communicable disease that is common in pregnant women.

_____ **8.** Genital herpes causes painless vesicular eruptions on the skin.

_____ **9.** An accumulation of fluid around the testicles is called "chancre."

_____ **10.** Orchitis is an inflammation of one or both of the testicles.

Definitions

Define each of the following words in one sentence.

1. testosterone: _____

2. ductus deferens: _____

3. glans penis: _____

4. rete testis: _____

5. scrotum: _____

6. vas deferens: _____

7. epispadias: _____

8. chancre: _____

9. impotence: _____

10. varicocele: _____

Abbreviations

Write the full meaning of each abbreviation.

Abbreviation	Meaning
1. STS	_____
2. GU	_____
3. PSA	_____
4. HPV	_____
5. PED	_____
6. STD	_____
7. HSV	_____
8. TSE	_____
9. VD	_____
10. DRE	_____

Matching – Terms and Definitions

Match each term with its correct definition by placing the corresponding letter on the line to its left.

_____ 1. corpus cavernosum

_____ 2. ejaculatory duct

_____ 3. ductus deferens

_____ 4. vas deferens

_____ 5. corpus spongiosum

_____ 6. glans penis

_____ 7. prepuce

_____ 8. seminiferous tubules

_____ 9. semen

_____ 10. rete testis

A. a structure composed of a fibrous network or mesh in the center of the testis

B. sensitive area at the tip of the penis

C. tiny tubules located in the testes that produce sperm

D. a combination of sperm, seminal fluid, prostaglandins, and enzymes

E. a loose fold of skin that covers the end of the penis

F. one of the cylinders of spongy tissue on the dorsum of the penis

G. a duct which begins at the vas deferens that passes through the prostate gland and empties into the urethra

H. the extension of the epididymis of the testis that ascends from the scrotum into the abdominal cavity and joins the seminal vesicle to form the ejaculatory duct

I. the erectile tissue that surrounds the urethra

J. the structure that carries sperm from the epididymis to the urethra

Spelling

Circle the correct spelling from each pairing of words.

1. scretum   scrotum

2. testicles   testiculs

3. purulent   perulent

4. epididimis   epididymis

5. chanker   chancre

6. peryneum   perineum

7. prepuce   perpuce

8. balanitis   balenitis

9. epyspadias   epispadias

10. chlamydia   chlamedia

CHAPTER 16

The Female Reproductive System

OBJECTIVES

Upon completion of this chapter, the reader should be able to:

1. Describe the parts of the female reproductive system and discuss the function of each part.
2. List and define the major pathological conditions of the female reproductive system.
3. Label a diagram of the female reproductive system and describe the function of each part.
4. List the hormones that are secreted from the female reproductive system and describe the function of each hormone.
5. Outline the events in the menstrual cycle.
6. Define, pronounce, and spell female reproductive system terms.
7. Recognize common drugs used in treating disorders of the female reproductive system.
8. Identify the meanings of related abbreviations.

STRUCTURE AND FUNCTION OF THE FEMALE REPRODUCTIVE SYSTEM

The female reproductive system is more complicated than the male reproductive system because of the cyclic nature of gamete production in the ovaries. The female external genitalia are known collectively as either the **vulva** or the **pudendum** (Figure 16-1). Starting at the periphery are the **labia majora**. Within the labia majora are the *labia minora*. The **clitoris** is a small bud of erectile, sensory tissue at the anterior end of the vulva, enclosed by the labia minora.

In females, the urethra opens to the external environment between the clitoris and the vagina. At birth, the external opening of the vagina is partially closed by a thin ring of tissue called the

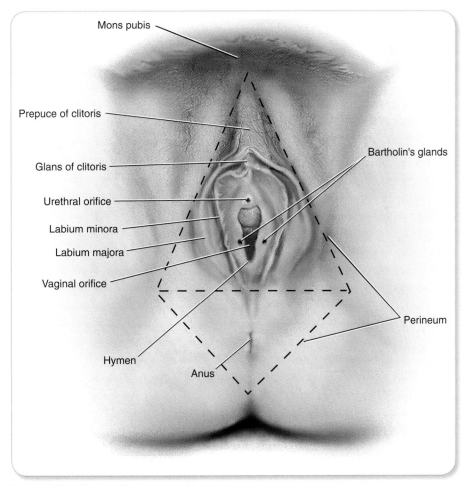

Figure 16-1 External female genitalia.

hymen. The uterus narrows to form the cervix (neck), which opens to the tubular **vagina**. The cervical canal is lined with mucous glands whose secretions create a barrier between the vagina and **uterus**. The uterus, or *womb*, is a hollow, muscular organ slightly smaller than a woman's clenched fist. It is the structure in which fertilized eggs are implanted, and where they develop during pregnancy. It is composed of three tissue layers: a thin, outer connective tissue covering (**perimetrium**), a thick middle layer of smooth muscle (*myometrium*), and an inner layer known as the **endometrium** (Figure 16-2) . The endometrium consists of an epithelium with glands that dip into a connective tissue layer below. The thickness and character of the endometrium vary during the menstrual cycle. Cells of the epithelial lining alternately proliferate and slough off, accompanied by a small amount of bleeding, in the process known as **menstruation**.

Sperm swimming upward through the uterus leave this cavity through openings into the two *Fallopian tubes* (Figure 16-3). The Fallopian tubes are 20 to 35 centimeters long, and about the diameter

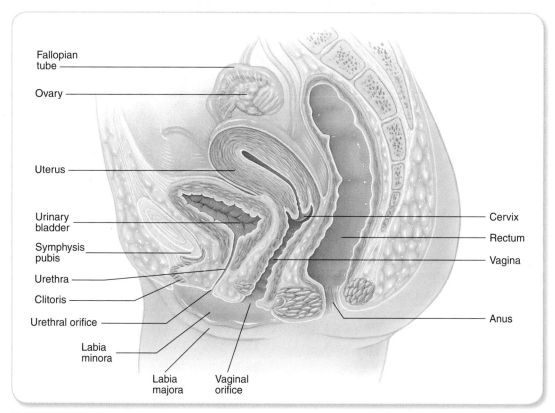

Figure 16-2 Structures of the female reproductive system.

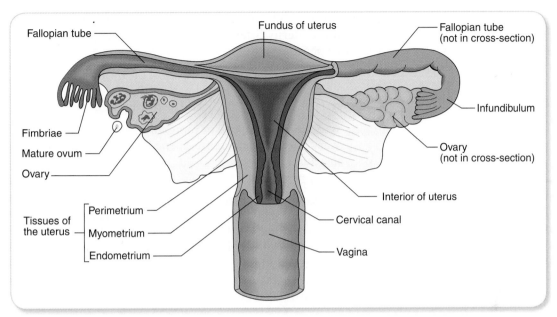

Figure 16-3 Anterior view of female reproductive organs.

of a drinking straw. Fluid movement created by the hair-like cilia, and aided by muscular contractions, transports an egg along one of the Fallopian tubes toward the uterus. If sperm moving up one of the tubes contacts an egg moving downward, fertilization may occur. The flared end of the Fallopian tubes divides into finger-like projections called **fimbriae**, which are held close to the adjacent ovary by connective tissue. This tissue helps ensure that the eggs released from the surface of the ovary will be swept into the tube rather than floating into the abdominal cavity.

Each ovary has an outer connective tissue layer and an inner connective tissue framework known as the **stroma**. Each ovary primarily consists of a thick outer *cortex* filled with ovarian follicles in various stages of development or decline. The small central *medulla* contains nerves and blood vessels.

The ovary, like the testis, produces both gametes and hormones. The ovaries function under the influence of follicle-stimulating hormone and luteinizing hormone from the anterior pituitary, producing both estrogen and progesterone.

Female humans produce gametes in monthly cycles (averaging 28 days, with a normal range of 24 to 35 days). These cycles are commonly called **menstrual cycles** because they are marked by a 3- to 7-day period of bloody uterine discharge known as the *menses* (or *menstruation*). The menstrual cycle includes changes that occur in the follicles of the ovary (**ovarian cycle**) and in the endometrial lining of the uterus (**uterine cycle**). The ovarian cycle is divided into three phases:

1. **follicular phase** – The first part of the ovarian cycle, this is a period of follicular growth in the ovary. It is the most variable phase in length, and lasts from 10 days to 3 weeks.

2. **ovulation** – Once one or more follicles have ripened, the ovary releases them; these ripened follicles are known as *oocytes*.

3. **luteal phase** – This is the final phase of the ovarian cycle, also known as the *postovulatory phase*. "Luteal phase" comes from the transformation of a ruptured follicle into a corpus luteum, named for its yellow pigment and lipid deposits. The corpus luteum secretes hormones that continue the preparations for pregnancy. If a pregnancy does not occur, the corpus luteum ceases to function after about two weeks, and the ovarian cycle begins again.

The endometrial lining of the uterus goes through its own cycle (the uterine cycle) and is regulated by ovarian hormones as follows:

1. **menses** – This is menstrual bleeding from the uterus, which corresponds with the beginning of the follicular phase in the ovary.

2. **proliferative phase** – The endometrium adds a new layer of cells in anticipation of pregnancy; this corresponds to the latter part of the ovary's follicular phase.

3. **secretory phase** – After ovulation, hormones from the corpus luteum convert the thickened endometrium into a secretory structure. Thus, this phase of the uterine cycle corresponds with the luteal phase of the ovarian cycle. If pregnancy does not occur, the superficial layers of the secretory endometrium are lost during menstruation, as the uterine cycle beings again.

The ovarian and uterine cycles are under the primary control of various hormones, which include:

- gonadotropin-releasing hormone (GnRH) from the hypothalamus
- FSH and LH from the anterior pituitary
- estrogen and progesterone from the ovaries; during the follicular phase, the dominant steroid is estrogen, while in the luteal phase, progesterone is dominant (although estrogen is still present)

The *mammary glands* are accessory organs of the female reproductive system that are specialized to secrete milk following pregnancy. They are in the subcutaneous tissue of the anterior thorax within elevations called *breasts* (Figure 16-4). The breasts lie over the *pectoralis major* muscles, extend from the send to the sixth ribs, and from the sternum to the axillae. A *nipple* is located near the tip of each breast at about the level of the fourth intercostal space. A circular area of pigmented skin, called the **areola**, surrounds each nipple.

A mammary gland is composed of 15 to 20 lobes. Each lobe contains glands (*alveolar glands*) and an *alveolar duct* that leads to a **lactiferous duct**, which in turn leads to the nipple and opens to the outside. Dense connective and adipose tissues separate the lobes. These tissues also support the glands and attach them to the fascia of the underlying pectoral muscles.

Following childbirth, in two or three days, prolactin hormone from the anterior pituitary gland stimulates the mammary glands to secrete milk. Meanwhile, the glands secrete a thin, watery fluid called **colostrum** that contains significant amounts of protein. Colostrum also contains antibodies from the mother's immune system that protect the newborn from certain infections.

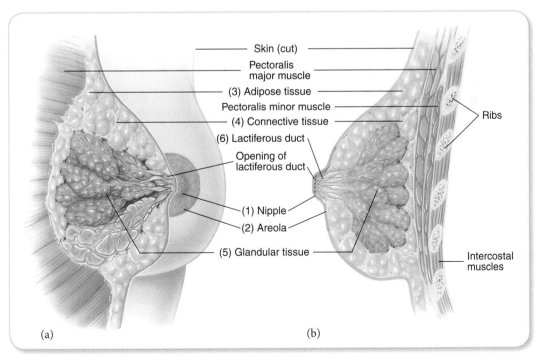

Skin (cut)
Pectoralis major muscle
(3) Adipose tissue
Pectoralis minor muscle
(4) Connective tissue
(6) Lactiferous duct
Opening of lactiferous duct
(1) Nipple
(2) Areola
(5) Glandular tissue
Ribs
Intercostal muscles

(a)   (b)

Figure 16-4 Structure of the breast (a) anterior view (b) sagittal view.

GENERAL TERMINOLOGY RELATED TO THE FEMALE REPRODUCTIVE SYSTEM

The following are common terms that relate to the female reproductive system.

Term	Pronunciation	Definition
abortion	ah-BOR-shun	the premature ending of a pregnancy
amnion	AM-nee-on	the innermost membrane of the sac surrounding the fetus during gestation
amniotic fluid	AM-nee-aw-tik FLOO-id	the fluid surrounding the fetus, contained within the amnion
areola	ah-REE-oh-lah	the darkened area surrounding the nipple on each breast
Bartholin's glands	BAR-toh-linz glands	two glands on either side of the vagina that secrete fluid into the vagina
cervix	SER-viks	the protective part of the uterus, located at the bottom, and protruding through the vaginal wall; contains glands that secrete mucus into the vagina
chorion	KOH-ree-on	the outermost membrane of the sac surrounding the fetus during gestation
climacteric	kly-MAK-teh-rik	the period of hormonal changes just prior to menopause
clitoris	KLIT-oh-ris	the primary organ of female sexual stimulation
coitus	KOH-ih-tus	sexual intercourse or copulation
colostrum	koh-LAW-strum	breast fluid that is secreted in the first few days after giving birth, before milk is produced
contraception	kon-trah-SEP-shun	a method of controlling conception by blocking access or interrupting reproductive cycles; birth control
copulation	kop-yoo-LAY-shun	sexual intercourse
diaphragm	DYE-ah-fram	a form of vaginal contraception
dyspareunia	dis-peh-ROO-nee-uh	painful sexual intercourse; usually due to dryness or inflammation in the female reproductive system
endometrium	en-doh-MEE-tree-um	the inner mucous layer of the uterus
estrogen	ESS-troh-jen	one of the primary female hormones produced by the ovaries
Fallopian tubes	fah-LOH-pee-an	one of two tubes that lead from the ovaries to the uterus; also called the *uterine tubes*
fertilization	fer-til-eye-ZAY-shun	the union of a male sperm and a female ovum
fimbriae	FIM-bree-ay	the hair-like ends of the uterine tubes that sweep the ovum into the uterus
foreskin	FOR-skin	the fold of skin at the top of the labia minora
fundus	FUN-dus	the top portion of the uterus

gamete	GAM-eet	a mature sex cell
gonad	GOH-nad	a male or female sex organ
gravida	GRAH-vih-da	a pregnant woman
hymen	HIGH-men	a fold of mucous membranes covering the vagina of a young female; it usually ruptures during first intercourse
intrauterine device	IN-trah-YOO-teh-rin dee-VYS	a contraceptive device consisting of a coil placed in the uterus to block implantation of a fertilized ovum; the most efficacious method of contraception on the market
isthmus	IS-mus	the narrow region at the bottom of the uterus which opens into the cervix
labia majora	LAY-bee-ah mah-JOR-ah	two folds of skin that form the borders of the vulva
labia minora	LAY-bee-ah mih-NOR-ah	two folds of skin between the labia majora
lactation	lak-TAY-shun	the secretion of milk from the mammary glands
lactiferous ducts	LAK-tih-feh-rus DUKTS	narrow tubular structures that transfer milk from the lobes of each breast to the nipple
leukorrhea	loo-koh-REE-uh	a white or yellowish discharge from the vagina
mammary glands	MAH-moh-ree GLANDZ	the glandular tissue that forms the breasts, which responds to cycles of menstruation and birth
mastectomy	mass-TEK-toh-mee	surgical removal of the breast as a treatment for breast cancer
menarche	men-AR-kee	the first menstrual period of a female
menopause	MEH-noh-pawz	the time when menstruation ceases; usually between the ages of 45 and 55
menorrhea	meh-noh-REE-ah	the normal discharge of blood and tissue from the uterus
menstruation	men-stroo-AY-shun	the cyclical release of the uterine lining through the vagina; usually occurs every 28 days
myometrium	my-oh-MEE-tree-um	the middle layer of muscle tissue of the uterus
nipple	NIH-pul	the projection at the apex of the breast through which milk flows during lactation
oocyte	OH-eh-syt	an immature ovum produced in the ovaries
ovary	OH-vah-ree	a female gonad
ovulation	ov-yu-LAY-shun	the release of an ovum from the ovary, occurring about 14 days prior to the beginning of menses
ovum	OH-vum	the mature female sex cell produced by the ovaries, which then travels to the uterus; if fertilized, it implants in the uterus; if not, it is released during menstruation to the outside of the body
para	PAH-rah	a woman who has given birth to one or more viable infants
parturition	par-cheh-RIH-shun	birth

(continues)

Term	Pronunciation	Definition
perimenopause	peh-ree-MEH-noh-pawz	a three- to five-year period of decreasing estrogen levels prior to menopause
placenta	plah-SEN-tah	a nutrient-rich organ that develops in the uterus during pregnancy; supplies nutrients to the fetus
progesterone	proh-JESS-ter-own	one of the primary female hormones
puberty	PYOO-ber-tee	a period during the early teenage years when secondary sex characteristics develop and menstruation begins
spermicide	SPER-mih-syd	a contraceptive chemical that destroys sperm; usually in cream or jelly form
sponge	SPUNJ	a polyurethane contraceptive device filled with spermicide and placed into the vagina near the cervix
umbilical	um-BIH-lih-kul	the cord that connects the placenta in the mother's uterus to the navel of the fetus during gestation for nourishment of the fetus
uterus	YOO-ter-us	the hollow, pear-shaped organ that houses the fertilized and implanted ovum as it develops throughout pregnancy
vagina	vah-JY-nah	the genital canal leading from the uterus to the vulva
vulva	VULL-vah	the external female genitalia
zygote	ZY-goat	a fertilized egg

PATHOLOGICAL CONDITIONS

The following are disorders and conditions of the female reproductive system.

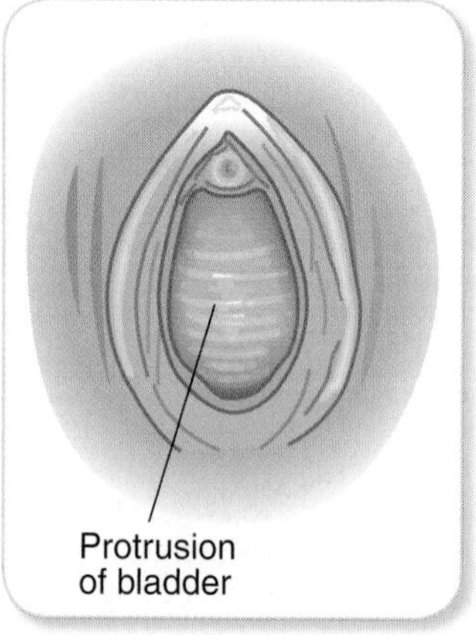

Protrusion
of bladder

Figure 16-5 Cystocele.

Abruptio placentae – the separation of the placenta from the uterine wall, requiring immediate delivery of the infant

Amenorrhea – the absence of menstruation; may result from a normal condition (pregnancy or menopause), or from an abnormal condition (such as excessive dieting or extremely strenuous exercise)

Breast cancer – a malignant tumor of the breast which is second only to lung cancer in causing cancer-related deaths among women in the United States; metastasizes readily through the lymph nodes and blood to other sites, such as the lung, bones, liver, and ovaries

Carcinoma in situ – cervical cancer that is often detected early with Pap smears before it can spread

Cervicitis – an inflammation of the uterine cervix

Cystocele – downward protrusion or herniation of the urinary bladder through the wall of the vagina (Figure 16-5)

Dysmenorrhea – a painful cramping associated with menstruation

Eclampsia – seizures in some patients who have preeclampsia; a serious complication of pregnancy (see *preeclampsia*)

Ectopic pregnancy – development of a fertilized egg outside of its normal position in the uterine cavity; although it may occur elsewhere in the abdominal cavity, an ectopic pregnancy usually occurs in the Fallopian tubes, resulting in a "tubal pregnancy"; salpingitis and endometriosis may lead to ectopic pregnancy by blocking passage of the ovum into the uterus; continued growth will rupture the Fallopian tube containing the ovum, causing dangerous hemorrhage

Endometrial cancer – a malignant tumor that occurs in the endometrium of the uterus

Endometriosis – a condition in which uterine tissue forms painful cysts outside of the uterus such as the pelvic cavity and intestine (Figure 16-6)

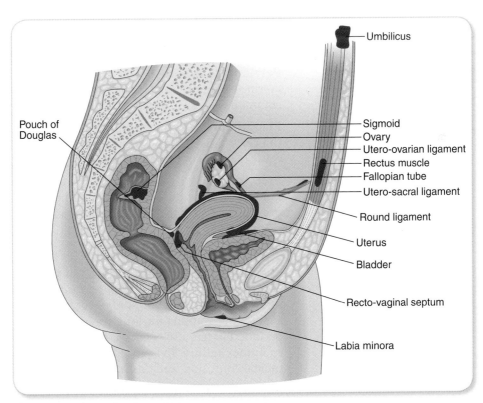

Figure 16-6 Sites of endometriosis.

Fibrocystic breast disease – the presence of single or multiple fluid-filled cysts that may be felt (palpated) during a breast examination

Fibroids – common benign tumors found in the uterus that may cause pain and bleeding

Leiomyoma – a smooth-muscle, benign uterine tumor that is often mislabeled as a fibroid tumor

Mastitis – an inflammation of the breast; commonly caused by *Staphylococcus* or *Streptococcus* bacteria that enter through the nipple

Menorrhagia – excessive menstrual bleeding

Metrorrhagia – uterine bleeding that occurs at times other than during the menstrual period

Miscarriage – loss of a fetus before the 20th week of pregnancy; in most cases, results from fetal malformation that is incompatible with life outside of the womb; also known as "spontaneous abortion"

Oligomenorrhea – abnormally light menstrual periods

Ovarian cancer – a malignant ovarian tumor, which is a potentially fatal cancer of the ovary; difficult to diagnose in its earliest stages, and often spreads to other organs before it is detected

Pelvic inflammatory disease (PID) – an infection of the uterine lining that may spread into the Fallopian tubes; the most common causes are gonorrhea and chlamydia

Placenta previa – the attachment of the placenta near or over the cervix instead of in the upper portion of the uterus; may cause bleeding in the later stages of pregnancy

Preeclampsia – development of serious hypertension along with fluid retention and loss of protein in the urine; develops in some pregnancies after the fifth month; symptoms resolve when the pregnancy ends

Salpingitis – an inflammation of the Fallopian tubes

Toxic shock syndrome – a rare but potentially fatal illness, caused by certain strains of *Staphylococcus aureas* that secrete a unique toxin; most commonly affects women who wear highly absorbent tampons for long intervals during their menstrual periods, but has also occurred in men and infants; may progress to kidney failure, liver impairment, unstable blood pressure, mental confusion, and death

Vaginitis – an inflammation of the mucous membrane of the vagina, usually due to infection; common causes include bacterial and yeast infections

ABBREVIATIONS

The following abbreviations are related to terms and procedures concerning the female reproductive system.

Abbreviation	Meaning
AB	abortion
AH	abdominal hysterectomy
BSE	breast self-examination
BV	bacterial vaginosis
CIS	carcinoma in situ
CS	caesarean section
Cx	cervix
D&C	dilation and curettage
DUB	dysfunctional uterine bleeding
ECC	endocervical curettage
EMB	endometrial biopsy
ERT	estrogen replacement therapy
FSH	follicle-stimulating hormone
G	gravida (pregnancy)
GYN	gynecology
HCG	human chorionic gonadotropin
HRT	hormone replacement therapy
HSG	hysterosalpingography
IUD	intrauterine device
LH	luteinizing hormone
LMP	last menstrual period
LSO	left salpingo-oophorectomy
OB	obstetrics
OCP	oral contraceptive pill
P	para (live births)
Pap smear	Papanicolaou smear
PID	pelvic inflammatory disease
PMP	previous menstrual period
PMS	premenstrual syndrome
RSO	right salpingo-oophorectomy
TAH	total abdominal hysterectomy
TSS	toxic shock syndrome
TVH	total vaginal hysterectomy
UC	uterine contractions

MEDICATIONS USED TO TREAT
FEMALE REPRODUCTIVE SYSTEM DISORDERS

The following are common medications used for female reproductive system disorders.

Drug Class	Generic Name	Pronunciation for Generic Name	Trade Name	Use
abortifacient (morning-after pill)	mifepristone	mih-FEH-prih-stone	Mifeprex®	to prevent implantation of an ovum
hormone replacement therapy	alendronate	ah-LEN-droh-nate	Fosamax®	to normalize body hormone levels
	estrogen	ES-troh-jen	Premarin®	
	estrogen / progestin	ES-troh-jen / pro-JES-tin	Prempro®	
	raloxifene	rah-LOK-sih-feen	Evista®	
hormones that are related to birth	oxytocin	ok-see-TOH-sin	Pitocin®	to induce or stop labor
	tocolytic agents (including nifedipine, ritodrine)	*toh-koh-LIH-tik* (ny-FEH-dih-peen), (ry-toh-DREEN)	(various, including Procardia,® Yutopar®)	

DRUG TERMINOLOGY

The following are common types of drugs used for female reproductive system conditions.

Drug Type	Pronunciation	Definition
abortifacients (morning-after pills)	ah-bor-tih-FAY-shunts	to prevent implantation of an ovum
birth control pills or implants	—	to control the flow of hormones, blocking ovulation
hormone replacement therapy (HRT)	—	to treat the body's stoppage or decreasing of normal hormone production
oxytocin	ok-sih-TOH-sin	to induce labor
tocolytic agents	toh-koh-LIH-tik	to stop labor

REVIEW EXERCISES

Multiple Choice

Select the best answer and write the letter of your choice to the left of each number.

1. The cervix is:

   A. the sensory tissue of the vagina
   B. a thin ring of tissue external from the vagina
   C. the neck of the uterus
   D. the lower portion of the birth canal

2. Which of the following organs provides mechanical protection and nutritional support for the developing embryo?

   A. the vagina
   B. the uterine tube
   C. the ovaries
   D. the uterus

3. Which of the following structures transports the ovum to the uterus?

   A. the myometrium
   B. the vagina
   C. the Fallopian tubes
   D. the cervix

4. A condition wherein uterine tissue forms painful cysts outside of the uterus is referred to as:

   A. endometritis
   B. salpingitis
   C. endometriosis
   D. benign cyst

5. A darkened area surrounding the nipple on a breast is called the:

   A. colostrum
   B. foreskin
   C. isthmus
   D. areola

6. Which of the following terms means "a fold of mucous membranes covering the vagina"?

   A. clitoris
   B. hymen
   C. labia minora
   D. labia majora

7. A rise in the blood levels of FSH at the beginning of the ovarian cycle is responsible for:

   A. follicle maturation
   B. ovulation
   C. menopause
   D. menstruation

8. Which of the following medical terms means "a period of hormonal changes just prior to menopause"?

   A. climacteric
   B. copulation
   C. ovulation
   D. parturition

9. Which of the following is the principal hormone secreted by the corpus luteum?

   A. estradiol
   B. estrogen
   C. FSH
   D. progesterone

10. Which of the following is the most effective method of contraception on the market?

    A. oral contraceptive pills
    B. an intrauterine device
    C. spermicide
    D. a diaphragm

11. A painful cramping associated with menstruation is called:

    A. oligomenorrhea
    B. menorrhagia
    C. dysmenorrhea
    D. amenorrhea

12. The first menstrual period is called:

    A. menarche
    B. menopause
    C. menorrhea
    D. menorrhagia

13. Which of the following is a potentially fatal cancer of the female reproductive system which is difficult to diagnose in its earliest stages?

    A. vaginal cancer
    B. carcinoma in situ
    C. uterine cancer
    D. ovarian cancer

14. An inflammation of the Fallopian tubes is referred to as:

   A. cervicitis
   B. mastitis
   C. salpingitis
   D. endometritis

15. Breast fluid that is secreted in the first few days after giving birth is called:

   A. leukorrhea
   B. colostrum
   C. milk let-out
   D. milk production

Fill in the Blank

Use your knowledge of medical terminology to insert the correct term from the list below into the appropriate statement.

contraception	zygote	menstruation
menopause	parturition	endometrium
fimbriae	ova	gamete
hymen	estrogen	ovulation
coitus	follicular	areola

1. The release of oocytes is called _____.

2. The term _____ means the process of giving birth.

3. Sexual intercourse is called _____.

4. The fertilized egg is properly referred to as a(n) _____.

5. The _____ are finger-like projections at the end of the uterine tube.

6. A darkened area around the breast nipple is known as the _____.

7. Birth control methods are also referred to as _____.

8. The term _____ means "the time when female menstrual cycles stop completely."

9. A substance produced by the ovaries is known as _____.

10. The term _____ describes the process of sloughing off the old functional layer of the endometrium.

Labeling – The Structures of the Female Reproductive System

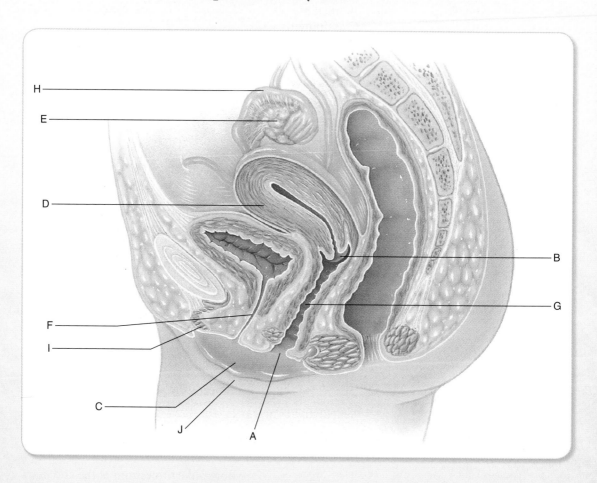

Write in the term below that corresponds with each letter on the figure above.

A. _____

B. _____

C. _____

D. _____

E. _____

F. _____

G. _____

H. _____

I. _____

J. _____

True / False

Identify each of the following statements as true or false by placing a "T" or "F" on the line beside each number.

_____ **1.** The union of a male sperm and a female ovum is called "gonad."

_____ **2.** The first menstrual period is known as "menorrhea."

_____ **3.** The outermost membrane of the sac surrounding the fetus during gestation is referred to as "chorion."

_____ **4.** The isthmus is a narrow region at the bottom of the vaginal opening to the outside of the body.

_____ **5.** Leukorrhea is a white or yellowish discharge from the vagina.

_____ **6.** The mammary glands consist of glandular tissue that forms the breasts.

_____ **7.** The clitoris is the primary organ of female sexual stimulation.

_____ **8.** The top portion of the uterus is called the "fimbriae."

_____ **9.** Surgical removal of the breast is referred to as "salpingotomy."

_____ **10.** Carcinoma in situ is often detected early with Pap smears.

Labeling – The Female Reproductive Organs

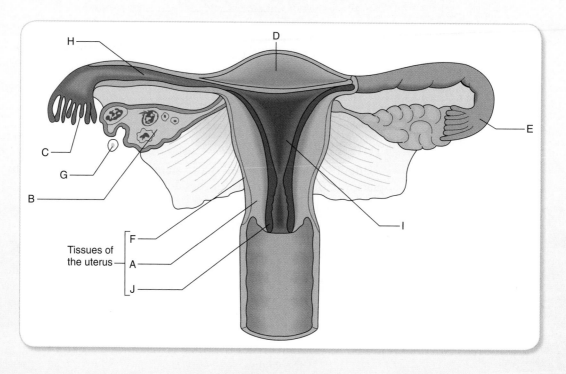

Write in the term below that corresponds with each letter on the figure above.

A. _____

B. _____

C. _____

D. _____

E. _____

F. _____

G. _____

H. _____

I. _____

J. _____

Definitions

Define each of the following words in one sentence.

1. menorrhea: _____

2. Fallopian tubes: _____

3. coitus: _____

4. menarche: _____

5. Bartholin's glands: _____

6. foreskin: _____

7. abortion: _____

8. sponge: _____

9. zygote: _____

10. oocyte: _____

Abbreviations

Write the full meaning of each abbreviation.

Abbreviation	Meaning
1. DUB	_____
2. PMP	_____
3. D&C	_____
4. IUD	_____
5. ERT	_____
6. OCP	_____
7. TSS	_____
8. PID	_____
9. EMB	_____
10. AB	_____

Matching – Terms and Definitions

Match each term with its correct definition by placing the corresponding letter on the line to its left.

_____ **1.** follicular

_____ **2.** ovulation

_____ **3.** luteal

_____ **4.** menses

_____ **5.** proliferative

_____ **6.** secretory

_____ **7.** zygote

_____ **8.** genitalia

_____ **9.** gonad

_____ **10.** ovary

A. general term for organs that produce gametes

B. a fertilized egg

C. the female gonad

D. increasing rates of secretion and gland enlargement

E. general term for external reproductive structures

F. formation of a new functional layer

G. formation of the corpus luteum

H. release of oocytes

I. sloughing off of the old functional layer

J. period of follicular growth

Spelling

Circle the correct spelling from each pairing of words.

1. fertillization   fertilization

2. menarkee   menarche

3. fimbriae   fimbria

4. diaphram   diaphragm

5. coitus   coites

6. isthmus   ismus

7. menorhea   menorrhea

8. colostrum   colestrum

9. lukorrhea   leukorrhea

10. zygote   zigote

SECTION III

TERMINOLOGY OF SPECIAL POPULATIONS

17 Terminology Related to Pediatrics

OBJECTIVES

Upon completion of this chapter, the reader should be able to:

1. Describe the periods of child development.
2. Define the three major domains of development.
3. List five congenital conditions in infants.
4. Define diseases commonly seen in pediatric patients.
5. Define, pronounce, and spell the medical terms related to children.
6. Interpret the meanings of the abbreviations presented in this chapter.

GROWTH AND DEVELOPMENT

Child development refers to the process of human development from conception to 18 years of age. It includes physical, cognitive, social, and emotional development. Child development is such a large and complex topic that it can be helpful to divide it into periods, such as infancy, childhood, and adolescence. It can also be divided into domains such as physical development and social development. Each period is unique. The periods of growth and development are listed below.

- *prenatal period* – This is the period from conception to birth during which a single fertilized cell grows into a living, breathing human baby. After five months, the developing organism is 1 inch long and weighs less than 1 ounce. By the end of nine months, the baby, on average, will be 18 inches long and weigh just over 7 pounds. In no other time of life is growth as rapid as it is during the prenatal period.

- *infancy and toddlerhood* (birth to 2 years of age) – At birth, babies cannot hold up their own heads, eat solid food, or sleep through the night. They do not yet have any social relationships. By the age of two years, they will have learned to walk and talk, eat at a table, and sleep through the night. They also will have formed close emotional bonds with their parents.

- *early childhood* (2 to 6 years of age) – During this period of life, children grow taller and stronger, they develop a conscience, and they have much stronger self-control.

- *middle childhood* (6 to 11 years of age) – Children develop as they contact more people outside the family, and their friendships become increasingly significant during this period.

- *adolescence* (11 to 18 years of age) – The transitions of **puberty** transform the bodies of children into adults. As their bodies change, so do their social roles. Teenagers struggle to become more **autonomous** to define their own goals and become independent of their parents. **Adolescents** become capable of more idealistic and abstract thought.

There are three major **domains** of development, which are listed below.

- *physical growth and health* – encompasses the phenomena of motor development (such as learning to sit, stand, and walk) as well as those of physical health and illness (such as common health issues, illnesses, and hazards)

- *cognitive development* – includes **cognitive growth** (such as learning mathematics, reading, science, speaking, writing, and comprehension of languages)
- *social and emotional development* – involves development of social relationships (such as those with parents, siblings, and friends) as well as the emotional growth that occurs (such as increasing conscience, self-control, and concern for others)

GENERAL TERMINOLOGY RELATED TO PEDIATRICS

The following are common terms that relate to pediatrics.

Term	Pronunciation	Definition
adolescent	ah-DOH-leh-sent	pertaining to adolescence or, a person in that stage of development
autonomous	aw-TAW-no-mus	occurring without direct control, or developing independently of the whole
cognitive	KOG-nih-tiv	pertaining to the mental activities associated with thinking, learning, and memory
congenital	kon-JEH-nih-tul	existing at the time of birth
deciduous teeth	deh-SID-yoo-us TEETH	the first or primary dentition
development	dee-VEH-lop-ment	the process of natural progression in physical and psychological maturation from a previous state
domain	doh-MAYN	an area of development, including physical growth and health, cognitive development, and social/emotional development
growth	—	an increase in the whole body or any of its parts
head circumference	HED sir-KUM-feh-rens	the measurement around the largest portion of the head of an infant
immunization	ih-myoo-nih-ZAY-shun	the procedure for inducing immunity
infant	IN-fant	a young child; some consider infancy to be the first 12 months of life, while others consider it to be the period from birth to the time when the child can assume an erect posture (usually 12 to 14 months); still others consider infancy to be the first 24 months of life
neonatologist	nee-oh-nay-TAW-loh-jist	a physician who specializes in treating newborn infants
neonatology	nee-oh-nay-TAW-loh-jee	the specialty concerned with diseases and abnormalities of newborn infants
newborn	NOO-born	an infant during its first 4 weeks of life

paroxysmal cough	pah-rok-SIZ-mul COFF	sudden, violent coughing
pediatrician	pee-dee-ah-TRIH-shun	a physician specializing in treating children
pediatrics	pee-dee-AH-triks	the medical specialty concerned with the study and treatment of children in health and diseases during development from birth through adolescence
prenatal	pre-NAY-tul	preceding birth
puberty	PYOO-ber-tee	the period of life at which the ability to reproduce begins
stillbirth	STILL-birth	the delivery of a fetus that died before or during the birthing process
wheezing	WEE-zing	a whistling, musical, or puffing sound made by air passing through the narrowed tracheobronchial airway in difficult breathing

PATHOLOGICAL CONDITIONS

The following are pathological conditions commonly seen during childhood.

Abortion – to expel an embryo or fetus before completion of pregnancy

Anencephaly – failure of the cephalic neural tube to close during the second or third week of prenatal development; more common in females; the fetus or infant lacks the cerebrum, cerebellum, and bones of the skull, and usually dies before birth, during the birth process, or shortly after parturition

Asthma – a respiratory condition characterized by difficulty exhaling, and by wheezing; caused by smooth muscle spasms in the airways, especially in the bronchi, that reduce airflow; causes inflammation and accumulation of mucus in the air passages; more common in children than in adults

Attention deficit disorder – a syndrome affecting children, adolescents, and adults characterized by short attention span, hyperactivity, and poor concentration; much more common in boys than in girls; may result from genetic factors, biochemical irregularities, and prenatal or postnatal injury or disease

Attention deficit hyperactivity disorder – a childhood mental disorder with onset before seven years of age and involving impaired or diminished attention and hyperactivity; also called *hyperactive child syndrome*

Bacteremia – the presence of bacteria in the blood

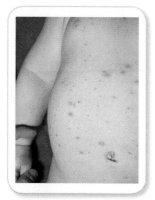

Figure 17-1 Varicella (chickenpox). *Courtesy of Robert A. Silverman, M.D., Pediatric Dermatology, Georgetown University*

Cerebral palsy – a group of congenital, usually non-progressive diseases characterized by major bilateral motor dysfunction

Chickenpox – a highly contagious, acute viral infection that is common in children and young adults; a systemic disease with superficial cutaneous lesions that begin as red macules, progressing to papules, and finally becoming vesicles that form crusts; lesions are first seen on the face or trunk, spreading over the extremities; also called *varicella* (Figure 17-1)

Cleft lip and palate – a congenital birth defect consisting of one or more clefts in the upper lip and a hole in the middle part of the roof of the mouth (Figure 17-2)

Clubfoot – an obvious, non-traumatic deformity of the foot of a newborn in which the anterior half of the foot is adducted and inverted

Coarctation of the aorta – this defect is characterized by a narrowed aortic lumen, causing a partial obstruction of the flow of blood through the aorta and resulting in increased left ventricular pressure and workload, with decreased blood pressure distal to the narrowing

Croup – a childhood disease involving a barking cough, difficult breathing, stridor, and laryngeal spasm

Cystic fibrosis – an inherited disorder of the exocrine glands, causing those glands to produce abnormally thick secretions of mucus and causing an elevation of sweat electrolytes; usually recognized in infancy or early childhood, chiefly among Caucasians; the most reliable diagnostic tool is the sweat test, which shows elevations of levels of both sodium and chloride

Diphtheria – a serious and acute contagious disease caused by the bacterium *Corynebacterium diphtheriae;* characterized by the production of a systemic toxin and affects the mucous membranes

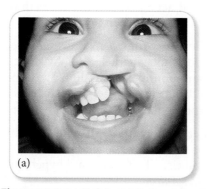

(a)

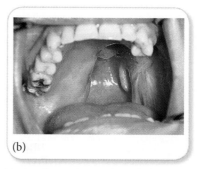

(b)

Figure 17-2 (a) Cleft lip (b) Cleft palate. *Courtesy of Dr. Joseph Konzelman, School of Dentistry, Medical College of Georgia*

of the throat; the toxin is particularly damaging to the tissue of the heart and central nervous system, and the dense pseudomembrane in the throat may interfere with eating, drinking, and breathing

Down syndrome – a congenital condition characterized by mild to severe mental retardation that occurs from a tripling of chromosome 21 (Figure 17-3)

Erythroblastosis fetalis – a blood disease in which maternal antibodies attack the developing red blood cells of the fetus

Esophageal atresia – an abnormal esophagus that ends in a blind pouch or narrows to a thin cord, thus not providing a continuous passage to the stomach; usually occurs as a congenital anomaly

Fetal alcohol syndrome – a set of congenital psychological, behavioral, and physical abnormalities that tend to appear in infants whose mothers consumed alcohol during pregnancy; characterized by typical craniofacial and limb defects, cardiovascular defects, intrauterine growth retardation, and retarded development

German measles – a contagious viral disease, resembling measles clinically, that has a shorter course and fewer complications; also called *rubella*

Hemophilia – a bleeding disease inherited from mothers on the X chromosome; usually appears in sons

Hyaline membrane disease – a severe impairment of respiration in newborns, especially those who are born prematurely or who are under 5 pounds in weight at birth; also called *respiratory distress syndrome* (*RDS*)

Hydrocephalus – a condition marked by an excessive accumulation of cerebrospinal fluid resulting in dilation of the cerebral ventricles and raised intracranial pressure; may also result in enlargement of the cranium and atrophy of the brain (Figure 17-4)

Impetigo – a streptococcal, staphylococcal, or combined infection of the skin beginning as focal erythema and progressing to pruritic vesicles and pustules; highly contagious through contact with the discharge from the lesions (Figure 17-5)

Kernicterus – yellow staining and degenerative lesions in the brain associated with high levels of bilirubin pigment in infants, as a consequence of erythroblastosis fetalis; also known as "bilirubin encephalopathy"

Klinefelter's syndrome – a condition of gonadal defects appearing in males after puberty, with an extra X chromosome in at least one cell line; characteristics are small, firm testis, long legs, gynecomastia (excessive breast development), subnormal

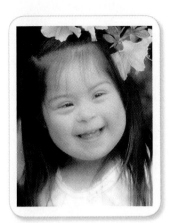

Figure 17-3 Down syndrome. *Marjorie Scott, Marijane's Designer Portraits, Down Right Beautiful 1996 Calendar*

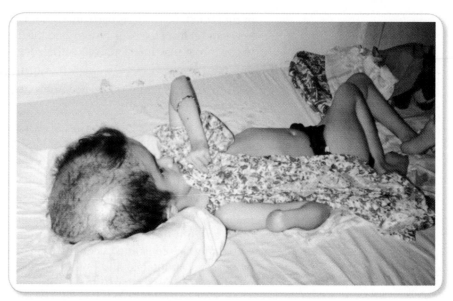

Figure 17-4 Untreated hydrocephalus. *Courtesy of Russell Cox, M.D., Gastonia, NC*

intelligence, and chronic pulmonary disease; the most common abnormality is a 47 XXY chromosome

Measles – an acute, highly contagious viral disease involving the respiratory tract, and characterized by a spreading maculopapular cutaneous rash; occurs primarily in young children who have not been immunized, and in teenagers or young adults who are inadequately immunized; also called *rubeola*

Meningocele – a sac-like protrusion of either the cerebral or spinal meninges through a congenital defect in the skull or the vertebral column; forms a hernial cyst that is filled with cerebrospinal fluid but does not contain neural tissue

Microcephalus – a congenital anomaly involving abnormal smallness of the head in relation to the rest of the body, and underdevelopment of the brain with some mental retardation

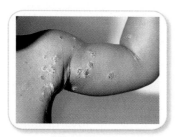

Figure 17-5 Impetigo. *Courtesy of Robert A. Silverman, M.D., Pediatric Dermatology, Georgetown University*

Mumps – acute viral disease of salivary (usually parotid) glands involving fever, swelling, and tenderness; also called *infectious parotitis* (Figure 17-6)

Myelomeningocele – a developmental defect of the central nervous system in which a hernial sac, containing a portion of the spinal cord, its meninges, and cerebrospinal fluid protrudes through a congenital cleft in the vertebral column

Omphalitis – an inflammation of the umbilical stump marked by redness, swelling, and purulent exudate in severe cases

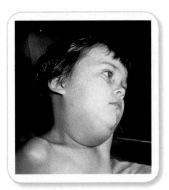

Figure 17-6 Mumps (parotitis).
Courtesy of the Centers for Disease Control and Prevention [CDC]

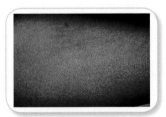

Figure 17-7 Scarlet fever.
Courtesy of the Centers for Disease Control and Prevention [CDC]

Omphalorrhea – a serous discharge from the umbilicus

Patent ductus arteriosus – a condition in which the normal channel between the pulmonary artery and the aorta fails to close at birth; one of the most common congenital cardiovascular anomalies associated with maternal rubella (German measles) during early pregnancy

Pertussis – an acute, highly contagious respiratory disease characterized by **paroxysmal coughing** that ends in loud, "whooping" inspiration; occurs primarily in infants and in children less than four years of age who have not been immunized; also called *whooping cough*

Phenylketonuria – abnormal presence of *phenylketone* and other metabolites of *phenylalanine* in the urine, characteristic of an inborn metabolic disorder caused by the absence of an enzyme responsible for the conversion of the amino acid phenylalanine into *tyrosine*; accumulation of phenylalanine is toxic to brain tissue; untreated individuals have very fair hair, eczema, a "mousy" odor of the urine and skin, and progressive mental retardation

Respiratory distress syndrome – the result of the absence, deficiency, or alteration of the components of pulmonary surfactant

Reye's syndrome – a metabolic disorder that primarily affects the central nervous system of children and adolescents; usually follows a viral infection, and has been associated with the use of aspirin; there is no specific treatment for this condition

Scarlet fever – an acute, contagious disease of childhood caused by an erythrotoxin-producing strain of group A hemolytic *Streptococcus*; characterized by sore throat, fever, facial flush, "strawberry" tongue, and petechiae on the body (Figure 17-7); also called *scarlatina*

Spina bifida occulta – defective closure of the laminae of the vertebral column in the lumbosacral region without hernial protrusion of the spinal cord or meninges

Sudden infant death syndrome – the unexpected and sudden death of an apparently normal and healthy infant that occurs during sleep, with no physical evidence of disease at autopsy; the most common cause of death in children between two weeks and one year of age; its origin is unknown

Talipes – a deformity of the foot and ankle, usually congenital, in which the foot is twisted and relatively fixed in an abnormal position

Tetanus – a potentially fatal infectious disease caused by *Clostridium tetani*, an organism that secretes a toxin that causes uncontrolled muscle contractions; can be prevented with immunization

Turner's syndrome – a chromosomal anomaly seen in females, characterized by the absence of one X chromosome, congenital ovarian failure, genital hypoplasia, cardiovascular anomalies, dwarfism, and underdeveloped breasts, uterus, and vagina

ABBREVIATIONS

The following abbreviations are related to terms and procedures concerning pediatrics.

Abbreviation	Meaning
ADD	attention deficit disorder
ADHD	attention deficit hyperactivity disorder
DPT	diphtheria, pertussis, and tetanus (vaccine)
DS	down syndrome
EA	esophageal atresia
FAS	fetal alcohol syndrome
HDN	hemolytic disease of the newborn (erythroblastosis fetalis)
HMD	hyaline membrane disease
NB	newborn
PDA	patent ductus arteriosus
PKU	phenylketonuria
RDS	respiratory distress syndrome
SIDS	sudden infant death syndrome

REVIEW EXERCISES

Multiple Choice

Select the best answer and write the letter of your choice to the left of each number.

1. Another name of pertussis is:

   A. diphtheria
   B. croup
   C. hyaline membrane disease
   D. whooping cough

2. Which of the following is characterized by typical craniofacial defects, limb defects, and intrauterine growth retardation?

   A. esophageal atresia
   B. Down syndrome
   C. fetal alcohol syndrome
   D. Turner's syndrome

3. Which of the following periods of growth and development has the most rapid growth?

   A. prenatal
   B. infancy
   C. toddlerhood
   D. middle childhood

4. Which of the following terms is defined as "existing at the time of birth"?

   A. cognitive
   B. congenital
   C. domain
   D. prenatal

5. A blood disease in which maternal antibodies attack the developing red blood cells of the fetus is known as:

   A. fetal alcohol syndrome
   B. Turner's syndrome
   C. hemophilia
   D. erythroblastosis fetalis

6. An infant during the first four weeks of life is called:

   A. prenatal
   B. newborn
   C. infant
   D. postnatal

7. The lack of the cerebrum and bones of the skull in an infant is known as:

   A. cerebral palsy
   B. hydrocephalus
   C. kernicterus
   D. anencephaly

8. A barking cough, difficult breathing, stridor, and laryngeal spasm are symptoms of:

   A. rubeola
   B. croup
   C. diphtheria
   D. asthma

9. Which of the following is the period of growth and development when a child is between two and six years of age?

   A. prenatal
   B. postnatal
   C. early childhood
   D. infancy

10. Which of the following is not included in child development?

    A. physical development
    B. social development
    C. spiritual development
    D. emotional development

11. The first, or primary, detention is referred to as:

    A. permanent teeth
    B. deciduous teeth
    C. decay of teeth
    D. newborn teeth

12. The first 12 months of life are called:

    A. newborn period
    B. early childhood
    C. toddlerhood
    D. infancy

13. A deformity of the newborn foot in which the anterior half of the foot is adducted and inverted is referred to as:

    A. clubfoot
    B. epispadias
    C. eruption foot
    D. talipes

14. Respiratory distress syndrome is also called:

    A. diphtheria
    B. croup
    C. impetigo
    D. hyaline membrane disease

15. A chromosomal anomaly seen in females, characterized by the absence of one X chromosome, is known as:

    A. Down syndrome
    B. coarctation of the aorta
    C. Turner's syndrome
    D. hyaline membrane disease

Fill in the Blank

Use your knowledge of medical terminology to insert the correct term from the list below.

head circumference	meningocele	microcephalus
congenital	cleft lip	mumps
neonatology	kernicterus	impetigo
pediatrician	chickenpox	German measles
anencephaly	erythroblastosis fetalis	myelomeningocele

1. Any defect that is present at the time of birth is referred to as _____.

2. A sac-like protrusion of the spinal column that is filled with cerebrospinal fluid only is called a _____.

3. The measurement around the largest portion of the skull of an infant is called _____.

4. A congenital anomaly involving abnormal smallness of the head in relation to the rest of the body is referred to as _____.

5. Another name for varicella is _____.

6. An acute viral disease of the salivary glands is called _____.

7. The specialty concerned with diseases and deformities of newborn infants is referred to as _____.

8. Another name for rubella is _____.

9. "Bilirubin encephalopathy" is also known as _____.

10. A contagious superficial skin infection which is caused by streptococcal or staphylococcal infection is called _____.

True / False

Identify each of the following statements as true or false by placing a "T" or "F" on the line beside each number.

_____ 1. Klinefelter's syndrome is seen mostly in females.

_____ 2. Rubella is a contagious viral disease resembling measles.

_____ 3. Turner's syndrome is an abnormality in which an individual has a 47 XXY chromosome.

_____ 4. Hemophilia is a bleeding disorder that usually appears in boys.

_____ 5. Cystic fibrosis is an inherited disorder of the exocrine glands.

_____ 6. An abnormal esophagus that ends in a blind pouch is called "esophageal varices."

_____ 7. Hemophilia is an inherited disorder of the digestive system.

_____ 8. Attention deficit disorder is more common in boys than in girls, and may result from genetic factors.

_____ 9. Bacteremia is an infection of the blood caused by bacteria.

_____ 10. Scarlet fever is also called "septicemia."

Definitions

Define each of the following words in one sentence.

1. stillbirth: _____

2. congenital: _____

3. abortion: _____

4. cognitive: _____

5. omphalitis: _____

6. hydrocephalus: _____

7. cleft lip: _____

    8. omphalorrhea: _____

    9. wheezing: _____

  10. talipes: _____

Abbreviations

Write the full meaning of each abbreviation.

Abbreviation	Meaning
1. ADD	_____
2. FAS	_____
3. DS	_____
4. RDS	_____
5. SIDS	_____
6. NB	_____
7. PDA	_____
8. HMD	_____
9. ADHD	_____
10. PKU	_____

Matching

Match each term with its correct definition by placing the corresponding letter on the line to its left.

_____ **1.** tetanus

_____ **2.** scarlet fever

_____ **3.** Reye's syndrome

_____ **4.** clubfoot

_____ **5.** cleft palate

_____ **6.** varicella

_____ **7.** rubeola

_____ **8.** diphtheria

_____ **9.** impetigo

_____ **10.** rubella

A. known as *German measles*

B. characterized by the production of a systemic toxin that affects the mucous membranes of the throat

C. a birth defect in which there is a hole in the middle part of the roof of the mouth

D. an acute, highly contagious viral disease involving the respiratory tract and also called "measles"

E. highly contagious disorder that may be caused by streptococcal or staphylococcal infection

F. usually follows a viral infection and has been associated with the use of aspirin

G. a potentially fatal infectious disease caused by *Clostridium tetani*

H. a deformity of the foot of a newborn

I. also called "chickenpox"

J. caused by an erythrotoxin produced by group A hemolytic *Streptococcus*

Spelling

Circle the correct spelling from each pairing of words.

1. meningosele   meningocele
2. kernicterus   kerrnicterus
3. omphallorrhea   omphalorrhea
4. attresia   atresia
5. parosysmal cough   paroxysmal cough
6. anencephaly   anancephaly
7. pertussis   pertussus
8. tallipes   talipes
9. imppetigo   impetigo
10. myelomeningocele   myellomeningocele

Terminology Related to Geriatrics

OBJECTIVES

Upon completion of this chapter, the reader should be able to:

1. Differentiate and describe primary and secondary age changes.
2. Explain two disorders in the elderly that may cause blindness.
3. List five common disorders or conditions that occur in elderly women.
4. List the most common malignant tumors in elderly men.
5. Define, pronounce, and spell common medical terms related to geriatrics.
6. Interpret the meanings of the abbreviations presented in this chapter.

THE AGING POPULATION

Today's health care system is under growing demand from the increasing numbers of elderly persons who live longer than ever before. The elderly have more illness and psychosocial difficulties than do younger people. As people age, they are more often affected by many different chronic disorders and disabilities, causing them to use more drugs than any other age group. Older persons are more vulnerable to environmental, pathological, and pharmacological illnesses.

Primary (physiological) age changes are difficult to differentiate from secondary (pathophysiological) and tertiary (sociogenic and behavioral) age changes. Age-related changes may be responsible for **atypical** diseases in elderly persons, including such conditions as depression, hyperthyroidism, rheumatoid arthritis, and uncontrolled diabetes mellitus. Aging may lessen or increase the severity of certain diseases, as the aging process affects all body systems on a physiological basis.

GENERAL TERMINOLOGY RELATED TO GERIATRICS

The following are common terms that relate to geriatrics.

Term	Pronunciation	Definition
agitation	ah-jih-TAY-shun	extreme emotional disturbance
alcoholism	AL-koh-haw-lih-zum	a disease characterized by the chronic abuse of alcohol
amnesia	am-NEE-zhuh	loss of memory, usually of a specific period of time
atypical	ay-TIH-pih-kul	unusual or irregular
benign	bee-NYN	capable of doing little or no harm; often used to describe a non-malignant tumor
B lymphocyte	BEE LIM-foh-syt	a type of white blood cell that performs a vital role in the immune system
capillary	KAH-pih-leh-ree	the smallest blood vessel in the cardiovascular system
coronary artery	KAW-roh-nair-ee AR-teh-ree	the blood vessel that provides blood supply for the heart
delusion	deh-LOO-zhun	an unshakable belief in a thing that cannot be true
dementia	dee-MEN-shuh	deterioration of intellectual faculties including memory, concentration, and judgment caused by organic disease or disorder of the brain
deterioration	dee-tee-ree-or-AY-shun	the diminishing or gradual worsening of strength or quality, commonly due to aging

diabetes mellitus	dy-uh-BEE-tees MEH-lih-tus	the inability to properly metabolize sugars; the predominant forms of this condition are Type I diabetes mellitus (occurring most often in children and adolescents), and Type II diabetes mellitus (which typically appears in middle age)
glaucoma	glauw-KOH-muh	an increased intraocular pressure, resulting in damage to the optic nerve, leading to blindness
hallucination	ha-loo-sih-NAY-shun	perception of visual, auditory, or other sensations during the waking state without an external stimulus; often due to brain illness or conditions
hip bone	—	the bone between the waste and thighs that is a common site of fracture in the elderly
hyperthyroidism	hy-per-thy-roy-DIH-zum	hyperactivity of the thyroid gland
hypothermia	hy-poh-THER-mee-uh	abnormally low body temperature, in which the oral temperature is lower than 95°F (35°C)
impotence	IM-poh-tens	an inability to achieve penile erection
insomnia	in-SOM-nee-uh	chronic inability to sleep or remain asleep throughout the night
insulin	IN-soo-lin	a hormone produced by the pancreas that lowers blood sugar by allowing the cells of the body to absorb glucose from the blood
ketone bodies	KEE-toan BAW-dees	organic compounds that are intermediate products of fat breakdown
ketosis	kee-TOH-sis	the accumulation of ketone bodies in the blood
malignant	mah-LIG-nent	the ability of a tumor to spread and invade other areas
menopause	MEH-noh-paws	the permanent end of menstruation and menstrual cycles; usually occurs between ages 45 and 55 when the ovaries stop producing estrogen
metabolic acidosis	meh-tah-BAW-lik ah-sih-DOH-sis	excess acid in the body fluids; also occurs when oxidation takes place without adequate oxygen
metabolize	meh-TAH-boh-lyz	the breaking down of carbohydrates, proteins, and fats into smaller units
metastasize	meh-TAH-stah-syz	the process of invading body cells by means of metastasis
neoplasm	nee-oh-PLAH-zum	an abnormal growth of new tissue that forms into a tumor; neoplasms may be either benign or malignant
osteoporosis	os-tee-oh-poh-ROH-sis	an abnormal decrease in bone density; causes bone shafts to thin and become more susceptible to fracture
paralysis	pah-RAH-lih-sis	loss of voluntary movement in a part of the body
pneumonia	noo-MOAN-yuh	an inflammation of the lungs characterized by fluid filling the alveoli and bronchioles

(continues)

Term	Pronunciation	Definition
presbyopia	prez-bee-OH-pee-ah	age-related difficulty in seeing or reading at close range; usually occurs after age 40
prostate	PRAW-stayt	a gland in males that lies at the base of the urinary bladder and surrounds the urethra
protozoa	pro-toh-ZOH-ah	a group of unicellular microorganisms that ingest food; include free-living forms such as amoebas
rickettsiae	rih-KET-see-ah or rih-KET-see-ay	small bacteria incapable of living free of a host; usually found in lice, fleas, ticks, and mites
spine	—	the column of 33 small bones (vertebrae) that form support for the back, ribs, and neck
symptom	SIMP-tum	a subjective, non-observable manifestation of a medical condition; symptoms can only be felt and reported by the person experiencing them
thromboembolism	throm-boh-EM-boh-lih-zum	a condition in which a blood vessel is obstructed by a clot carried in the bloodstream from its site of formation
thrombolytic	throm-boh-LIH-tik	a drug that dissolves blood clots
thrombus	THROM-bus	a blood clot that forms in the cardiovascular system; thrombi may form in a blood vessel or in a chamber of the heart, and a thrombus that breaks away from its site of formation and floats through the bloodstream is called an *embolus*
tremor	TREH-mor	an uncontrollable rhythmic shaking or trembling; tremors may affect either the limbs or the trunk

PATHOLOGICAL CONDITIONS

Certain disorders occur almost exclusively in elderly persons. Others occur in all ages but are more prevalent in the elderly. The following are pathological conditions commonly seen in the elderly.

Accidental hypothermia – body temperature below 35°C (95°F) or lower that continues to fall slowly; may cause death if the situation is not corrected; develops over many hours to several days; more common during the winter

Alcoholism – a disorder consisting of physical and psychological dependence on alcohol, which may be on a daily or otherwise regular basis; often associated with anxiety, depression, **impotence**, behavioral disorders, and **insomnia**, both before and during intoxication; **amnesia** often occurs after intoxication, and repeated heavy drinking of alcohol produces symptoms and signs in nearly every organ system

Alzheimer's disease – a progressive degenerative disease of the brain that produces a loss of mental and physical functioning; the most common cause of **deterioration** in intellectual capacity, or *dementia*; most common in people older than 65, and its incidence increases in people older than 80

Basal cell carcinoma – the most common type of skin cancer; early tumors are so small that they are not clinically apparent; does not usually invade blood or lymph vessels, and therefore does not **metastasize** beyond the skin, but grows by direct extension to adjacent structures; the greatest risk factor for basal cell carcinoma is sunlight exposure upon fair-skinned individuals; lesions are seen most often in regions of the world that have intense sunlight, on the areas of the skin that are most exposed, such as the face and neck (Figure 18-1)

Benign prostatic hypertrophy – a non-malignant enlargement of the prostate gland that becomes problematic as prostatic tissue compresses the urethra where it passes through the prostate; results in frequent lower urinary tract symptoms; greater than half of men older than 60 have prostatic enlargement

Breast cancer – the most common cancer in American women; the leading cause of death in women after age 40; the second most common killer of women of all ages after lung cancer; lifetime risk of breast cancer increases due to the aging process; risk factors and possible causes of breast cancer are environmental, familial, and hormonal

Cataract – an opacity or loss of transparency in the **crystalline lens** of the eyes; cataracts may be congenital, and usually occur in individuals after the age of 60; significant correlations exist between aging and the occurrence of lens opacities

Chronic lymphocytic leukemia – a **neoplasm** that usually involves the **B lymphocytes**; a slowly progressing disease; the median age at diagnosis is 60 years, usually affecting males

Colorectal cancer – a cancer of the lower intestinal tract, it is the third most common cause of cancer death in the United States for both males and females; occurs primarily in individuals older than 50 years, and is rare in children

Decubitus ulcers – erosions of connective tissue, muscle, and skin caused by staying too long in a single position while in bed; occur when the body's weight pressed against a mattress restricts blood flow through the **capillaries**; if not periodically relieved by turning the body, pressure on the tissues in the affected area causes tissue death because of lack of oxygen and nutrition

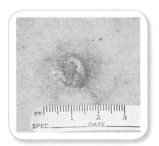

Figure 18-1 Basal cell carcinoma. *Courtesy of Robert A. Silverman, M.D., Pediatric Dermatology, Georgetown University*

Degenerative osteoarthritis – a type of arthritis caused by cartilage breakdown in one or more joints; also known simply as *osteoarthritis*, this condition is the most common form of arthritis, and occurs more frequently due to aging; commonly affects the feet, hands, large weight-bearing joints (such as the hips and knees), and the spine; affects both males and females in differing degrees due to specific ages

Dementia – a long-term deterioration of intellectual function; an irreversible and permanent condition; most common varieties are Alzheimer's disease and multi-infarct dementia

Depression – a psychological state characterized by feelings of doom, inability to sense pleasure, and lack of self-worth; anxiety and depression often exist simultaneously, and are the two most common mental disorders

Diabetic coma – a life-threatening condition occurring in persons with **diabetes mellitus**; caused by undiagnosed diabetes, inadequate treatment, excessive food intake, failure to take prescribed insulin, surgery, trauma, or other stressors that increase the body's need for insulin; without insulin to **metabolize** glucose, fats are used for energy, resulting in **ketone** waste accumulation and **metabolic acidosis**

Glaucoma – a condition of increased fluid pressure inside the eye that compresses the end of the optic nerve; failure to treat the condition adequately leads to blindness

Herpes zoster – an infection caused by the varicella-zoster virus, which also causes *chickenpox*; people who have had chickenpox previously continue to harbor the virus in their nervous systems, where it may develop during times of physical stress, or when the immune system is impaired, into herpes zoster; once reactivated, the virus inflames nerves in the abdomen and trunk, causing blisters and severe pain (a condition also known as *shingles*)

Hip fracture – falling is a common cause of hip fractures in the elderly; occurs most often because of trauma to the hip bone in women over age 60 who have osteoporosis; usually, an outward rotation along with a shortening of the affected extremity is seen

Lung cancers – these tumors arise from the epithelium of the respiratory tract, and are also known as *bronchogenic carcinomas*, hence the term "lung cancer," excluding other pulmonary tumors; occurs in epidemic proportions in the United States, and is the most common cause of cancer death; cigarette smoking is the leading cause of lung cancer, with approximately 1 in every 10 smokers developing the disease

Myocardial infarction – sudden death of a section of heart muscle caused by an abrupt interruption of blood flow to a part of the heart; most often caused by a blood clot that occludes a coronary artery; the occlusion cuts off blood flow and oxygen supply, resulting in the section of the heart that is affected dying if **thrombolytic** medications are not started within a few hours; can range from relatively small, causing few long-term effects, to massive, which can cause immediate death

Osteoporosis – an abnormal decrease in bone density; causes bone shafts to become thin and more susceptible to fracture, and is much more common in women than men; about 30 percent of women are affected, with the condition developing in susceptible women after **menopause**; occurs because of the inability of bone to regenerate itself, and is more likely to occur in individuals (both males and females) who are immobilized, inactive, or on long-term corticosteroid therapies

Parkinson's disease – a chronic, progressive, degenerative central nervous system condition characterized by muscle stiffness and **tremors**; as it progresses, causes difficulty in speaking and walking

Pneumonia – inflammation of the lungs characterized by fluid filling the alveoli and bronchioles; may be caused by fungi, **protozoa**, **rickettsiae**, or viruses

Polymyalgia rheumatica – an inflammatory disorder characterized by widespread muscle aches and stiffness; can either appear overnight or develop gradually; aging and immune system factors appear to be the cause

Prostate cancer – among the most common cancers affecting males, and is the most common cancer affecting American males; its cause is poorly understood, and its incidence is much higher beginning at age 65, though it also commonly occurs beginning at age 50

Psychosis – a mental disorder characterized by loss of contact with reality; symptoms may include depression, **hallucination**, **agitation**, anxiety, social isolation, and **delusions**

Pulmonary embolism – an occlusion of a portion of the pulmonary vascular bed by an embolus, which can be a tissue fragment, **thrombus**, an air bubble, or a mass of **lipids**; the most common emboli are **thrombi** dislodged from deep veins located in the thighs, but they can also originate in the pelvis, most commonly of pregnant women; although overall incidence of pulmonary embolism has declined, it remains a serious cause of death, especially in elderly and hospitalized persons; trauma (usually fractures of the lower extremities,

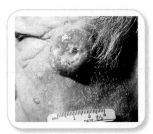

Figure 18-2 Squamous cell carcinoma. *Courtesy of Robert A. Silverman, M.D., Pediatric Dermatology, Georgetown University*

spine, or pelvis as well as head injuries) increases the risks for venous **thromboembolism**; emboli are the third leading cause of death in the United States

Squamous cell carcinoma – a tumor of the epidermis characterized by an invasive nature, being significantly more **malignant** if left untreated; usually caused by exposure to sunlight, with the most commonly affected areas being the hands, head, and neck (Figure 18-2)

Stroke – a neurological problem caused by sudden blockage of a blood vessel in the brain, or sudden hemorrhage of a blood vessel with bleeding into the brain; can lead to death of brain tissue, resulting in problems that may be mild, severe, or even life-threatening; complications of a stroke include difficulty with speech, **paralysis, dementia**, and visual disturbances; also known as *cerebrovascular accident*

Suicide – depression is a significant condition in older adults that frequently leads them to attempt killing themselves; geriatric suicide is common within a short period after these patients visit their doctors; therefore, reliable assessment of suicide risk in older adults is critical

Thyrotoxicosis – a condition caused by excessive amounts of thyroid hormone; a form of thyrotoxicosis known as **hyperthyroidism** is characterized by excessive amounts of thyroid hormones being secreted from the thyroid gland

ABBREVIATIONS

The following are common abbreviations that relate to geriatrics.

Abbreviation	Meaning
AD	Alzheimer's disease
BCC	basal cell carcinoma
BPH	benign prostatic hypertrophy
CLL	chronic lymphocytic leukemia
CV	cardiovascular
CVA	cerebrovascular accident (stroke)
DM	diabetes mellitus
DU	decubitus ulcer
fx	fracture
HF	hip fracture
MI	myocardial infarction
PSA	prostatic-specific antigen
TH	thyroid hormone

REVIEW EXERCISES

Multiple Choice

Select the best answer and write the letter of your choice to the left of each number.

1. Accumulation of which of the following substances in the blood may result in diabetic coma?

   A. urea
   B. catecholamine
   C. bilirubin
   D. ketone waste

2. Herpes zoster infection is the same virus that causes:

   A. the common cold
   B. chickenpox
   C. smallpox
   D. influenza

3. Tremors and muscle stiffness are seen in which of the following disorders?

   A. diabetic coma
   B. thyrotoxicosis
   C. osteoporosis
   D. Parkinson's disease

4. Small bacteria incapable of living free of a host that may be found in ticks or mites are known as:

   A. protozoa
   B. fungi
   C. rickettsiae
   D. staphylococci

5. Which of the following is the most common emboli in the lungs?

   A. tissue fragment
   B. thrombus
   C. a piece of fat
   D. kidney stone

6. A sudden blockage of a blood vessel in the brain is called:

   A. thyrotoxicosis
   B. pulmonary embolism
   C. acute leukemia
   D. stroke

7. Which of the following is the most common type of skin cancer?

   A. basal cell carcinoma
   B. squamous cell carcinoma
   C. melanoma
   D. lipoma

8. Which of the following terms means "loss of memory"?

   A. delusion
   B. dementia
   C. deterioration
   D. amnesia

9. Increased intraocular pressure is called:

   A. pneumonia
   B. glaucoma
   C. presbyopia
   D. polymyalgia

10. Which of the following usually occurs in women between ages 45 and 60 when they are unable to produce estrogen?

    A. diabetes mellitus
    B. glaucoma
    C. thromboembolism
    D. menopause

11. Hallucinations, agitation, and anxiety are symptoms of which of the following disorders or conditions?

    A. suicide
    B. stroke
    C. dementia
    D. psychosis

12. Which of the following causes prostate cancer in the elderly?

    A. The cause is not known
    B. too much testosterone
    C. the aging process
    D. cigarette smoking

13. An inflammatory disorder characterized by widespread muscle aches and stiffness is referred to as:

    A. degenerative osteoarthritis
    B. osteoporosis
    C. polymyalgia rheumatica
    D. stroke

14. Which of the following is the third most common cause of cancer death in the United States for both males and females?

    A. skin cancer
    B. colorectal cancer
    C. breast cancer
    D. prostate cancer

15. Which of the following disorders is the most common cause of deterioration in intellectual capacity?

    A. thyrotoxicosis
    B. alcoholism
    C. Alzheimer's disease
    D. Parkinson's disease

Fill in the Blank

Use your knowledge of medical terminology to insert the correct term from the list below.

ketosis	impotence	hypothermia
insomnia	presbyopia	thrombus
menopause	amnesia	delusion
tremor	dementia	amnesia
agitation	hallucination	malignant

1. Age-related difficulty in reading at close range is called _____.

2. An unshakable belief in a thing that cannot be true is referred to as a(n) _____.

3. An extreme emotional disturbance is defined as _____.

4. A perception of a visual or auditory sensation during the waking state without an external stimulus is known as a(n) _____.

5. A tumor that spreads and invades other areas of the body is called _____.

6. A blood clot that forms in the cardiovascular system is referred to as a(n) _____.

7. The accumulation of ketone bodies in the blood is called _____.

8. Inability to sleep during the night is known as _____.

9. An uncontrollable rhythmic shaking or trembling is called a(n) _____.

10. An inability to achieve penile erection is referred to as _____.

True / False

Identify each of the following statements as true or false by placing a "T" or "F" on the line beside each number.

_____ 1. Excessive use of alcohol is often associated with impotence, depression, and insomnia.

_____ 2. Body temperature below 37.8°C may cause death if the situation is not corrected.

_____ 3. The greatest risk factor for basal cell carcinoma is chewing tobacco.

_____ 4. Risk factors and possible causes of breast cancer are hormonal, environmental, and familial.

_____ 5. Chronic lymphocytic leukemia is a slowly progressing disease that usually affects males.

_____ 6. Decubitus ulcers occur when the body's weight presses upon the knees or hips.

_____ 7. Shingles is also called *herpes zoster*.

_____ 8. Failure to treat glaucoma adequately leads to dementia.

_____ 9. Myocardial infarction is caused by a blood clot that occludes the aorta.

_____10. Prostate cancer is the most common cancer affecting American males, and commonly occurs beginning at age 50.

Definitions

Define each of the following words in one sentence.

1. atypical: _____

2. capillary: _____

3. insulin: _____

4. metastasize: _____

5. neoplasm: _____

6. agitation: _____

7. B lymphocyte: _____

8. amnesia: _____

9. paralysis: _____

10. ketosis: _____

Abbreviations

Write the full meaning of each abbreviation.

Abbreviation	Meaning
1. MI	_____
2. PSA	_____
3. CVA	_____
4. CLL	_____
5. HF	_____
6. BPH	_____
7. AD	_____
8. DU	_____
9. TH	_____
10. BCC	_____

Matching

Match each term with its correct definition by placing the corresponding letter on the line to its left.

_____ 1. dementia

_____ 2. amnesia

_____ 3. presbyopia

_____ 4. insomnia

_____ 5. paralysis

_____ 6. malignant

_____ 7. impotence

_____ 8. symptom

_____ 9. neoplasm

_____ 10. tremor

A. uncontrollable rhythmic shaking

B. inability to achieve penile erection

C. the ability of a tumor to spread and invade other areas

D. a subjective, non-observable manifestation of a medical condition

E. an abnormal growth of new tissue

F. deterioration of intellectual faculties including memory and concentration, caused by an organic disorder of the brain

G. loss of voluntary movement in a part of the body

H. age-related difficulty in seeing or reading at close range

I. loss of memory, usually of a specific period of time

J. chronic inability to sleep or remain asleep during the night

Spelling

Circle the correct spelling from each pairing of words.

1. ricketsiae   rickettsiae
2. protozoa   protoza
3. thromboembulism   thromboembolism
4. halucination   hallucination
5. benign   beinign
6. deterioration   deteroration
7. metastasise   metastasize
8. kytosis   ketosis
9. tremor   tremer
10. menopause   menopauze

Oncology

OBJECTIVES

Upon completion of this chapter, the reader should be able to:

1. Describe benign and malignant tumors.
2. Identify the most common types of cancer.
3. Classify cancers, discussing major pathological conditions.
4. Describe predisposing factors for cancer.
5. List common pharmacological agents used in treating cancer.
6. Interpret the meanings of the abbreviations presented in this chapter.
7. Define, pronounce, and spell the terms listed in this chapter.

OVERVIEW AND CLASSIFICATION OF NEOPLASMS

The study of tumors is called **oncology**. A tumor falls into one of two broad categories. It is said to be **benign** if its growth is relatively slow and the tumor remains localized. A malignant tumor, by contrast, is characterized by more rapid, disorderly growth, and by aggressive invasion into normal tissues. The term **cancer**, from the Latin word that means "crab," refers to malignant tumors in general. The invasiveness of a malignant tumor is usually accompanied by spread to other distant points in the body. This process is called **metastasis**.

The suffix "-oma" may be used to designate any tumor. In naming benign tumors, a root word indicating the type of tissue that has become *neoplastic* is used. For example, where glandular tissue is involved, the benign tumor is called an **adenoma**.

Malignant tumors arising in epithelial tissues are known as **carcinomas**. Generally, carcinomas are malignant tumors of the skin and the epithelial linings of the alimentary canal and respiratory passages. Malignant glandular tumors are included with the carcinomas and are called **adenocarcinomas**. If a benign adenoma contains pockets of tumor secretions (cysts), it is called a **cystadenoma**. A highly malignant tumor that begins in connective tissue is called a **sarcoma**. Specific sarcoma terminology makes reference to the particular tissue of origin. For example, tumors of cartilage and fibrous connective tissue are called *chondrosarcomas* and *fibrosarcomas*.

There are a few cases in which traditional but less precise usage persists. For example, one may think that a **melanoma, lymphoma,** or **hepatoma** is benign because of its name, but all three are actually quite malignant. The more accurate terms are *malignant melanoma, lymphosarcoma,* and *hepatocellular carcinoma*. When the cells in the deepest layer become neoplastic, the tumor is called a **basal cell carcinoma**. If cells nearer the surface of the skin or other epithelia are involved, the term **squamous cell carcinoma** is used.

RISK FACTORS

Risk factors associated with geographic areas or ethnic groups may relate to environmental influences or diet as well as genetic variations. Some risk factors, such as foods, can be avoided. Other factors, such as genetic predisposition, cannot be avoided, but can be addressed by encouraging frequent screening, and therefore, early diagnosis. Risk factors are summarized in Table 19-1.

TABLE 19-1   Risk Factors for Cancer

Factors	Examples
genetic factors	breast cancer, retinoblastoma
viruses	hepatic cancer, cervical cancer, Kaposi's sarcoma
radiation (sun, x-ray)	skin cancer, leukemia (radiation exposure)
chemicals	lung cancer (asbestos, nickel); leukemia (benzene); and bladder cancer (aniline dyes)
biologic factors	colon cancer, oral cancer
age (increasing)	many cancers are more common in older persons
diet	colon cancer (high-fat diet); gastric cancer (smoked foods)
hormones	endometrial cancer (estrogen)

STAGING OF CANCER

Staging of cancer is a classification process applied to a specific malignant tumor at the time of diagnosis. The staging at a certain time therefore provides a basis for treatment and **prognosis**. Staging systems are based on the:

- size of the primary tumor (T)
- extent of involvement of regional lymph nodes (N)
- spread (invasion or metastasis) of the tumor (M)

GENERAL TERMINOLOGY RELATED TO ONCOLOGY

The following are common terms that relate to oncology.

Term	Pronunciation	Definition
anaplastic	ah-nuh-PLAH-stik	pertaining to anaplasia
antineoplastic	an-ty-nee-oh-PLAS-tik	pertaining to a substance, procedure, or measure that prevents the proliferation of cells
benign	beh-NYN	a non-cancerous tumor, and therefore not an immediate threat
cancer	KAN-ser	a neoplasm characterized by the uncontrolled growth of anaplastic cells that tend to invade surrounding tissue, and to metastasize to distant body sites
carcinogen	kar-SIH-no-jen	an agent or a substance that produces cancer
chemotherapy	kee-moh-THAIR-uh-pee	treatment of a medical condition with a chemical agent; most often applies to drug treatments for cancer

(continues)

Term	Pronunciation	Definition
differentiation	dih-feh-ren-she-AY-shun	a process in development in which unspecialized cells become specialized
encapsulated	en-KAP-suh-lay-ted	enclosed within a fibrous or membranous site or sheath, referring to organisms that form a protective capsule
immunosuppression	ih-myoo-no-suh-PREH-shun	the process of preventing formation of the immune response
invasive	in-VAY-siv	pertaining to the spreading process of a cancer into normal tissue
ionizing radiation	EYE-oh-ny-zing ray-dee-AY-shun	high-energy electromagnetic waves (such as x-rays and gamma rays) that directly affect living organisms by killing cells or retarding their development
malignant	mah-LIG-nent	a tumor that spreads cancer from one area of the body to another
metastasis	meh-TAH-stuh-sis	the spreading process of cancer from a primary site to a secondary site
mutation	myoo-TAY-shun	the process by which the genetic structure is changed
neoplasm	NEE-oh-plah-zum	an abnormal growth of tissue that may be malignant or benign; a tumor
oncogenes	ONG-koh-jens	cancer-causing genes in a virus that can induce tumor formation
papillary	PAH-pih-leh-ree	pertaining to a papilla or papilloma
precancerous	pree-KAN-ser-us	pertaining to the state of a growth or condition before the onset of cancer
prognosis	prog-NO-sis	expected course of a disease or the chance of recovery
proliferation	pro-lih-feh-RAY-shun	the process of rapid production
radiation	ray-dee-AY-shun	the waves of energy emitted by an atom
relapse	REE-laps	return of the symptoms or signs of cancer after a period of improvement or even remission
remission	ree-MIH-shun	lessening in the severity of disease or even the complete disappearance of disease, particularly one that fluctuates in intensity; in cancer, a long remission may be an indication of a cure
tumor	TOO-mer	an abnormal growth of cells or tissues

PATHOLOGICAL CONDITIONS

The following are commonly seen pathological conditions related to cancer.

Adenocarcinoma – any one of a large group of malignant, epithelial cell tumors of the glands

Adenoma – a benign tumor composed of glandular tissue

Anaplasia – a change in the structure and orientation of cells, characterized by a loss of differentiation and reversion to a more primitive form

Astrocytoma – a primary tumor of the brain composed of astrocytes (a type of nerve cell) and characterized by slow growth, cyst formation, invasion of surrounding structures, and, often, development of a highly malignant tumor

Basal cell carcinoma – a malignant epithelial cell tumor which is rarely metastasized; the most common form of skin cancer; most commonly, this lesion occurs between the hairline and the upper lip; the primary known cause of this cancer is excessive exposure to the sun or to radiation

Breast cancer – the most common type of cancer in females, and the second leading cause of their cancer deaths in the United States; a malignant neoplastic disease of the breast tissue; risk factors include certain genetic abnormalities, a family history of breast cancer, nulliparity (never giving birth), exposure to ionizing radiation, early menarche, late menopause, obesity, diabetes, hypertension, chronic cystic disease of the breast, and, possibly, post-menopausal estrogen therapy; metastasis through the lymphatic system to axillary lymph nodes and to the bones, lungs, brain, and liver is common

Burkitt's lymphoma – a malignant neoplasm composed of lymphoreticular cells that cause destruction of the jaw; seen chiefly in Central Africa, and is associated with the Epstein-Barr virus

Carcinoid tumor – a small yellow tumor derived from particular cells in the gastrointestinal mucosa that secrete a chemical substance known as *serotonin*; carcinoid tumors spread slowly locally, but may metastasize widely

Carcinoma – a malignant tumor arising in epithelial tissue

Carcinoma in situ – a premalignant neoplasm that has not invaded the basement membrane but signifies cancer; frequently occurs on the uterine cervix and in the anus, bronchi, buccal mucosa, esophagus, eye, lip, penis, and vagina

Chondrosarcoma – a malignant neoplasm of cartilaginous cells that occurs most frequently in long bones, the pelvis, and the scapula (shoulders); appears as a large, smooth growth

Dysplasia – any abnormal development of tissues or organs

Ewing's sarcoma – a malignant tumor that develops from bone marrow, usually in long bones, or the pelvis; occurs most frequently in adolescent boys

Glioma – any of the largest group of primary tumors of the brain, composed of malignant glial cells

Hodgkin's disease – a malignant disorder characterized by painless, progressive enlargement of lymphoid tissue; usually first evident in cervical lymph nodes and splenomegaly

Hyperplastic – abnormal increase in number of cells causing enlargement

Hypoplastic – abnormal decrease in number of cells causing incomplete development

Kaposi's sarcoma – a malignant neoplasm that begins as soft brownish or purple papules on the feet and slowly spreads in the skin, metastasizing to the lymph nodes and viscera; occurs most often in men and is associated with diabetes, malignant lymphoma, and acquired immunodeficiency

Leiomyosarcoma – a sarcoma that contains unstriated muscle cells

Leukemia – a broad term given to a group of malignant diseases characterized by diffuse replacement of bone marrow with increased production of immature leukocytes in circulation, and infiltration of the lymph nodes, spleen, and liver; males are affected twice as frequently as females; the origin is not clear, but it may result from genetic predisposition plus exposure to ionizing radiation, benzene, or other chemicals that are toxic to bone marrow; the risk of the disease increases in individuals with Down syndrome; classified as *acute* or *chronic*; there are four major types of leukemia, named for how quickly they progress and the type of white blood cell they affect; acute leukemias progress rapidly; chronic leukemias progress slowly; lymphocytic leukemia affects lymphocytes, while myeloid (myelocytic) leukemias affect myelocytes

Leukoplakia – a precancerous, slowly developing change in a mucous membrane characterized by thickened, white, firmly attached patches that are slightly raised and sharply circumscribed; may occur on the lips and the buccal mucosa, and are associated with pipe smoking; may also appear on the penis or vulva

Liposarcoma – a malignant growth of primitive fat cells; also called *lipoma sarcomatodes*

Lung cancer – a pulmonary malignancy attributable in the majority of cases to cigarette smoking; other predisposing factors are exposure to arsenic, asbestos, coal products, ionizing radiation, mustard gas, and petroleum; the most common cause of cancer deaths worldwide for both men and women; the four major histological types of lung cancer include squamous cell carcinoma, adenocarcinoma, large cell carcinoma, and small cell carcinoma; the first three types are often collectively referred to as *non–small cell lung cancer* because they behave and are treated similarly; small cell lung cancer occurs almost exclusively in smokers, has a rapid growth rate, and metastasizes early in the disease process

Lymphadenopathy – an enlargement of the lymph nodes

Lymphoma – a malignant cancer of the lymphatic system; normally appears first as a single, painless, enlarged lymph node, usually in the neck; lymphomas are usually categorized as *Hodgkin's* or *non-Hodgkin's* lymphomas

Medulloblastoma – a tumor consisting of neoplastic cells that resemble undifferentiated cells; medulloblastomas are usually located in the cerebellum and occur most frequently in children

Malignant melanoma – a skin cancer derived from cells that are capable of forming the pigment *melanin* (Figure 19-1); may form on any part of the body, and are most commonly associated with exposure to the sun or ultraviolet radiation from tanning booths

Myeloma – a tumor arising in the bone marrow

Myosarcoma – a malignant tumor of muscular tissue

Neuroblastoma – a malignant neoplasm of the kidney occurring in young children (usually before age 5); slightly more common among females than males, and among African-American children than Caucasian children; also called *Wilms' tumor*

Osteosarcoma – a malignant cancer of the bones, also called *osteogenic sarcoma*

Ovarian cancer – a type of cancer with a very poor prognosis, ranking high in mortality rates; hidden in the peritoneal cavity, and is a "silent" tumor; hormonal and genetic factors appear to play a role in development of this cancer; spreads easily by means of the lymphatic vessels

Papilloma – a benign epithelial neoplasm characterized by a branching or lobular tumor

Prostatic cancer – a slowly progressive adenocarcinoma of the prostate that affects an increasing proportion of American

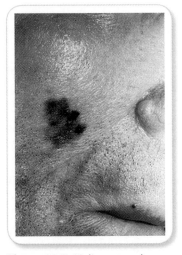

Figure 19-1 Malignant melanoma. *Courtesy of Robert A. Silverman, M.D., Pediatric Dermatology, Georgetown University*

males after 50 years of age; the third leading cause of cancer deaths in the United States; cause is unknown, but it is believed to be hormone-related; may cause no direct symptoms, but can be detected in the course of diagnosing bladder or urethral obstruction, humaturia, or pyuria; can spread to cause bone pain in the pelvis, ribs, or vertebrae; commonly detected by a prostate-specific antigen test and digital rectal examination, followed by core-needle biopsy

Retinoblastoma – a congenital hereditary neoplasm developing from retinal germ cells; characteristic signs are diminished vision and retinal detachment; the rapidly growing tumor may invade the brain and metastasize to distant sites

Rhabdomyosarcoma – a highly malignant tumor derived from primitive striated muscle cells that occurs most frequently in the head and neck, and is also found in the genitourinary tract; in some cases, the onset is associated with trauma

Sarcoma – a highly malignant tumor that begins in connective tissue, such as that in muscle or bone; the specific type of tumor is usually named after the tissue of origin (for example, *osteogenic sarcoma original*)

Seminoma – a malignant tumor of the testis; the most common testicular tumor, believed to arise from the seminiferous epithelium of the testis

Squamous cell carcinoma – a slow-growing malignant tumor of the squamous epithelium, frequently found in the lungs and skin, and also occurring in the anus, cervix, larynx, nose, and bladder

Teratoma – a malignant tumor of the ovary or testis which is contained in embryonic tissue of the hair, bones, muscles, or teeth

Testicular cancer – a malignant neoplastic disease of the testis occurring most frequently in men between 20 and 35 years of age; an undescended testicle is often involved; patients with early testicular cancer are often asymptomatic, and metastases may be present in lymph nodes, the lungs, and the liver before the primary lesion is palpable; tumors develop more often in the right than in the left testis

Thyroid cancer – a neoplasm of the thyroid gland, usually characterized by slow growth and a slower and more prolonged clinical course than that of other malignancies; women are nearly three times more likely to develop thyroid cancer than are men; the four main types of thyroid cancer are papillary, follicular, medullary, and anaplastic; papillary and follicular carcinomas are the most common

ABBREVIATIONS

The following are common abbreviations that relate to oncology.

Abbreviation	Meaning
ALL	acute lymphocytic leukemia
AML	acute myelogenous leukemia
BMT	bone marrow transplantation
bx	biopsy
CA	carcinoma
CEA	carcinoembryonic antigen
chemo	chemotherapy
CLL	chronic lymphocytic leukemia
CML	chronic myelogenous leukemia
DES	diethylstilbestrol
DNA	deoxyribonucleic acid
DRE	digital rectal exam
ER	estrogen receptor
METS, mets	metastases
NHL	non-Hodgkin's lymphoma
PR	progesterone receptor
PSA	prostate-specific antigen
RNA	ribonucleic acid
RT	radiation therapy
TNM	tumor, nodes, metastasis
Tx	treatment
XRT	x-ray or radiation therapy

DRUG CATEGORIES

Basic treatment measures for cancer include surgery, chemotherapy, radiation, or a combination thereof, depending on the specific cancer. Not all cancer cells are sensitive to radiation or chemotherapy. For example, leukemia is treated by chemotherapy and solid tumors are frequently removed by surgery, which is then followed by chemotherapy, radiation, or both. The most common drug categories for the treatment of cancers are listed in the following table.

Drug Category	Description	Examples
alkylating drugs	a chemical reaction substitutes an alkyl group for a hydrogen molecule, breaking DNA strands in the cancerous cell	Cytoxan®, Emcyt®
antiemetic drugs	used to treat the side effects of chemotherapy (nausea and vomiting)	Compazine®, Phenergan®
antimetabolite drugs	blocking folic acid (used to form some amino acids in cancer cell DNA) or directly blocking DNA from being able to use amino acids	fluorouracil (5-FU), methotrexate
chemotherapy – antibiotics	binding to DNA strands and inhibiting enzymes that split DNA to stop cell division	bleomycin, doxorubicin
chemotherapy – enzymatics	breaking down asparagine (an amino acid) which cancer cells cannot synthesize	Elspar®, Oncaspar®
hormonal drugs	producing hormonal conditions that cancer cannot reproduce in	Nolvadex®, tamoxifen
mitosis inhibitors	breaking DNA strands in cancerous cells during cell division	Camptosar®, VePesid®
monoclonal antibodies	binding to cancer cell antigens to destroy the cell	Campath®, Herceptin®
platinum-containing drugs	creating links to DNA strands that prevent cancer cell division	cisplatin, Platinol-AQ®

REVIEW EXERCISES

Multiple Choice

Select the best answer and write the letter of your choice to the left of each number.

1. Which of the following is a malignant tumor?

   A. cystadenoma
   B. lipoma
   C. papilloma
   D. hepatoma

2. The second leading cause of cancer deaths among women in the United States is:

   A. lung cancer
   B. ovarian cancer
   C. breast cancer
   D. cervical cancer

3. The process by which the genetic structure is changed is referred to as:

   A. mutation
   B. myeloma
   C. oncogene
   D. teratoma

4. Which of the following terms is referred to as a change in the structure and orientation of cells?

   A. neoplasm
   B. metastasis
   C. dysplasia
   D. anaplasia

5. Sarcoma is a highly malignant tumor that begins in which of the following tissues?

   A. connective tissue
   B. nerve tissue
   C. muscle tissue
   D. epithelial tissue

6. Astrocytoma is a primary tumor of the:

   A. lungs
   B. kidneys
   C. brain
   D. liver

7. Which of the following malignant epithelial cell tumors occurs between the hairline and the upper lip?

    A. glioma
    B. astrocytoma
    C. Burkitt's lymphoma
    D. basal cell carcinoma

8. Which of the following cancers occurs most often in men and is associated with diabetes, malignant lymphoma, and acquired immunodeficiency syndrome?

    A. Ewing's sarcoma
    B. Kaposi's sarcoma
    C. Burkitt's lymphoma
    D. Hodgkin's disease

9. Malignant glial cells are found in which of the following organs?

    A. brain
    B. heart
    C. kidneys
    D. bones

10. Which of the following malignant diseases is seen in individuals with Down syndrome?

    A. osteosarcoma
    B. leukoplakia
    C. leiomyosarcoma
    D. leukemia

11. Which of the following malignant cancers is called a "silent" tumor?

    A. neuroblastoma
    B. malignant melanoma
    C. ovarian cancer
    D. testicular cancer

12. Seminoma is a malignant tumor of the:

    A. testicle
    B. ovary
    C. kidney
    D. gallbladder

13. Which of the following terms means "pertaining to the state of a growth or condition before the onset of cancer"?

    A. proliferation
    B. neoplasm

C. dysplasia
D. precancerous

14. A premalignant neoplasm that has not invaded the basement membrane, but shows some characteristics of cancer is called:

A. encapsulated
B. carcinoma in situ
C. remission
D. relapse

15. Osteosarcoma is also called:

A. neuroblastoma
B. malignant melanoma
C. osteomyelitis
D. osteogenic sarcoma

Fill in the Blank

Use your knowledge of medical terminology to insert the correct term from the list below.

medulloblastoma	hepatoma	carcinoma
osteosarcoma	testicular cancer	antineoplastic
oncology	prostatic cancer	dysplasia
retinoblastoma	ovarian cancer	hypoplastic
carcinogen	oncogenes	mutation

1. Cancer-causing genes in a virus that can induce tumor formation are referred to as _____.

2. A type of cancer with a very poor prognosis is _____.

3. The study of malignant tumors is called _____.

4. The process by which the genetic structure is changed is called _____.

5. A malignant cancer of the bones is known as _____.

6. A slowly progressive adenocarcinoma that affects males after 50 years of age, and is the third leading cause of cancer deaths in the United States, is known as _____.

7. Any abnormal development of tissue or organs is called _____.

8. A malignant tumor of the liver is called _____.

9. A malignant tumor arising in epithelial tissue is referred to as _____.

10. A congenital hereditary neoplasm developing from retinal germ cells is called _____.

True / False

Identify each of the following statements as true or false by placing a "T" or "F" on the line beside each number.

_____ 1. Neoplasms are always malignant.

_____ 2. Sarcomas grow rapidly and show anaplasia.

_____ 3. Leukemia can be acute or chronic.

_____ 4. Kaposi's sarcoma most often affects patients with leukemia.

_____ 5. Astrocytoma is a primary tumor of the testes.

_____ 6. Leukoplakia is a precancerous condition in a mucous membrane that is associated with pipe smoking.

_____ 7. A malignant growth of primitive fat cells is referred to as "liposarcoma."

_____ 8. Prostatic cancer affects an increasing proportion of American males after 30 years of age.

_____ 9. Wilms' tumor is a malignant neoplasm of the ovaries.

_____ 10. A congenital hereditary neoplasm developing from retinal germ cells is called "rhabdomyosarcoma."

Definitions

Define each of the following words in one sentence.

1. carcinoma: _____

2. benign: _____

3. sarcoma: _____

4. Burkitt's lymphoma: _____

5. Ewing's sarcoma: _____

6. glioma: _____

7. leiomyosarcoma: _____

8. liposarcoma: _____

9. osteosarcoma: _____

10. seminoma: _____

Abbreviations

Write the full meaning of each abbreviation.

	Abbreviation	Meaning
1. CEA	_____	_____
2. DRE	_____	_____
3. XRT	_____	_____
4. PSA	_____	_____
5. ER	_____	_____
6. PR	_____	_____
7. BMT	_____	_____
8. AML	_____	_____
9. bx	_____	_____
10. RNA	_____	_____

Matching

Match each term with its correct definition by placing the corresponding letter on the line to its left.

_____ 1. lymphadenopathy

_____ 2. neoplasm

_____ 3. relapse

_____ 4. adenocarcinoma

_____ 5. malignant melanoma

_____ 6. myeloma

_____ 7. myosarcoma

_____ 8. teratoma

_____ 9. dysplasia

_____ 10. mutation

A. cancer of the muscles

B. contained in embryonic tissue of the hair

C. any abnormal development of tissues or organs

D. a tumor arising in the bone marrow

E. the process by which the genetic structure is changed

F. a malignant tumor arising in a glandular organ

G. most commonly associated with exposure to the sun

H. an abnormal growth of tissues

I. enlarged lymph nodes

J. return of the signs and symptoms of cancer after a period of improvement

Spelling

Circle the correct spelling from each pairing of words.

1.	ostosarcoma	osteosarcoma
2.	medulloblastoma	meduloblastoma
3.	leukoplakia	leucoplakia
4.	chondrrosarcoma	chondrosarcoma
5.	carcinoid	carcenoid
6.	glyoma	glioma
7.	astrocytoma	astrocitoma
8.	skuamous cell	squamous cell
9.	benian	benign
10.	rhabdomyosarcoma	rabdomyosarcoma

SECTION IV

TERMINOLOGY RELATED TO THE PHARMACY PROFESSION

Pharmacological Vocabulary

OBJECTIVES

Upon completion of this chapter, the reader should be able to:

1. Describe the sources and types of drugs.
2. List various names of drugs.
3. Classify various drug names.
4. Define symbols and the meaning of related abbreviations.
5. Describe some of the ways in which drugs affect the body.
6. List the basic parts of prescriptions.
7. Explain the general principles of pharmacology.

OUTLINE

THE FIELD OF PHARMACOLOGY

Pharmacology is one of the most challenging aspects of study for pharmacy technician students. In today's health care, drug therapy is of the utmost importance, but is also a complicated area of understanding. A fundamental understanding of pharmacology begins with learning medical terminology. Therefore, pharmacy students must know pharmacological vocabulary and abbreviations as well as understand the interactions of drugs within the body. A knowledge of the sources, forms, classifications, interactions, dosage ranges, desired effects, and adverse effects of drugs is essential. A working knowledge of medical terms helps in comprehending newly encountered drug names and is beneficial to everyone.

PRESCRIPTION DRUGS

Prescription drugs are also known as **legend drugs**, and may only be dispensed by certain individuals. These include pharmacists, pharmacy technicians who are being directed to do so by a pharmacist, and actual prescribers of prescriptions. Prescription drugs require a prescription, or written order, from a physician or another individual who is licensed to prescribe. Though the Food and Drug Administration designates which drugs require a prescription in general, individual states also designate certain drugs (and devices) as requiring prescriptions.

A prescription has four basic parts, as follows:

- *superscription* – the date, patient's full name and address, date of birth, and the symbol "℞" (which means "take thou" in Latin)
- *inscription* – the name of the drug, its amount, and its concentration
- *subscription* – the directions to the pharmacist
- *signature* – the patient instructions (also called the *transcription*)

Other items included in a prescription include:

- physician's name, office address, telephone number, and DEA registration number
- physician's signature
- the number of times the prescription can be refilled
- an indication of whether the pharmacist may substitute a generic version of a trade name drug at the patient's request

Nonprescription Drugs

Nonprescription drugs are also known as **over-the-counter** drugs. They do not require a physician's order and can be purchased directly by adult patients. Over-the-counter drugs demonstrate wide margins of safety, and it is generally considered that patients can safely treat themselves with these drugs as long as they follow the enclosed instructions carefully. It is important to remember that OTC drugs can still have serious adverse effects if taken incorrectly.

Drug Sources

There are basically five drug sources, though new drug sources are being created today via the use of continually developing chemicals and research of human tissue therapies. The five basic drug sources are as follows:

- *animal sources* – Drugs are obtained from the body fluids and glands of animals, including enzymes (including pancreatin and pepsin) and hormones (thyroid hormone and insulin).

- *engineered sources* – This new area, which includes genetic engineering and gene splicing, has produced new types of insulin, growth hormones, cancer drugs, HIV drugs, and tissue plasminogen activator. An emerging type of genetic engineering focuses on gene replacement.

- *mineral sources* – Naturally occurring minerals, found in soil and deeper into the earth's crust, are **inorganic** sources of drugs. These include iron, potassium, gold, silver, sodium chloride (table salt), and coal tar.

- *plant sources* – These drug sources are organized via their chemical and physical properties, including **organic** compounds such as alkaloids. Examples of drugs obtained from plant sources include morphine, atropine, digoxin, and nicotine.

- *synthetic sources* – These drug sources may come from both living, organic sources or non-living, inorganic sources. Also called *manufactured drugs*, they are not found in nature, but are created through chemical and biological methods. Synthetic drugs include meperidine, oral contraceptives, and sulfonamides. Penicillin is an organic, semi-synthetic drug made by alteration of its elements, while propylthiouracil (an antithyroid hormone) is both organic and inorganic.

DRUG NAMES

A drug usually has a chemical name, a generic name, and a trade (brand) name. The *chemical name* of a drug describes the chemicals that make up the drug product, using precise biochemical or zoological terminology. A *generic name* (also called the *nonproprietary* or *official name*) is simpler than the chemical name, and encouraged to be used over trade names in order to avoid confusion. Usually, a generic drug is cheaper than a trade name drug. A *trade name* is legally registered by the drug manufacturer, and is a copyrighted name, becoming the legal property of the manufacturer. It is also known as the *proprietary name*.

DRUG CLASSIFICATIONS

Various drugs are used for many different diseases or conditions that may affect the organs or systems of the body. They are classified according to their pharmacologic activities on the human body. These categories are listed in the following table.

Classification	Purpose	Generic Name	Trade Name
analgesic	relieves pain	acetylsalicylic acid (aspirin) acetaminophen	— Tylenol®
anesthetic	partially or completely numbs or eliminates sensitivity, with or without loss of consciousness	lidocaine	Xylocaine®
antacid	neutralizes stomach acid	calcium carbonate and magnesium	Rolaids®
antianginal	dilates coronary arteries to increase blood flow and reduce angina	nitroglycerin	Nitrocot®
antianxiety	relieves anxiety	alprazolam lorazepam	Xanax® Ativan®
antiarrhythmic	controls cardiac arrhythmias	amiodarone	Cordarone®
antibiotic	destroys or inhibits the growth of harmful microorganisms	phenoxymethyl-penicillin trimethoprim-sulfamethoxazole	Pen-Vee-K® Bactrim®
anticoagulant	prevents clot formation	heparin warfarin	Calcilean® Coumadin®
anticonvulsant	inhibits convulsions	phenobarbital diazepam	Luminal® Sodium® Valium®

(continues)

Classification	Purpose	Generic Name	Trade Name
antidepressant	prevents or alleviates symptoms of depression	amitriptyline imipramine	Elavil® Tofranil®
antidiabetic	lowers blood sugar	chlorpropamide tolazamide	Diabinese® Tolinase®
antidiarrheal	prevents or treats diarrhea	diphenoxylate-atropine loperamide	Lomotil® Imodium®
antidiuretic	suppresses urine formation	vasopressin	Pitressin®
antiemetic	prevents or relieves nausea and vomiting	chlorpromazine meclizine	Thorazine® Bonine®
antifungal	destroys or inhibits fungal growth	miconazole nystatin	Monistat® Mycostatin®
antihistamine	slows allergic reactions by counteracting histamines	diphenhydramine brompheniramine	Benadryl® Dimetane®
antihypertensive	controls high blood pressure	nadolol furosemide	Corgard® Lasix®
anti-infective	destroys or inhibits the growth of infection-causing microorganisms	amoxicillin doxycycline	Amoxil® Vibramycin®
anti-inflammatory	counteracts inflammation	nabumetone naproxen	Relafen® Aleve®
antineoplastic	destroys malignant cells	fluorouracil methotrexate	Adrucil® Rheumatrex®
antiparkinson	controls symptoms of Parkinson's disease	levodopa biperiden	Sinemet® Akineton®
antipsychotic	controls symptoms of schizophrenia and some psychoses	risperidone olanzapine	Risperdal® Zyprexa®
antitubercular	decreases growth of microorganisms that cause tuberculosis	ethambutol isoniazid rifampin	Myambutol® Laniazid® Rifadin®
antitussive	relieves cough due to various causes	dextromethorphan pseudoephedrine-guaifenesin	Vick's® Formula 44® Robitussin® PE®
anti-ulcer	heals ulcers	ranitidine nizatidine	Zantac Axid®
antiviral	controls the growth of viruses	acyclovir vidarabine	Zovirax® Vira-A®
bronchodilator	dilates bronchial passages	theophylline aminophylline	Bronkodyl® Truphyllin®
decongestant	reduces nasal congestion and swelling	pseudoephedrine	Drixoral®, Sudafed®

diuretic	increases excretion of urine	furosemide bumetanide	Lasix® Bumex®
hemostatic	controls or stops bleeding	aminocaproic acid	Amicar®
hormone	treats abnormally low hormone levels	conjugated estrogen glucagon	Premarin® Glucagon®
hypnotic	induces sleep	pentobarbital secobarbital sodium	Nembutal® Seconal®
laxative	promotes easy bowel emptying	docusate bisacodyl	Surfak® Dulcolax®
lipid-lowering agent	reduces blood fat (lipid) levels	niacin lovastatin	Nicobid® Mevacor®
sedative	exerts soothing or tranquilizing effects	diazepam flurazepam	Valium® Dalmane®
skeletal muscle relaxant	relieves muscle tension	dantrolene carisoprodol	Dantrium® Soma®
vasodilator	decreases blood pressure by relaxing blood vessels	benazepril hydralazine	Lotensin® Apresoline®
vitamin	prevents and treats vitamin deficiencies	vitamins A, D, E (etc.) ascorbic acid	— Vitamin C®

GENERAL TERMINOLOGY RELATED TO PHARMACOLOGY

The following are common terms that relate to pharmacology.

Term	Definition
adverse reaction	any unexpected or dangerous reaction to a drug
agonist	a drug that produces a functional change in a cell
allergy	a state of hypersensitivity induced by exposure to a particular antigen
anaphylactic reaction	a severe, life-threatening allergic reaction to a drug
antagonist	a drug that blocks a functional change in a cell
antimetabolite	a substance that is produced to alter the actions of liver enzymes
bactericidal	killing bacterial growth
bacteriostatic	suppressing bacterial growth by triggering a mechanism that blocks folic acid synthesis, thereby forcing bacteria to form their own folic acid
bioavailability	measurement of the rate of absorption and total amount of a drug that reaches the systemic circulation
biotransformation	the conversion of a drug within the body; also known as *metabolism*
brand name	the name under which a drug is sold by its manufacturer

(continues)

Term	Definition
chemical name	a drug's full name; refers to its complete chemical makeup
chemotherapy	drugs that have intended, deadly effects on specific diseases such as cancer
cumulation	a drug level that accumulates in the body with repeated doses due to incomplete excretion of the previous doses
desired effect	the intended effect of a drug
drug	a substance used to diagnose, cure, treat, or prevent disease; any substance or product that is used to modify or explore the physiological system or pathological states for the benefit of the recipient
drug absorption	the movement of a drug from its site of administration into the bloodstream
drug action	how a drug produces changes within the body
drug clearance	elimination rate over time divided by a drug's concentration
drug contraindication	conditions under which a drug is not indicated and should not be administered
drug effect	a change that takes place in the body as a result of drug action
drug facts and comparisons	a reference book that provides drug information according to their therapeutic classifications
drug interaction	an increase or decrease in the effectiveness and/or adverse effects of two or more drugs being used
drug metabolism	the conversion of a drug within the body; also known as *biotransformation*
drug toxicity	the degree to which a drug can be harmful
druggist	a pharmacist
efficacy	measure of a drug's effectiveness
excretion	the process whereby the undigested residue of food and waste products of metabolism are eliminated
filtration	the movement of water and dissolved substances from the glomerulus to the Bowman's capsule in the kidney
first dose	an initial dose
first-dose effect	an undesired medication effect that occurs from 30 to 90 minutes after the first dose is administered
first-pass effect	process whereby the liver has metabolized nearly all of a drug before it passes into the general circulation
generic name	a drug not protected by a trademark, but regulated by the FDA; also called the *official name*
genetic engineering	techniques wherein genes from one organism are spliced into the chromosomes of another organism; also known as *recombined DNA technology*
half-life	length of time it takes for the plasma concentration of a drug to be reduced by 50 percent
hepatotoxicity	a serious adverse reaction that occurs in the liver
hospital formulary	a reference book listing all drugs commonly stocked in hospital pharmacies

idiosyncrasy	an unexpected drug reaction; also known as *idiosyncratic reaction*
initial dose	the first dose of a medication
inorganic	a substance that is of a mineral, and not biological, origin
legend drug	a drug that is required by state or federal law to be dispensed via a prescription only; prescriptions must be written for a legitimate medical condition, and issued by a practitioner authorized to prescribe
local effect	a response to a medication that is confined to a specific body part
maintenance dose	a dose of medication that keeps the concentration of the medication in the bloodstream at the desired level
mechanism of action	the manner in which a drug produces its effects
metabolite	the product of drug metabolism; metabolites may be inactivated drugs or active drugs with equal or greater activity than the parent drug
nephrotoxicity	a serious adverse effect that occurs in the kidneys
official name	the generic name of a drug
onset of action	the time it takes a drug to reach the concentration necessary to produce a therapeutic effect
organic	a substance considered to be of a biological origin
over-the-counter	a drug that may be obtained without a prescription
package insert	a leaflet that is placed inside a prescription drug package or container required by the FDA to contain specific drug information
peak effect	the maximum drug effect product by a drug; it is achieved once the drug has reached its maximum concentration in the body
pharmacist	a person who is licensed to prepare and dispense drugs
pharmacodynamics	the study of the biochemical and physiological effects of drugs
pharmacognosy	the science dealing with the biologic and biochemical features of natural drugs and their constituents; the study of drugs of plant and animal origins
pharmacokinetics	the study of the absorption, distribution, metabolism, and excretion of drugs
pharmacology	the science concerned with drugs and their sources, appearance, chemistry, actions, and uses
pharmacotherapy	the use of drugs in the treatment of disease
pharmacy	the part of a drugstore or other store where drugs are dispensed by a pharmacist
Physicians' Desk Reference	a thick reference guide to all prescription drugs available in the United States; abbreviated as *PDR*
potency	the measure of the amount of drug required to produce a response; it is the effective dose concentration
potentiation	to enhance or increase the effect of a drug
reabsorption	the movement of water and selected substances from the tubules to the peritubular capillaries
side effect	a secondary, usually adverse effect of a drug or therapy

(continues)

Term	Definition
standards	established rules to control the strength, quality, and purity of medications
systemic effect	a generalized response to a drug by the entire body via the bloodstream
therapeutic dose	a dose of a medication that achieves the desired effect
therapeutic index	the ratio of the effective dose to the lethal dose
tolerance	reduced responsiveness of a drug because of adaptation to it
toxicology	the science dealing with the study of poisons
trade name	the brand name given to a drug by its manufacturer (such drugs are marked with the symbol "®"); also called *proprietary* or *brand name*
tubular secretion	a process that is important for the regulation of hydrogen and potassium in the kidneys
United States Pharmacopoeia	a publication (by the U.S. Pharmacopoeial Convention) containing formulas and information about the preparation and dispensation of drugs

ABBREVIATIONS

The following are common abbreviations that relate to the pharmacological vocabulary.

Abbreviation	Meaning
ADR	adverse drug reaction
ARA	aldosterone receptor antagonist
ARB	angiotensin receptor blocker
BC	birth control
BZD	benzodiazepine
CCB	calcium channel blocker
Cx	contraindicated
DMARD	disease-modifying antirheumatic drug
MOA	mechanism of action
NMBA	neuromuscular blocking agents
NSAID	nonsteroidal anti-inflammatory drug
OTC	over-the-counter
PDR	*Physician's Desk Reference*
PPI	proton pump inhibitor
TCA	tricyclic antidepressants
TI	therapeutic index
T½	half-life
USP	*United States Pharmacopoeia*
USP/NF	*United States Pharmacopoeia / National Formulary*

SYMBOLS USED IN MEDICINE

Symbols are objects or marks that stand for specific terms. In medicine, symbols may consist of graphical shapes, punctuation marks, numbers, letters, and characters from the Greek and Latin alphabets. The definitions of apothecary symbols are not absolute. Many of them have more than one meaning when used in different contexts. The symbols used most commonly in medicine are shown in the table below.

Symbol	Meaning
Ⓛ	left
Ⓡ	right
>	greater than
<	less than
=	equal to
↑	increase
↓	decrease
Ø	none
Δ	change
'	minutes
"	seconds
°	hours
1°	primary
2°	secondary
ℨ	dram
♏	minim
#	pound
×	times (as in "two times a week," or "multiplied by")
♀	female
♂	male
:	ratio

Review Exercises

Multiple Choice

Select the best answer and write the letter of your choice to the left of each number.

1. Which of the following terms in a prescription means "the directions to the pharmacist"?

   A. signature
   B. subscription
   C. inscription
   D. superscription

2. Which of the following substances is an example of drugs obtained from plant sources?

   A. silver
   B. insulin
   C. oral contraceptives
   D. atropine

3. Which of the following terms is also called the "nonproprietary name"?

   A. generic name
   B. trade name
   C. brand name
   D. chemical name

4. Which of the following drugs inhibits the growth of harmful microorganisms?

   A. hemostatic
   B. laxative
   C. antibiotic
   D. antianginal

5. Which of the following agents induces sleep?

   A. vasodilator
   B. skeletal muscle relaxant
   C. bronchodilator
   D. hypnotic

6. Which of the following is defined as "the time it takes a drug to produce its effects"?

   A. metabolic
   B. first-pass effect
   C. first-dose effect
   D. mechanism of action

7. Drug metabolism is also known as:

   A. drug toxicity
   B. maintenance dose
   C. biotransformation
   D. pharmacognosy

8. The ratio of the effective dose to the lethal dose is referred to as the:

   A. therapeutic dose
   B. therapeutic index
   C. first-dose effect
   D. first-pass effect

9. The study of the absorption, distribution, metabolism, and excretion of drugs is called:

   A. pharmacotherapy
   B. pharmacognosy
   C. pharmacodynamics
   D. pharmacokinetics

10. Which of the following classes of drugs relieves coughing due to various causes?

    A. antitussives
    B. antitubercular agents
    C. antivirals
    D. hypnotics

11. Which of the following drugs is an example of a sedative?

    A. ranitidine (Zantac)
    B. diazepam (Valium)
    C. ascorbic acid (Vitamin C)
    D. furosemide (Lasix)

12. Which of the following agents is the mechanism of action for antidiabetics?

    A. to increase blood calcium
    B. to increase blood potassium
    C. to increase blood sugar
    D. to decrease blood sugar

13. Which of the following classes of drugs is able to destroy malignant cells?

    A. antidiuretics
    B. antiparkinson agents
    C. antineoplastics
    D. antiemetics

14. Synthetic drug sources are also called:

    A. engineered sources
    B. manufactured sources
    C. animal sources
    D. plant sources

15. Prescription drugs are also known as:

    A. legend drugs
    B. generic drugs
    C. initial drugs
    D. reference drugs

Fill in the Blank

Use your knowledge of medical terminology to insert the correct term from the list below.

adverse reaction	efficacy	toxicology
antagonist	half-life	potentiation
bacteriostatic	metabolite	side effect
cumulation	bactericidal	potency
desired effect	peak effect	tolerance

1. The length of time it takes for the plasma concentration of a drug to be reduced by 50 percent is called

    _____.

2. The measure of the amount of drug required to produce a response is referred to as _____.

3. A drug level that accumulates in the body with repeated doses due to incomplete excretion of the previous doses is called _____.

4. An agent that suppresses bacterial growth is described as

    _____.

5. The measure of a drug's effectiveness is referred to as

    _____.

6. The enhancing of the effect of a drug is called _____.

7. The maximum drug effect produced by a drug is known as

    _____.

8. A drug that blocks a functional change in a cell is called a(n) _____.

9. Reduced responsiveness of a drug because of adaptation to it is known as _____.

10. Any unexpected reaction to a drug is called a(n) _____ reaction.

True / False

Identify each of the following statements as true or false by placing a "T" or "F" on the line beside each number.

_____ 1. An agent that controls the growth of viruses is an "antitubercular."

_____ 2. An antipsychotic controls symptoms of schizophrenia.

_____ 3. An antitussive relieves nasal congestion and swelling of the bronchi.

_____ 4. A laxative promotes urination, but causes nausea and vomiting.

_____ 5. An antineoplastic counteracts inflammation.

_____ 6. An antihistamine slows allergic reactions.

_____ 7. A drug that produces a functional change in a cell is called an *agonist*.

_____ 8. Drug clearance is elimination rate over time divided by a drug's concentration.

_____ 9. A serious adverse effect that occurs in the kidneys is referred to as *hepatotoxicity*.

_____10. An initial dose is called the first-dose effect.

Definitions

Define each of the following words in one sentence.

1. agonist: _____

2. desired effect: _____

3. drug effect: _____

4. efficacy: _____

5. over-the-counter: _____

6. pharmacodynamics: _____

7. initial dose: _____

8. laxative: _____

9. antifungal: _____

10. pharmacokinetics: _____

Abbreviations

Write the full meaning of each abbreviation.

Abbreviation	Meaning
1. ADR	_____
2. Cx	_____
3. OTC	_____
4. TI	_____
5. USP	_____
6. MOA	_____
7. NSAID	_____
8. BC	_____
9. T½	_____
10. TCA	_____

Matching

Match each term with its correct definition by placing the corresponding letter on the line to its left.

_____ 1. vasodilator

_____ 2. hemostatic

_____ 3. antiemetic

_____ 4. antacid

_____ 5. diuretic

_____ 6. analgesic

_____ 7. decongestant

_____ 8. anticoagulant

_____ 9. brand name

_____ 10. antibiotic

A. destroys or inhibits the growth of harmful microorganisms

B. the title under which a product is sold by its manufacturer

C. reduces nasal congestion and swelling

D. increases excretion of urine

E. prevents or relieves nausea and vomiting

F. prevents clot formation

G. relieves pain

H. controls or stops bleeding

I. neutralizes stomach acid

J. decreases blood pressure by relaxing blood vessels

Spelling

Circle the correct spelling from each pairing of words.

1. anaphilactic   anaphylactic
2. bactericidal   bacterisidal
3. hepatotoxicity   hepattotoxicity
4. idiocyncrasy   idiosyncrasy
5. pharmacognosy   pharmacognocy
6. potenciation   potentiation
7. bioavaillability   bioavailability
8. pharmacokinetics   pharmacokenetics
9. druggest   druggist
10. hemostatic   hemestatic

Terminology Used in Administering Medications

OBJECTIVES

Upon completion of this chapter, the reader should be able to:

1. Identify the different types of dosage forms.
2. List the various routes of drug administration.
3. Explain oral and parenteral drugs.
4. Summarize the methods of administering medications.
5. Distinguish solid drugs from semisolid drugs and give examples.
6. Define *sublingual*, *buccal*, and *oral routes*.
7. Explain the significance of medication errors.
8. List different routes of parenteral administration.

OVERVIEW

Medications come from a variety of drug sources, and are available in many different forms. They have the potential to cause serious harm to the patient. Therefore, the process of dispensing and administering medications must be performed carefully. Students studying to be pharmacists or pharmacy technicians should understand different forms of drugs and their routes of administration to prevent medication errors while they are dispensing, preparing, and compounding.

DOSAGE FORMS OF DRUGS

Drug dosage forms are classified according to their physical state and chemical composition. Drug dosage forms include solids (Figure 21-1), semisolids (Figure 21-2), liquids (Figure 21-3), and gases. Some drugs can undergo a change of state, from solids to liquids (melting), or from liquids to gases (vaporization). Drugs may be soluble in water, alcohol, or mixtures or liquids.

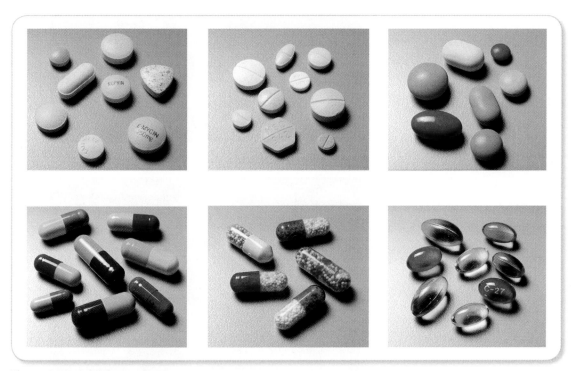

Figure 21-1 Solid dosage forms.

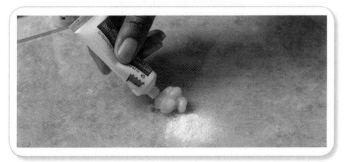

Figure 21-2 Semisolid dosage forms.

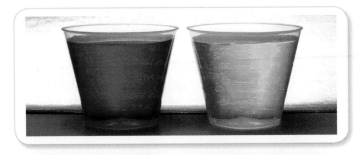

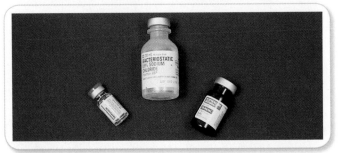

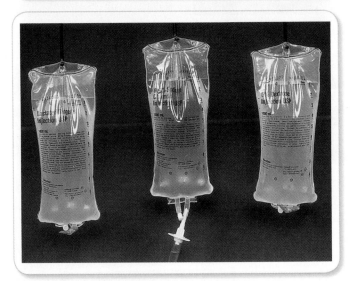

Figure 21-3 Liquid dosage forms.

ROUTES OF DRUG ADMINISTRATION

The *route* of a drug refers to how it is administered to a patient. The rate and intensity of a drug's effect is determined by the chosen route of drug administration. Each drug route requires different dosage forms. A drug that is prepared for one route may not have any effect if administered via another route, or may potentially be dangerous. Certain medications can be administered by more than one route, but others must be administered via a specified route.

The method of administration is selected according to the drug's solubility, pathophysiology, intended therapies, and the simplicity of the route of administration. The major delivery systems are the mouth (oral), injection (parenteral), inhalation (usually via the mouth), and topical (absorbed through the skin or a mucous membrane). A drug intended to have *systemic effects* is usually administered either by oral (enteral), parenteral, or inhalation methods, while a drug intended to have *localized effects* is administered topically.

Oral dosage forms must be dissolved and disintegrated before they can be absorbed and distributed throughout the body. Sublingual tablets (dissolved under the tongue) and buccal tablets (dissolved in the cheek pouch) are shown in Figures 21-4 and 21-5. The oral route is the safest and most convenient route chosen for most medications. Medications taken by mouth include solids (such as capsules) and liquids (such as syrups). Disadvantages of this method include variable absorption rates, the presence of food in the stomach, acid and enzyme actions, and decreased *bioavailability* (how readily a drug is absorbed and distributed to the site of the body in which it is intended to act).

Parenteral dosage forms are preferred if a patient is unconscious, cannot swallow, is nauseous, is vomiting, or better absorption of the drug is required. Parenteral dosage forms include subcutaneous (Figure 21-6), intradermal (Figure 21-7, see p. 397), intramuscular

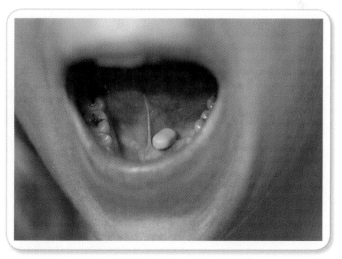

Figure 21-4 Sublingual medication administration.

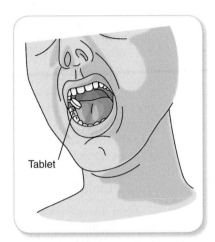

Figure 21-5 Buccal medication administrations.

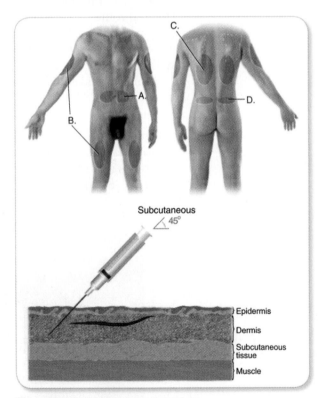

Figure 21-6 Subcutaneous injection.

(Figure 21-8), and intravenous injections (Figure 21-9). It is easier to control the exact amount of a drug throughout the body by using the parenteral method of administration. However, *aseptic*

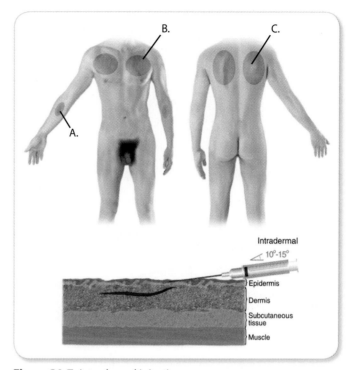

Figure 21-7 Intradermal injection.

technique must be used when preparing and administering these dosage forms due to the higher possibility of causing infection.

Inhaled dosage forms quickly deliver drugs to the respiratory tract and general circulation. In this method, drugs are easily absorbed and side effects may be lessened. Respiratory disorders such as asthma are commonly treated via the inhalation method, and general anesthetics may also be given in this manner (Figure 21-10).

Topical dosage forms are generally used for localized effects, and offer less potential for side effects, which usually occur only in the immediate area of the medication's application. Other forms considered "topical" are those that use the mucous membranes for application. Other drugs may be applied to the skin that are intended for systemic effects, via a method known as "transdermal administration." Common transdermal drugs, often administered via a "transdermal patch," include estrogen, nitroglycerin, and testosterone (Figure 21-11).

Other routes of drug administration include the ophthalmic (Figure 21-12), otic (Figure 21-13), nasal (Figure 21-14), vaginal, and rectal (Figure 21-15) routes.

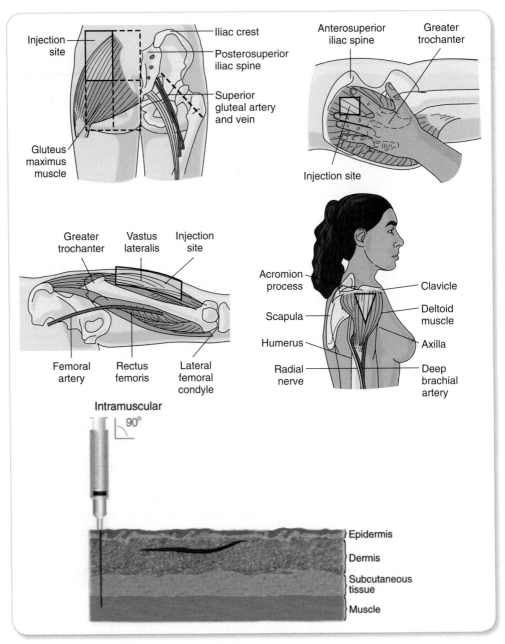

Figure 21-8 Intramuscular injection.

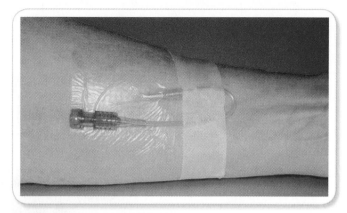

Figure 21-9 Intravenous injection.

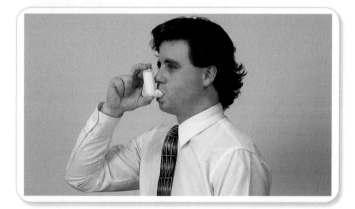

Figure 21-10 Inhaled medication.

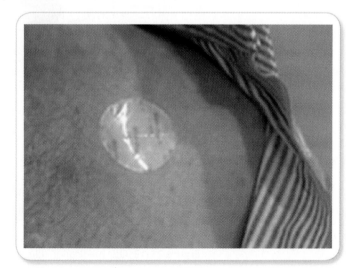

Figure 21-11 Topical medication administration. *Courtesy of 3M Pharmaceuticals*

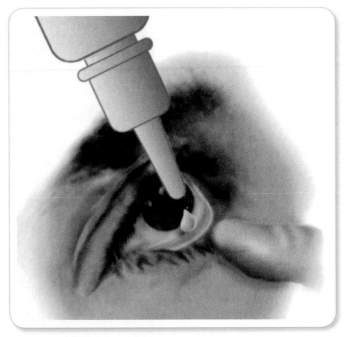

Figure 21-12 Ophthalmic medication administration.

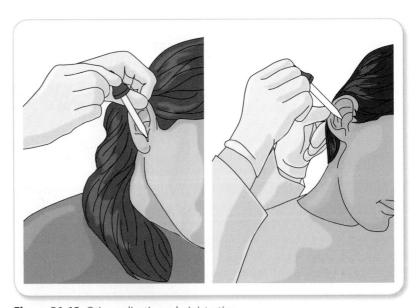

Figure 21-13 Otic medication administration.

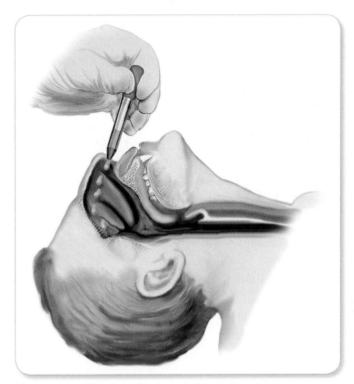

Figure 21-14 Nasal medication administration.

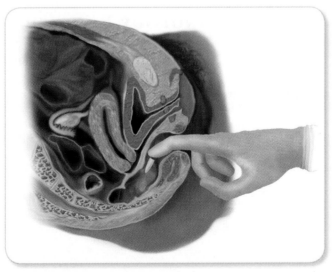

Figure 21-15 Rectal medication administration.

EQUIPMENT FOR DRUG ADMINISTRATION

The following are common terms that relate to equipment used in drug administration.

Term	Pronunciation	Definition
ampule	AM-pyool	a sealed glass container usually containing a single dose of medication; its top is broken off prior to use
gauge	GAYJ	the outside diameter of a needle
hypodermic	hy-poh-DER-mik	relating to the skin layer just below the epidermis
implant	IM-plant	an object inserted into the body for prosthetic, therapeutic, diagnostic, or experimental reasons
injector pen	in-JEK-tor PEN	an injection device designed for subcutaneous or intramuscular injection that dispenses a premeasured dose of medication
needle	NEE-dul	the steel shaft attached to the end of a syringe through which substances may be injected into the body
prefilled	PREE-fild	a syringe or similar device containing a predetermined amount of medication
pump system	—	a system of medication delivery that uses an electronic or manual pump
syringe	SRINJ	a hollow cylinder of glass or plastic with a tightly fitting plunger, with which substances may be injected through a hollow needle
vial	VY-ul	a small glass or plastic bottle containing medication; its top is punctured to withdraw the medication within

GENERAL TERMINOLOGY RELATED TO DOSAGE FORMS

The following are common terms that relate to dosage forms of drugs.

Term	Pronunciation	Definition
aerosol	EH-roh-sol	particulates of medication contained with a gaseous spray
anesthetic gas	ah-nes-THEH-tik GAS	an inhaled vapor that possesses anesthetic properties
aromatic water	ah-roh-MAH-tik WAW-ter	sweetened solution of alcohol and water used to deliver a medication
buffered tablet	BUH-ferd TAH-blet	a medicated tablet with a coating that neutralizes stomach acid
caplet	CAH-plet	a smooth, coated medicine tablet shaped like a capsule
capsule	CAP-sool	a solid dosage form with the drug enclosed in a hard or soft shell of soluble material
cream	CREEM	a semisolid emulsion intended for topical use

dosage form	DOH-sej FORM	the manner in which a dose of medication is administered; common dosage forms include solids, semisolids, liquids, and gases
dose	DOHS	a quantity of medication to be administered at one time
elixir	ee-LIK-sir	a sweetened hydro-alcoholic liquid intended for oral use
emulsion	ee-MUL-shun	a system containing two liquids that cannot be mixed together; one is dispersed in the form of small globules throughout the other
enteric-coated tablet	en-TEH-rik KOH-ted TAH-blet	a coated tablet that is protected from stomach acid, allowing it to dissolve in the intestines
fluidextract	floo-id-EK-strakt	a liquid preparation of filtered vegetable medications, containing alcohol as a solvent, preservative, or both
gel	JEL	a jelly or solid/semisolid colloidal solution
gelcap	JEL-kap	an oil-based medication enclosed in a soft gelatin capsule
granule	GRAN-yool	a gelatin- or sugar-coated small pill, containing a drug to be given in a small dose
liniment	LIH-nih-ment	a liquid preparation for external use, usually applied by using friction onto the skin
lozenge	LAW-zenj	a small, disk-shaped tablet of solidifying paste with a drug intended for local treatment of the mouth or throat where it is intended to be dissolved; a troche
mixture	MIKS-cher	an incorporation of two or more substances that do not unite chemically; it retains the physical characteristics of each component
ointment	OYNT-ment	a semisolid preparation that usually contains medicinal substances intended for external application
patch	PACH	an adhesive pad placed on the skin to deliver a controlled, timed-release dose of medication
pill	PIL	a small, globular mass of soluble material, containing a medicinal substance to be swallowed
plaster	PLAS-ter	a solid preparation that can be spread when heated; it becomes adhesive at body temperature
powder	POW-der	a dry mass of minute separate particles
semisolid drug	SEH-mee-saw-lid DRUG	a soft, pliable drug form such as a gel, ointment, or suppository
solid drug	SAW-lid DRUG	a hardened drug form such as a tablet, capsule, or powder
solution	soh-LOO-shun	a liquid dosage form in which active ingredients are dissolved in a liquid vehicle
spirits	SPEAR-its	alcoholic or hydro-alcoholic solutions of volatile substances
spray	SPRAY	liquid medication consisting of a mass of dispersed droplets
suppository	suh-paw-sih-TOH-ree	a small, semisolid dosage form to be introduced into a body orifice (usually, the rectum) that melts at body temperature

(continues)

Term	Pronunciation	Definition
suspension	sus-PEN-shun	a liquid dosage form containing solid drug particles that float in a liquid medium; it must be shaken well before use
sustained release	sus-TAYND ree-LEES	a capsule with a controlled release of the dosage over a special period of time
syrup	SEAR-up	a liquid preparation in a highly concentrated aqueous solution of a sugar used for medicinal purposes, or to add flavor to a substance
tablet	TAH-blet	a solid dosage form containing medication with or without diluents
tincture	TINK-chur	an alcoholic solution prepared from vegetable sources or chemical substances
total parenteral nutrition	TOH-tul pah-REN-teh-rul noo-TRIH-shun	an injected solution of required nutrients that is introduced into the vena cava; often used when patients cannot eat or are unconscious
troche	TROH-kee	a lozenge

GENERAL TERMINOLOGY RELATED TO ROUTES OF ADMINISTRATION

The following are common terms that relate to routes of administration.

Term	Pronunciation	Definition
buccal	BUH-kul	pertaining to the inside of the cheek
enteral	EN-teh-rul	given orally for absorption via the stomach and intestines; the enteral route means that the medication must be swallowed (therefore, this does not include sublingual or buccal medications)
gavage	gah-VAZH	feeding with a stomach tube
intradermal injection	in-truh-DER-mul in-JEK-shun	injection between the layers of the skin; the intradermal route is used for allergy testing or tuberculin testing
intramuscular injection	in-truh-MUS-kyoo-lar in-JEK-shun	injection inside a muscle
intravenous injection	in-truh-VEE-nus in-JEK-shun	injection into a vein
oral	OH-rul	pertaining to the mouth; a medication that is intended to be swallowed
parenteral	pah-REN-teh-rul	administration of a medication without use of the gastrointestinal tract; it typically includes all forms of injections
subcutaneous injection	sub-kyoo-TAY-nee-us in-JEK-shun	injection into the layer of fat and blood vessels beneath the skin

sublingual	sub-LING-wul	pertaining to the area under the tongue
topical	TAW-pih-kul	pertaining to a drug applied to the surface of the skin
transdermal	trans-DER-mul	pertaining to passage through the skin; for example, transdermal patches are dosage forms that release minute amounts of a drug at a consistent rate; as the drug is released from the patch, it is absorbed into the skin and carried off by the capillary blood supply
Z-track method	ZEE-trak MEH-thud	an intramuscular injection method wherein the skin is pulled to one side before the tissue is grasped for injection; it is used when a drug is highly irritating to the subcutaneous tissues or can permanently stain the skin

ABBREVIATIONS

The following are common abbreviations that relate to dosage forms and routes of administration.

Abbreviation	Meaning
cap	capsule
dil	dilute
DW	distilled water
D_5LR	dextrose 5% in lactated Ringer's
D_5NS	dextrose 5% in normal saline (0.9% sodium chloride)
D_5W	dextrose 5% in water
$D_{10}W$	dextrose 10% in water
elix	elixir
ex aq.	in water
f. or fl.	fluid
gl. aq.	glass of water
ID	intradermal
IM	intramuscular
iso	isotonic
IV	intravenous
IVP	intravenous push
IVPB	intravenous piggyback
mix	mixture
N.S. or NS	normal saline
½ NS	half-strength normal saline
NTG	nitroglycerin

(continues)

Abbreviation	Meaning
oint.	ointment
p.o.	by mouth
pulv.	powder
SL	sublingual
sol.	solution
sup. or supp.	suppository
susp.	suspension
syr.	syrup
tab	tablet
top.	topically
TPN	total parenteral nutrition
ung.	ointment
vol.	volume

MEDICATION ERRORS

A medication error is a preventable event that leads to inappropriate use of a medication, and possible patient harm. They occur because of actions of consumers, health care professionals, or patients, and can happen at any time in clinics, homes, hospitals, and pharmacies.

Medication errors are assuredly one of the most common yet avoidable causes of harm to patients. They may occur at three critical points, as follows:

- prescribing
- dispensing
- administering

Prevention of medication errors must be the ultimate priority of health care professionals. These individuals, including pharmacists and pharmacy technicians, must educate patients in order to prevent further medication errors.

The use of a controlled vocabulary, reduced use of abbreviations, careful use of decimal points, and proper use of leading or terminal zeroes are encouraged to help in reducing medication errors. The following table constitutes a "do not use list" of abbreviations prone to causing medication errors.

Do Not Use	Potential Problem	Use Instead
U (unit)	mistaken for "0" (zero), the number "4" (four) or "cc"	write "unit"
IU (international unit)	mistaken for "IV" (intravenous) or the number "10" (ten)	write "International Unit"
Q.D., QD, q.d., qd (daily), Q.O.D., QOD, q.o.d., qod (every other day)	mistaken for each other; the period after the Q may be mistaken for "I" and the "O" may be mistaken for "1"	write "daily" or "every other day"
trailing zero (X.0 mg) or lack of leading zero (.X mg)	decimal point is missed	write "X mg" or "0.X mg"; a trailing zero may be used only where required to demonstrate the level of precision of the value being reported, but not in medication orders or other medication-related documentation
MS	can mean "morphine sulfate" or "magnesium sulfate"	write "morphine sulfate" or "magnesium sulfate"
MSO^4 and $MgSO^4$	may be confused for each other	
> (greater than) or < (less than)	may be misinterpreted as the number "7" (seven) or the letter "L," or confused for each other	write "greater than" or "less than"
abbreviations for drug names	may be misinterpreted due to similar abbreviations for multiple drugs	write drug names in full
apothecary units	may be unfamiliar to many practitioners or confused with metric units	use metric units
@ (at)	may be mistaken for the number "2" (two)	write "at"
cc (cubic centimeters)	may be mistaken for "U" (units) when poorly written	write "mL" or "milliliters" instead of using "cc"
Mg	may be mistaken for "mg" (milligrams) resulting in a one thousand–fold overdose	write "mcg" or "micrograms"

The following is another list of error-prone abbreviations that should *never* be used when communicating medical information in any form.

Abbreviation	Intended Meaning	Potential Problem	Use Instead
AD, AS, AU	right ear, left ear, each ear	may be mistaken as "OD," "OS," "OU" (right eye, left eye, each eye)	use "right ear," "left ear," or "each ear"
BT	bedtime	may be mistaken as "BID" (twice daily)	use "bedtime"
D/C	discharge or discontinue	premature discontinuation of medications if D/C (intended to mean "discharge") has been misinterpreted as "discontinued" when followed by a list of discharge medications	use "discharge" or "discontinue"
HS	half-strength	may be mistaken as "bedtime"	use "half-strength"
hs	at bedtime, or hours of sleep	may be mistaken as "half-strength"	use "bedtime"
i/d	one daily	may be mistaken as "tid" (three times daily)	use "1 daily"
IJ	injection	may be mistaken as "IV" or "intrajugular"	use "injection"
IN	intranasal	may be mistaken as "IM" or "IV"	use "intranasal" or "NAS"
OJ	orange juice	may be mistaken as "OD" or "OS" (right or left eye); drugs meant to be diluted in orange juice may be administered into the eye	use "orange juice"
o.d. or OD	once daily	may be mistaken as "right eye" (OD – oculus dexter), leading to oral liquid medications administered into the eye	use "once daily"
OD, OS, OU	right eye, left eye, each eye	may be mistaken as "AD," "AS," or "AU" (right ear, left ear, each ear)	use "right eye," "left eye," or "each eye"
per os	by mouth, or orally	"os" may be mistaken as "left eye" (OS – oculus sinister)	use "PO," "by mouth," or "orally"
q.d. or QD	every day	may be mistaken as "q.i.d.," especially if the period after the "q" or the tail of the "q" is misunderstood as an "i"	use "every day" or "daily"
qhs	nightly at bedtime	may be mistaken as "qhr" or "every hour"	use "nightly" or "nightly at bedtime"
qn	nightly or at bedtime	may be mistaken as "qh" (every hour)	use "nightly" or "at bedtime"

q.o.d. or QOD	every other day	may be mistaken as "q.d." (daily) or "q.i.d." (four times daily) if the "o" is poorly written	use "every other day"
q1d	daily	may be mistaken as "q.i.d." (four times daily)	use "daily"
q6PM, etc.	every evening at 6 PM	may be mistaken as "every 6 hours"	use "6 PM nightly" or "6 PM daily"
SC, SQ, sub q	subcutaneous	sc may be mistaken as "SL" (sublingual); SQ may be mistaken as "5 every"; the "q" in "sub q" may be mistaken for "every"	use "subcut" or "subcutaneously"
ss	sliding scale (insulin) or ½ (apothecary)	may be mistaken as "55"	spell out "sliding scale"; use "one-half" or "1/2"
SSI	sliding scale insulin	may be mistaken as "Strong Solution of Iodine" (Lugol's)	write out "sliding scale insulin"
SSRI	sliding scale regular insulin	may be mistaken as "selective serotonin reuptake inhibitor"	spell out "sliding scale (insulin)"
TIW or tiw	3 times a week	may be mistaken as "3 times a day" or "twice in a week"	use "3 times weekly"

REVIEW EXERCISES

Multiple Choice

Select the best answer and write the letter of your choice to the left of each number.

1. Medication placed between the gum and cheek until absorbed into the mucous membranes signifies which of the following routes?

   A. oral
   B. sublingual
   C. nasal
   D. buccal

2. Transdermal medications are absorbed through:

   A. the mucous membranes
   B. the lungs
   C. the skin
   D. the eyes

3. Which of the following routes of administration is appropriate for allergy testing?

   A. intravenous
   B. intradermal
   C. subcutaneous
   D. intramuscular

4. A semisolid preparation that is usually white, non-greasy, and has a water base is called a(n):

   A. suppository
   B. ointment
   C. troche
   D. cream

5. A liquid preparation for external use, usually applied by friction to the skin, is referred to as (a):

   A. liniment
   B. spirits
   C. solution
   D. suspension

6. Which of the following dosage forms is described as a small, disk-shaped tablet composed of solidifying paste containing an antiseptic used for local treatment of the mouth or throat?

   A. pill
   B. tincture

C. troche
D. liniment

7. Which of the following types of syringes is used intradermally for small quantities of drugs?

A. insulin syringe
B. hypodermic syringe
C. tuberculin syringe
D. disposable syringe

8. An oil-based medication that is enclosed in a soft gelatin capsule is called a:

A. caplet
B. gelcap
C. granule
D. capsule

9. A drug dosage form that consists of a high concentration of a sugar in water is called a(n):

A. elixir
B. spirit
C. solution
D. syrup

10. Which of the following dosage forms usually is intended for a local effect at the site of insertion?

A. suppository
B. tincture
C. liniment
D. emulsion

11. A tube inserted through the nose into the stomach in order to feed a patient is a method called:

A. pump system
B. total parenteral nutrition
C. sustained release
D. gavage

12. Which of the following abbreviations should *never* be used when communicating medical information in any form?

A. HS
B. Mg
C. MS
D. IU

13. Which of the following pertains to passage through the skin?

    A. topical
    B. transdermal
    C. Z-track method
    D. sublingual

14. Which type of injection is given "between the layers of skin"?

    A. intrathecal
    B. intramuscular
    C. subcutaneous
    D. intradermal

15. A solid preparation that can be spread when heated that becomes adhesive at body temperature is a:

    A. powder
    B. pill
    C. plaster
    D. liniment

Fill in the Blank

Use your knowledge of medical terminology to insert the correct term from the list below.

topical	enteral	gauge
parenteral	buffered tablet	liniment
aseptic	gavage	plaster
prefilled	aerosol	gelcap
injector pen	caplet	ointment

1. A semisolid preparation that usually contains medicinal substances intended for external application is called a(n) _____.

2. A syringe that contains a predetermined amount of medication is referred to as _____.

3. A term that pertains to a drug applied to the surface of the skin is _____.

4. Feeding with a stomach tube is referred to as _____.

5. Particulates of medication contained within a gaseous spray is known as a(n) _____.

6. An oil-based medication enclosed in a soft gelatin capsule is referred to as a(n) _____.

7. An injection device designed for subcutaneous or intramuscular injections that dispenses a premeasured dose of medication is called a(n) _____.

8. A medicated tablet with a coating that neutralizes stomach acid is referred to as a(n) _____.

9. A solid preparation that can be spread when heated, becoming adhesive at body temperature, is known as a(n) _____.

10. The outside diameter of a needle is called the _____.

True / False

Identify each of the following statements as true or false by placing a "T" or "F" on the line beside each number.

_____ 1. One of the disadvantages of oral dosage forms is the acid and enzyme actions in the stomach.

_____ 2. Inhaled dosage forms quickly deliver drugs to the digestive tract and then to the general circulation.

_____ 3. The term "hypodermic" relates to the skin layer just below the dermis.

_____ 4. Aromatic water is a sweetened solution of alcohol and water used to deliver a medication.

_____ 5. A granule is a small coated tablet that is protected from stomach acid.

_____ 6. A lozenge is a small, disk-shaped tablet of solidifying paste with a drug intended for local treatment of the mouth or throat.

_____ 7. An injected solution of required nutrients that is introduced into the vena cava is called "sustained release."

_____ 8. An intravenous injection is an injection flowing into a small artery.

_____ 9. The term "sublingual" pertains to the area under the skin.

_____10. A troche is also called a *lozenge*.

Definitions

Define each of the following words in one sentence.

1. transdermal: _____

2. subcutaneous injection: _____

3. tincture: _____

4. buccal: _____

5. fluidextract: _____

6. semisolid drug: _____

7. intradermal injection: _____

8. sublingual: _____

9. vial: _____

10. implant: _____

Abbreviations

Write the full meaning of each abbreviation.

Abbreviation	Meaning
1. ID	_____
2. TPN	_____
3. SL	_____
4. susp.	_____
5. IVP	_____
6. D_5W	_____
7. fl.	_____
8. IVPB	_____
9. pulv.	_____
10. sup.	_____

Matching

Match each term with its correct definition by placing the corresponding letter on the line to its left.

_____ 1. mixture

_____ 2. granule

_____ 3. spray

A. a small glass or plastic bottle containing medication

_____ 4. emulsion

_____ 5. aerosol

_____ 6. ampule

_____ 7. liniment

_____ 8. cream

_____ 9. tincture

_____ 10. vial

B. particulates of medication contained within a gaseous spray

C. a semisolid emulsion intended for topical use

D. a liquid preparation for external use

E. liquid medication consisting of a mass of dispersed droplets

F. an alcoholic solution prepared from vegetable sources or chemical substances

G. a gelatin- or sugar-coated small pill

H. a sealed glass usually containing a single dose of medication

I. a system containing two liquids that cannot be mixed together

J. an incorporation of two or more substances that do not unite chemically

Spelling

Circle the correct spelling from each pairing of words.

1. anesthetic   anisthetic

2. losenge   lozenge

3. emolsion   emulsion

4. liniment   leniment

5. suppository   supository

6. truche   troche

7. parenteral   parinteral

8. guvage   gavage

9. bufered tablet   buffered tablet

10. spirits   spyrits

The Practice of Pharmacy

OBJECTIVES

Upon completion of this chapter, the reader should be able to:

1. Explain the major roles of a pharmacy technician in pharmacy practice.
2. Describe national certification for pharmacy technicians.
3. Explain why the field of pharmacy needs pharmacy technicians.
4. Describe the roles of the pharmacist in pharmacy practice today.
5. List various types of professional organizations.
6. Interpret the meaning of the abbreviations presented in this chapter.
7. Differentiate between pharmacy technician certification, registration, and licensure.

OVERVIEW

Pharmacy practice generally deals with preparing medications, **dispensing**, and providing drug-related information to the public. It also focuses on interpreting prescription orders, selecting drug products, compounding, labeling, conducting drug use reviews, monitoring patients, and providing services related to the use of medications and medical devices.

The practice of pharmacy has changed and expanded in the last two or three decades. Pharmacists focus more on customer education than they do on physical compounding and dispensing of medications. Pharmacists and pharmacy technicians focus on matters concerning the health and well-being of the patients for whom they dispense medications. The field of pharmacy is highly useful on a social basis, and is a sought-after profession. Technology has revolutionized the field of pharmacy. Many different pharmacy settings exist, requiring a variety of different pharmacist and pharmacy technician roles and specialized training. Professional pharmacy is supported by many different organizations and laws with which pharmacy personnel must be familiar. Every pharmacy technician must be comfortable with the many aspects of pharmacy practice.

PHARMACISTS

A **pharmacist** is a person trained to formulate and dispense medications, and also to provide clinical information about drugs and medications to patients and health professionals. A pharmacist must complete a university program of at least four years' duration, usually followed by an additional two years of study, resulting in a **Pharm.D** degree. After this, they must pass state and federal **licensing** exams in order to practice. A pharmacist seeking to practice in any state in the U.S. must register with that state's **Board of Pharmacy**, which will issue his or her license. Today, the practice of pharmacy has become more specialized, requiring individual training in different areas of expertise. These include ambulatory care, drug information, community practice, managed care, long-term care, home health care, **oncology**, nutritional support, and pharmacy administration. The pharmacist retains the ultimate responsibility over the pharmacy technicians whom he or she supervises.

Education

The Pharm.D degree usually requires six years of study in order to qualify an individual to be able to practice. There are currently more than 85 colleges of pharmacy in the U.S., with most accredited by the Accreditation Council for Pharmaceutical Education. Prior to beginning the course of study for a Pharm. D degree, students should take prerequisite courses, which include mathematics, physical sciences, and biological sciences. When studying for the Pharm.D degree, students will learn about general education topics, as in most areas of study, followed by specialized professional courses. These professional courses include chemistry, pharmacology, **biopharmaceutics**, and pharmaceutics. Following this is an **externship** in a clinical pharmacy, with additional coursework in social pharmacy, **administrative pharmacy**, and pharmacy law. Common areas of minor study include hospital (**institutional**) **pharmacy**, management, **nuclear pharmacy**, and research specialties.

Licensure

The Board of Pharmacy (or similar group in each state) controls regulation over the license to practice pharmacy. Applicants must be of good moral character, have graduated from an accredited degree program, be at least 21 years of age, and have passed their state pharmacy examination. Candidates for licensure must have proven practical experience or internship under a licensed pharmacist. Some states allow license transfers when practitioners move between one state and another. Accredited continuing education to assure **competency** over time must be completed in order to maintain licensure status.

Graduate Education

Pharmacists may study **industrial pharmacy**, pharmaceutics, pharmacology, pharmaceutical or medicinal chemistry, **pharmacognosy**, and social/administrative pharmacy as part of intended graduate study programs. For a pharmacist who wishes to become a researcher, a **master's degree** or PhD in pharmacy or a similar field is usually necessary. Administrative/faculty pharmacy positions usually require either a Pharm.D, **Master of Science**, or PhD degree. Pharmacy residency programs usually last between 1 and 2 years, and involve intensive postgraduate training in specific areas of practice.

PHARMACY TECHNICIANS

Pharmacy technicians practice in many pharmacy settings, including: community pharmacies, institutional pharmacies, extended-care facilities, home health care agencies, mail-order pharmacies, and **ambulatory clinics**. Pharmacy technicians have larger roles in the practice of pharmacy than ever before. They work under the supervision of licensed pharmacists, assisting with many technical activities. These activities require pharmacy technicians to have sufficient levels of education and training in order to handle their increasing responsibilities. Some states refer to pharmacy technicians as "pharmacy aides" or "pharmacy technologists."

The requirements of pharmacy technicians have grown more rapidly in the last 10 years than in any time before. As a result, there has been an increased focus on regulating the activities of pharmacy technicians to a national standard. This is being accomplished through the establishment of nationalized pharmacy technician training programs and standardized examinations. As the roles of pharmacists have become more focused on drug use review and **patient counseling**, the roles of pharmacy technicians have expanded to include many activities traditionally only done by licensed pharmacists.

The individual state Boards of Pharmacy and similar organizations dictate what tasks the pharmacy technicians in their state can legally perform. The states have this regulating authority over all forms of pharmacy practice regardless of setting. Pharmacy technicians regularly enter medication orders into computer systems, fill medication doses, stock shelves, and do nearly everything formerly handled by licensed pharmacists except for patient counseling and giving advice about medical products to patients.

Prior to taking a certification exam, pharmacy technicians usually must complete 6 to 24 months of **vocational** or technical coursework, which includes internship programs at pharmacy facilities. Further training may be required for pharmacy technician students wishing to work in more complicated settings, such as nuclear pharmacy. Continuing education is required upon the beginning of practice. These credits help to assure continued expansion of knowledge and greater competency in the field as the pharmacy technician is employed.

Certification

The Pharmacy Technician Certification Board was developed to offer an examination requiring technicians to meet basic levels of skill in order to become certified. In order to take the exam, a student must at least have a high school diploma or general equivalency **diploma**, and have never been convicted of a drug-related felony. However, it is not advisable that a student bypass a focused college degree or diploma program if he or she desires to become a pharmacy technician. A fully qualified pharmacy technician must have a thorough background of specialized training in the area of pharmacy in which he or she wishes to work, followed by passing the certification exam. Once certified, pharmacy technicians can practice for two years and then must apply for **re-certification**.

Various Pharmacy Settings

Pharmacy technicians may practice in a variety of specialties, with each of these requiring specific training and skills. The main responsibilities of pharmacy technicians in different pharmacy settings are listed below.

In the home infusion pharmacy, pharmacy technicians handle many compounding tasks, including:

- cleaning and disinfecting areas and equipment, and completing **cleaning logs**
- completing **compounding** records
- compounding of sterile products
- disposing of hazardous wastes
- **labeling** sterile products and medications
- maintaining patient information and other computer data

- ordering, receiving, and **stocking** medications, equipment, and supplies
- performing **quality control**
- processing home infusion equipment and supply orders
- programming **infusion devices**

In the hospice pharmacy, the pharmacy technician's duties are similar to those in both retail and home infusion pharmacies, and include:

- dispensing prescriptions for terminally ill patients, including the assembly of "**starter kits**"
- maintaining patient records, plans of care, and coordinating weekly team reports for meetings
- performing **extemporaneous** and sterile compounding

In the long-term care pharmacy, pharmacy technicians handle many dispensing tasks, including:

- billing and invoicing
- entering and maintaining computer data, files, and records
- labeling medications
- maintaining equipment
- ordering medications and supplies
- packaging and **repackaging** medications
- performing general pharmacy maintenance
- processing returned medications to be re-used
- receiving and stocking medications and supplies
- transporting medications

In the mail-order pharmacy, pharmacy technicians perform many dispensing, data entry, and production tasks, such as:

- assisting the pharmacist with specific prescription orders that require phone calls to obtain **authorization** to fill them
- entering written orders into the computer
- filling, dispensing, packaging, and labeling prescription orders
- maintaining the computer system
- ordering, receiving, and stocking medications and supplies
- training other pharmacy technicians about their duties in this type of pharmacy

In the managed-care pharmacy, pharmacy technicians do not perform dispensing activities, but are responsible for many administrative and clerical duties, such as:

- assisting, conducting, or participating in the auditing of the pharmacy to ensure **compliance** with the prescription drug benefit plan

- handling all data collection, correspondence, benefit information, committee meetings, educational programs, providers, and pharmacist appointments

- receiving and properly handling calls from members, physicians, and pharmacists

- referring people to the pharmacist when their calls are outside the scope of the pharmacy technician's training

In the nuclear pharmacy, pharmacy technicians must have specialized skills allowing them to work with **radiopharmaceuticals**. Their duties include:

- accepting verbal orders for diagnostic radiopharmaceuticals

- completing compounding records

- handling, creating, and printing labels, shipping papers, delivery tags, reports, drug information requests, and other materials

- maintaining the nuclear pharmacy with various safety monitoring techniques

- measuring unit-doses of radiopharmaceuticals

- packaging and labeling radiopharmaceuticals

- performing quality control tests

- performing radiopharmaceutical calculations

- working with **radionuclide generators**

PROFESSIONAL ORGANIZATIONS

The following pharmacy organizations and associations have been created to advance knowledge and improve the quality of pharmacy practice:

- **American Association of Colleges of Pharmacy** – represents all U.S. colleges and schools, focusing on the interests of pharmaceutical educators; it publishes many journals, including the *American Journal of Pharmaceutical Education*

- **American Association of Pharmaceutical Scientists** – represents pharmaceutical scientists in many areas of research; it publishes many journals, including *Pharmaceutical Research*

- **American Association of Pharmacy Technicians** – represents pharmacy technicians and encourages them to become certified; it has also established a *Code of Ethics for Pharmacy Technicians*

- **American College of Clinical Pharmacy** – a society of scientific professionals providing advocacy, education, leadership, and resources for clinical pharmacists

- **American Council on Pharmaceutical Education** – accredits pharmacy education programs in the U.S. that are recognized by the Secretary of Education

- **American Pharmacists Association** – the largest national pharmacy organization, with three academies; it publishes several journals including the *Journal of the American Pharmacists Association*, and operates a political action committee

- **American Society of Health-System Pharmacists** – represents institutional pharmacists and accredits pharmacist and pharmacy technician training programs; it also publishes the *American Journal of Health-System Pharmacy*

- **Pharmacy Technician Certification Board** – offers the Pharmacy Technician Certification Examination (PTCE), which may be taken voluntarily by any pharmacy technician wishing to become certified in the U.S.; it also oversees re-certification of pharmacy technicians

- **Pharmacy Technician Educators Council** – consists of educators who instruct pharmacy technicians, and publishes the *Journal of Pharmacy Technology*

- **United States Pharmacopoeia** – a non-profit organization that sets standards for drug product identity, quality, purity, packaging, labeling, and strength

THE ROLE OF AUTOMATION

In the pharmacy, automated machinery may be used to package, store, compound, dispense, and distribute medications. Automated systems can perform efficient tasks at a much faster rate than humans are capable of. Correct use of automated pharmacy systems saves time, and allows pharmacists and pharmacy technicians to concentrate on more effective tasks in the day-to-day pharmacy activities.

Automation helps to improve documentation, enhance security, increase authorized access to information and medications, and reduce medication errors. Automated pharmacy systems are commonly used today to count, package, and label dosage forms, as well as document every step of each process. These systems may be centralized in the pharmacy, or used on a de-centralized basis for long-term care facilities, other health care facilities, and nursing units.

In automated pharmacy systems, an order is input into a pharmacy computer system, which communicates with the automated machinery. The machinery can print bar-coded labels and receipts, select proper prescription containers, label the containers, select the medication, count the medication, fill the container with the medication, and cap it correctly. Mail-order pharmacies commonly use automated machinery to speed up their ability to distribute medications.

GENERAL TERMINOLOGY RELATED TO THE PRACTICE OF PHARMACY

The following are general terms that relate to the practice of pharmacy.

Term	Pronunciation	Definition
administrative	ad-mih-nih-STRAY-tiv	relating to the management of an organization
ambulatory clinic	AM-byoo-lah-toh-ree KLIH-nik	a clinic that treats patients who can walk and are not bedridden
authorization	aw-thor-ih-ZAY-shun	the power to give orders or make decisions
automation	aw-toh-MAY-shun	machinery used to perform tasks otherwise performed by humans; automation commonly involves robotics
biopharmaceutics	by-oh-far-mah-SOO-tiks	the study of physical and chemical drug properties and their proper dosage related to onset, duration, and intensity of drug action
Board of Pharmacy	BORD UV FAR-mah-see	usually, the state board charged with regulating the practice of pharmacy within that state
certification	ser-tih-fih-KAY-shun	in pharmacy, the recognition of competency in providing safe and effective patient care
cleaning log	KLEE-ning LOG	a record of cleaning or maintenance activities undertaken in the workplace
competency	KOM-peh-ten-see	being qualified to do a specific type of work

(continues)

Term	Pronunciation	Definition
compliance	kum-PLY-ans	the following of qualified instructions
compounding	kum-POWN-ding	mixing, reconstituting, and packaging a drug
diploma	dih-PLOH-mah	a document issued by an educational institution testifying to an individual's earning a degree or completing a specific course of study
dispensing	dih-SPEN-sing	preparing and distributing medications
extemporaneous	ex-tem-poh-RAY-nee-us	a type of compounding wherein medications are mixed in a pharmacy for a specific patient
externship	EK-stern-ship	a training program that is part of a course of study from an educational institution; an externship is usually conducted in a place of business relating to the program of study
industrial pharmacy	in-DUH-stree-ul FAR-mah-see	the area of pharmacy concerned with research and development of new drug products
infusion devices	in-FYOO-zhun dee-VY-ses	devices that regulate intravenous solutions as they flow into the body
institutional pharmacy	in-stih-TOO-shuh-nal FAR-mah-see	the area of pharmacy contained with hospitals and other health care settings
labeling	LAY-beh-ling	applying a printed adhesive label signifying a container's contents to the outside of the container
licensing	LY-sen-sing	the giving of legal approval to conduct business in a specified manner
licensure	LY-sen-shur	the act or instance of granting a license, usually to practice a profession
Master of Science	MAS-ter UV SY-ens	a postgraduate academic master's degree awarded by universities covering various sciences
master's degree	MAS-ters deh-GREE	a degree proving mastery of a specific field of study or area of professional practice
nuclear pharmacy	NOO-clee-ar FAR-mah-see	the area of pharmacy concerned with preparing radioactive materials used for diagnoses and treatments
oncology	on-KAW-loh-jee	the study of cancer
patient counseling	PAY-shent KOWN-seh-ling	the sharing of information about a patient's health condition and therapies, including medications
pharmacist	FAR-mah-sist	a person who is licensed to dispense drugs and counsel patients

pharmacognosy	far-mah-KAWG-noh-see	the study of medicines derived from natural sources
pharmacy technician	FAR-mah-see tek-NIH-shun	a person who is trained to assist a pharmacist in many activities
Pharm.D	FARM DEE	a "doctor of pharmacy" degree enabling an individual to practice, after taking the licensing examination, as a pharmacist
quality control	KWAH-lih-tee kun-TROL	a system designed to ensure that products or services meet or exceed customer requirements
radionuclide generators	ray-dee-oh-NOO-klyd geh-neh-RAY-tors	devices that produce radionuclides (atoms that have unstable nuclei), used in radiopharmaceutical preparation
radiopharmaceuticals	ray-dee-oh-far-mah-SOO-tih-kuls	radioactive drugs used to diagnose or treat diseases
re-certification	ree-ser-tih-fih-KAY-shun	renewal of certification
registration	reh-jih-STRAY-shun	a professional record of qualification
repackaging	ree-PAH-kuh-jing	placing bulk medications or other forms of prescription drugs into unit doses or more patient-specific packages
starter kits	STAR-ter KITS	a collection of specific medications designed for hospice patients to "start" treatment for the most urgent conditions that can develop during the final weeks of life
stocking	STAW-king	supplying a certain amount of a specified product, substance, device, piece of equipment, or other entity
vocational	voh-KAY-shuh-nal	relating to a job, occupation, or trade

ABBREVIATIONS

The following are common abbreviations used in pharmacy practice.

Abbreviation	Meaning
AACP	American Association of Colleges of Pharmacy
AAPS	American Association of Pharmaceutical Scientists
AAPT	American Association of Pharmacy Technicians
ACCP	American College of Clinical Pharmacy
ACPE	American Council on Pharmaceutical Education
APhA	American Pharmacists Association
ASHP	American Society of Health-System Pharmacists
BOP	Board of Pharmacy
PTCB	Pharmacy Technician Certification Board
PTCE	Pharmacy Technician Certification Examination
PTEC	Pharmacy Technician Educators Council
USP	United States Pharmacopoeia

REVIEW EXERCISES

Multiple Choice

Select the best answer and write the letter of your choice to the left of each number.

1. Which of the following professional organizations publishes many journals, including *Pharmaceutical Research*?

    A. United States Pharmacopoeia
    B. Pharmacy Technician Educators Council
    C. American Society of Health-System Pharmacists
    D. American Association of Pharmaceutical Scientists

2. Which of the following professional organizations represents institutional pharmacists and accredits pharmacy technician training programs?

    A. Pharmacy Technician Educators Council
    B. American Society of Health-System Pharmacists
    C. Pharmacy Technician Certification Board
    D. American Pharmacists Association

3. The giving of legal approval to conduct business in a pharmacy is referred to as:

    A. licensing
    B. compounding
    C. registering
    D. certification

4. A collection of specific medications designed for hospice patients to begin treatment for the most urgent conditions is called a:

    A. generator kit
    B. diagnostic kit
    C. palliative kit
    D. starter kit

5. A pharmacist must complete a university program of at least:

    A. 2 years
    B. 3 years
    C. 4 years
    D. 6 years

6. The *Journal of Pharmacy Technology* is published by which of the following organizations?

   A. Pharmacy Technician Educators Council
   B. Pharmacy Technician Certification Board
   C. American Pharmacists Association
   D. American Council on Pharmaceutical Education

7. Today, pharmacists focus primarily on which of the following activities?

   A. counseling patients
   B. diagnosing disorders
   C. educating customers
   D. both A and C

8. Being qualified to do a specific type of work is referred to as:

   A. certified
   B. competent
   C. authorized
   D. administrative

9. The study of malignant tumors is called:

   A. cytology
   B. microbiology
   C. oncology
   D. biology

10. The study of medicine derived from natural sources is known as:

    A. pharmacognosy
    B. pharmacology
    C. pharmacodynamics
    D. pharmacopoeia

11. Which of the following terms means "placing bulk medications into unit doses"?

    A. dispensing
    B. registering
    C. repackaging
    D. labeling

12. Which of the following terms means "mixing and packaging a drug"?

    A. certifying
    B. licensing
    C. re-certifying
    D. compounding

13. Which of the following areas of pharmacy is concerned with research and development of new drug products?

    A. retail pharmacy
    B. institutional pharmacy
    C. industrial pharmacy
    D. nuclear pharmacy

14. The study of physical and chemical drug properties and their proper dosage related to onset, duration, and intensity of drug action is referred to as:

    A. biopharmaceutics
    B. pharmacognosy
    C. radioactivity
    D. radiopharmaceuticals

15. Which of the following terms is defined as "a system designed to ensure that products or services meet or exceed customer requirements"?

    A. repackaging
    B. quality control
    C. patient counseling
    D. cleaning log

Fill in the Blank

Use your knowledge of medical terminology to insert the correct term from the list below.

stocking	starter kits	quality control
licensure	dispensing	extemporaneous
labeling	authorization	certification
externship	cleaning log	ambulatory clinic
oncology	infusion devices	compounding

1. The study of cancer or malignant tumors is called
   _____.

2. The preparation and distribution of medications is referred to as _____.

3. Reconstituting, mixing, and packaging a drug is known as
   _____.

4. The recognition of competency in providing safe and effective patient care is called _____.

5. A system designed to ensure that products or services meet or exceed customer requirements is referred to as _____.

6. The power to give orders or make decisions is called _____.

7. The act of granting a license, usually to practice a profession, is known as _____.

8. A training program that is part of a course of study from an educational institution is called a(n) _____.

9. A type of compounding wherein medications are mixed in a pharmacy for a specific patient is referred to as _____ compounding.

10. Pieces of equipment that regulate intravenous solutions as they flow into the body are called _____.

True / False

Identify each of the following statements as true or false by placing a "T" or "F" on the line beside each number.

_____ 1. The Board of Pharmacy in each state regulates licenses to practice pharmacy.

_____ 2. For a pharmacist who wishes to become a researcher, a master's degree or PhD in pharmacy is usually required.

_____ 3. Pharmacy technicians practice only in community pharmacies or institutional pharmacies.

_____ 4. The pharmacy technician retains the ultimate responsibility over the pharmacy practice.

_____ 5. Pharmacy technicians have larger roles in the practice of pharmacy than ever before.

_____ 6. The national boards of pharmacy dictate which tasks pharmacy technicians can legally perform within their states.

_____ 7. Pharmacy technicians regularly fill medication doses and stock shelves.

_____ 8. In the home infusion pharmacy, pharmacy technicians handle intravenous administration to patients.

_____ **9.** The American Association of Pharmacy Technicians offers an examination requiring technicians to meet basic levels of skill in order to become certified.

_____**10.** Continuing education is required for technicians upon beginning practice.

Definitions

Define each of the following words in one sentence.

1. administrative: _____

2. compliance: _____

3. licensing: _____

4. Pharm.D: _____

5. vocational: _____

6. stocking: _____

7. registration: _____

8. quality control: _____

9. dispensing: _____

10. competency: _____

Abbreviations

Write the full meaning of each abbreviation.

Abbreviation	Meaning
1. UPS	_____
2. PTCE	_____
3. BOP	_____
4. AAPS	_____
5. ACPE	_____
6. AAPT	_____
7. APhA	_____
8. PTEC	_____
9. AACP	_____
10. ACCP	_____

Matching

Match each term with its correct definition by placing the corresponding letter on the line to its left.

_____ **1.** institutional pharmacy

_____ **2.** nuclear pharmacy

_____ **3.** industrial pharmacy

_____ **4.** ambulatory clinic

_____ **5.** patient counseling

_____ **6.** stocking

_____ **7.** radionuclide generators

_____ **8.** Board of Pharmacy

_____ **9.** extemporaneous

_____ **10.** oncology

A. supplying a certain amount of specified products or devices

B. devices that produce radionuclides

C. a type of compounding wherein medications are mixed in a pharmacy for a specific patient

D. in charge of regulating the practice of pharmacy within the state in which it is located

E. the study of cancer

F. the area of pharmacy concerned with preparing radioactive materials

G. the area of pharmacy concerned with research and development of new drug products

H. treats patients who can walk and are not bedridden

I. the sharing of information about a patient's health condition and therapies

J. the area of pharmacy contained within hospitals and other health care settings

Spelling

Circle the correct spelling from each pairing of words.

1. extempuraneous   extemporaneous
2. compitency   competency
3. institutional   institotional
4. pharmacoknosy   pharmacognosy
5. oncology   oncollogy
6. licensure   lisensure
7. dispensing   dispencing
8. radionucleide   radionuclide
9. vocasional   vocational
10. compliance   complianse

23 Advanced Pharmacy

OBJECTIVES

Upon completion of this chapter, the reader should be able to:

1. Describe nursing home settings and long-term care.
2. Explain pharmacy's role in long-term care.
3. Define *home health care*.
4. Describe a hospice pharmacy.
5. Explain nuclear pharmacy practice.
6. Interpret the meaning of the abbreviations presented in this chapter.
7. Define *telepharmacy* and its various types.
8. Describe federal pharmacy.

OVERVIEW

The practice of pharmacy has grown into new, non-traditional areas. These include home health care, long-term care, home infusion pharmacy, managed care, and hospice care. Other less familiar pharmacy practice areas include mail-order pharmacy, nuclear pharmacy, federal pharmacy, and telepharmacy. Each setting is unique, offering patients advanced pharmaceutical services. Pharmacy technicians may find employment in any of these practice settings, and advanced pharmacy offers expanded roles with increased levels of responsibility. It requires advanced knowledge and skills that are beyond the levels required in traditional community pharmacy practice settings.

TYPES OF SPECIAL PHARMACY SETTINGS

Advanced pharmacy settings require pharmacy technicians to have additional skills and familiarities with the types of work required. Different types of pharmacy settings are described below.

- *long-term care* – This is special care provided for an extended period of time. Long-term care patients include children with congenital conditions, adults recovering from trauma, those with chronic diseases, and those with mental or physical impairments. The goal of long-term care is to enable patients to maintain the ultimate possible level of functional independence.

- *ambulatory care* – This term includes outpatient pharmacies, emergency care facilities, primary care and specialty clinics, ambulatory care centers, and family practice groups. Ambulatory patients are able to walk and can obtain, store, and self-administer their own medications.

- *home health care* – This term relates to services and health-related products provided to a patient in his or her home. Home care services include drug therapy, nursing care, physical therapy, respiratory therapy, counseling, occupational therapy, hospice care, and the use of durable medical equipment. *Home care pharmacy* is a specialized area of pharmacy focused on treating patients in their own homes, usually coordinated by nurses or other home care personnel, often involving the use of intravenous drugs. Drugs commonly used in this setting include intravenous antibiotics, cancer chemotherapy, narcotics, hydration fluids, and either enteral or total parenteral nutrition.

- *home infusion* – Home infusion is a unique practice wherein infusion therapies are prepared and dispensed to a patient in his or her home. Home infusion pharmacy services include intravenous solution preparation, other injectable drug preparation, and enteral nutrition therapy.

- *hospice care* – Originally a facility usually found within a hospital that was designed to care for the terminally ill, particularly to offer emotional support, physical comfort and counseling, and social and spiritual support to these patients, a hospice pharmacy dispenses medications to patients either at home or in institutions. Hospice care focuses on making patients as comfortable as possible rather than trying to cure them.

- *mail-order* – A mail-order pharmacy is a licensed pharmacy that dispenses maintenance medications to members via delivery through the mail or overnight carriers and parcel services. Mail-order pharmacies operate at high volume, serving patients throughout the U.S. They often contract with insurance companies and offer prescriptions at discounted rates for members of insurance plans.

- *managed-care* – A system that provides both financing and delivery of health care services, managed-care pharmacy practice involves clinical and administrative activities within a managed-care organization, by a pharmacist. Prescriptions are coordinated through these organizations via approval boards.

- *nuclear* – A pharmacy that is specially licensed to work with radioactive materials, a nuclear pharmacy prepares, stores, and dispenses radiopharmaceuticals. Nuclear pharmacies tag radioactive elements to other drugs or chemicals for use in nuclear medicine. Previously, a "nuclear pharmacy" was known as a *radiopharmacy*.

- *telepharmacy* – Telepharmacy is the provision of pharmaceutical care to patients at a distance via the use of telecommunication and information technology. Pharmacy technicians fill prescriptions from remote pharmacies under the direction of pharmacists at a "base" pharmacy location, but without direct supervision.

GENERAL TERMINOLOGY RELATED TO ADVANCED PHARMACY

The following terms are used in advanced pharmacy practice settings.

Term	Pronunciation	Definition
adulterated drug	ah-DUHL-teh-ray-ted DRUG	a drug that is not pure
ambulatory infusion pump	AM-byoo-luh-toh-ree in-FYOO-zhun PUMP	an infusion device that is portable, and worn by the patient
breakdown area	BRAYK-down EH-ree-uh	the area in a nuclear pharmacy where empty or unused radiopharmaceutical containers are returned and dismantled to be re-used
chart review	CHART ree-VYOO	a drug regimen review
chemical impurity	KEH-mih-kul im-PYOO-rih-tee	the presence of a foreign chemical in a radiopharmaceutical
closed-shop pharmacy	KLOHZD-SHAWP FAR-muh-see	a pharmacy for only long-term care facility residents

compounding record	kum-POWN-ding REH-kord	the form used to record compounding activities in a home infusion pharmacy
consultant pharmacist	kun-SUHL-tant FAR-muh-sist	one who has special training to provide long-term pharmaceutical care
dose calibrator	DOHS KAH-lih-bray-tor	an instrument that measures radioactivity of a sample radionuclide during compounding of a radiopharmaceutical
dosimeter	doh-SIH-mih-ter	a personal monitoring device that measures radiation exposure to the individual
enteral nutrition	EN-teh-rul noo-TRIH-shun	nutrition delivered through a tube into the gastrointestinal tract
e-prescribing	EE-preh-SCRY-bing	transmission of a prescription, by using an electronic medium, between a physician and a pharmacist
federal pharmacist	FEH-deh-rul FAR-muh-sist	a licensed pharmacist who works as part of the federal government
feeding tube	FEE-ding TOOB	a hollow tube that passes food into the stomach
fume hood	FYOOM HOOD	a work station for compounding radiopharmaceuticals; also known as a *laminar-airflow hood*
infusion device	in-FYOO-zhun dee-VYS	a device that controls the infusion of intravenous solutions
in-house pharmacy	IN-HOWS FAR-muh-see	a closed-shop pharmacy inside a long-term care facility
Internet pharmacy	IN-ter-net FAR-muh-see	an established, commercial Web site allowing patients to obtain medications via the Internet
non-resident pharmacy	NON-REH-zih-dent FAR-muh-see	a pharmacy that mails, ships, or delivers prescriptions to patients from other states than where it is located
nursing facility	NER-sing fah-SIH-lih-tee	an institutional long-term care facility staffed by nurses
open-shop pharmacy	OH-pen-SHAWP FAR-muh-see	one that dispenses medications for both long-term care facility residents and for regular retail pharmacy patients
outpatient pharmacy	OUT-pay-shent FAR-muh-see	a pharmacy that serves outpatients
parenteral nutrition	pah-REN-teh-rul noo-TRIH-shun	nutrition provided through a vein directly into the bloodstream
pharmacy network	FAR-muh-see NET-werk	a group of pharmacies contracted to provide services to pharmacy members in exchange for a specified reimbursement
radioactive	ray-dee-oh-AK-tiv	releasing radiation
radioactive decay	ray-dee-oh-AK-tiv dee-KAY	the disintegration of a radionuclide as it returns to a stable state
radiopharmaceutical	ray-dee-oh-far-muh-SOO-tih-kul	a radioactive drug for the diagnosis and treatment of disease

ABBREVIATIONS

The following are common abbreviations related to advanced pharmacy.

Abbreviation	Meaning
DRR	drug regimen review
EN	enteral nutrition
GI	gastrointestinal
IV	intravenous
TPN	total parenteral nutrition

REVIEW EXERCISES

Multiple Choice

Select the best answer and write the letter of your choice to the left of each number.

1. Which of the following pharmacy settings is designed to care for terminally ill patients?

   A. home infusion
   B. home health care
   C. ambulatory care
   D. hospice care

2. A personal monitoring device that measures radiation exposure to an individual is referred to as a(n):

   A. endoscope
   B. dosimeter
   C. pacemaker
   D. microscope

3. A closed-shop pharmacy is a facility that serves:

   A. hospice residents
   B. ambulatory care patients
   C. mail-order patients
   D. long-term care facility residents

4. A group of pharmacies contracted to provide services to pharmacy members in exchange for a specified reimbursement is called a(n):

   A. pharmacy network
   B. non-resident pharmacy
   C. Internet pharmacy
   D. in-house pharmacy

5. A pharmacy that mails, ships, or delivers prescriptions to patients from other states than where it is located is referred to as a(n):

   A. in-house pharmacy
   B. outpatient pharmacy
   C. open-shop pharmacy
   D. non-resident pharmacy

6. Which type of pharmacy is also called *radiopharmacy*?

   A. telepharmacy
   B. nuclear pharmacy

    C. managed-care pharmacy
    D. mail-order pharmacy

7. Home infusion pharmacy services include:

    A. enteral nutrition therapy
    B. injectable drug preparation
    C. intravenous solution preparation
    D. all of the above

8. The disintegration of a radionuclide as it returns to a stable state is referred to as:

    A. radiopharmaceutical
    B. radioactive
    C. radioactive decay
    D. radiopharmacy

9. A federal pharmacist is a licensed pharmacist who works in:

    A. a mail-order pharmacy
    B. a pharmacy network
    C. a non-resident pharmacy
    D. a part of the federal government

10. The area in a nuclear pharmacy where empty radiopharmaceutical containers are dismantled to be re-used is called:

    A. the breakdown area
    B. the clean room
    C. the anteroom
    D. the open-shop area

Fill in the Blank

Use your knowledge of medical terminology to insert the correct term from the list below.

chart review	outpatient pharmacy	infusion device
adulterated drug	radioactive	dose calibrator
dosimeter	enteral nutrition	Internet pharmacy
e-prescribing	pharmacy network	in-house pharmacy
feeding tube	internet pharmacy	fume hood

1. A work station for compounding radiopharmaceuticals is called a(n) _____.

2. An instrument that measures radioactivity of a sample radionuclide is referred to as a(n) _____.

3. A drug regimen review is called a(n)

   _____.

4. Substances that release radiation are known as

   _____.

5. A closed-shop pharmacy inside a long-term care facility is called a(n) _____.

6. A pharmacy that serves outpatients is known as a(n)

   _____.

7. Transmission of a prescription by using an electronic medium is called _____.

8. A personal monitoring device that measures radiation exposure to an individual is referred to as a(n)

   _____.

9. A commercial Web site allowing patients to obtain medications via the Internet is called a(n)

   _____.

10. A drug that is not pure is referred to as a(n)

    _____.

True / False

Identify each of the following statements as true or false by placing a "T" or "F" on the line beside each number.

_____ 1. Nutrition provided through a vein directly into the bloodstream is known as *enteral nutrition*.

_____ 2. One who has special training to provide mail-order pharmacy services is called a *consultant pharmacist*.

_____ 3. A pharmacist who is licensed to work with radioactive materials is called a *nuclear pharmacist*.

_____ 4. A radioactive drug used for the diagnosis of diseases is referred to as a *radiopharmaceutical*.

_____ 5. The presence of a foreign chemical in a radiopharmaceutical is called *contamination*.

_____ 6. E-prescribing is transmission of a prescription by a federal pharmacist.

_____ 7. A device that controls the infusion of intravenous drugs is called an *infusion device*.

_____ **8.** An infusion device that is portable and worn by the patient is referred to as an *ambulatory infusion pump*.

_____ **9.** A compounding record is a form used to record medication errors in a home infusion pharmacy.

_____ **10.** A pharmacy that services as an in-house pharmacy is known as an *outpatient pharmacy*.

Definitions

Define each of the following words in one sentence.

1. long-term care pharmacy: _____

2. hospice care pharmacy: _____

3. nuclear pharmacy: _____

4. telepharmacy: _____

5. mail-order pharmacy: _____

6. nursing facility: _____

7. chemical impurity: _____

8. feeding tube: _____

9. infusion device: _____

10. breakdown area: _____

Abbreviations

Write the full meaning of each abbreviation.

Abbreviation	Meaning
1. IV	_____
2. GI	_____
3. DRR	_____
4. TPN	_____
5. EN	_____

Matching

Match each term with its correct definition by placing the corresponding letter on the line to its left.

_____ 1. non-resident pharmacy

_____ 2. in-house pharmacy

_____ 3. dose calibrator

_____ 4. pharmacy network

_____ 5. enteral nutrition

_____ 6. fume hood

_____ 7. radioactive

_____ 8. Internet pharmacy

_____ 9. open-shop pharmacy

_____ 10. dosimeter

A. a work station for compounding radiopharmaceuticals

B. nutrition delivered through a tube into the gastrointestinal tract

C. a personal monitoring device that measures radiation exposure to an individual

D. releasing radiation

E. an established, commercial Web site allowing patients to obtain medications via the Internet

F. dispenses medications for both long-term care facility residents and retail pharmacy customers

G. a closed-shop pharmacy inside a long-term care facility

H. a pharmacy that mails, ships, or delivers prescriptions to patients in states other than the one in which it is located

I. a group of pharmacies contracted to provide services to pharmacy members in exchange for a specified reimbursement

J. measures radioactivity of a sample radionuclide during compounding of a radiopharmaceutical

Spelling

Circle the correct spelling from each pairing of words.

1. hospice   hospise
2. telopharmacy   telepharmacy
3. radiopharmacy   radiapharmacy
4. ambuletory   ambulatory
5. terminaly   terminally
6. dosemeter   dosimeter
7. reimbursement   reimbursment
8. nucular   nuclear
9. radionuclide   radionucleide
10. addulterated   adulterated

Pharmacy Laboratory Procedures

OBJECTIVES

Upon completion of this chapter, the reader should be able to:

1. Describe graduates, compounding slabs, beakers, and their uses.
2. Explain the various types of compounding.
3. Describe the clean room in the pharmacy setting, and its purpose.
4. Describe sterile products and aseptic technique.
5. Define *class A prescription balances* and *counter balances*.
6. Explain laminar-airflow hoods.
7. Interpret the meaning of the abbreviations presented in this chapter.
8. Describe extemporaneous compounding.

OVERVIEW

Compounding means "the preparation, mixing, assembling, packaging, or labeling of a drug or device." Compounded prescriptions are medicines that must be prepared by a pharmacist. Compounded prescriptions may be lotions, ointments, suppositories, capsules, solutions, or other forms. Today, pharmacy technicians play important roles in compounding. They must receive special training and education to assist pharmacists in compounding activities.

COMPOUNDING PRACTICES

Pharmacy technicians maximize the therapeutic effects of drugs by using drug knowledge and patient information. They must understand drug action and how prescriptions are structured. To prepare and package drugs correctly, they must be familiar with many different prescription and non-prescription drugs, drug references, drug classifications, drug routes, and various drug forms. Pharmacy technicians must be aware of various factors that affect compounding, because they play assistive roles in the preparation and dispensing of compounded medications.

Pharmaceutical compounding is increasing due to a limited number of dosage forms and drug strengths, a shortage of drug products and combinations, increasing special patient populations, and growing home health care and hospice environments. Compounding may involve oral liquids, topical creams, ointments, and suppositories. It may require conversion of dosage forms, preparation of dosage forms from bulk chemicals, and preparation for the use of various drug administration devices. Intravenous admixtures, parenteral nutrition solutions, pediatric dosage forms, and radioactive isotopes are all commonly compounded in pharmacies.

EQUIPMENT AND SUPPLIES FOR COMPOUNDING

Each type of equipment used in medication compounding must be correct and appropriate in design, size, and location for ease of use. They must be able to be easily cleaned and maintained. Pharmacy technicians should be familiar with the pieces of equipment that are necessary for compounding drugs. The following are types of equipment and supplies used in extemporaneous compounding and for sterile products.

Antimicrobial preservatives – substances that keep solutions and other mixtures free from infiltration by microbes; common antimicrobial preservatives include phenol and benzyl alcohol

Aseptic technique – specific practices and techniques performed under controlled conditions to minimize contamination by pathogens

Auxiliary labels – labels that indicate specific information about a pharmacy product, such as route of administration, expiration information, dietary information, usage instructions, warnings, pricing, legal information, dosage information, etc.

Beaker tongs – devices resembling ice tongs; used for transporting beakers without allowing them to come in contact with the hands or potential contaminants

Beakers – simple liquid containers, usually cylindrical in shape, with flat bases; primarily used to mix and melt substances

Blenders – electrical appliances with rotating blades for mixing; used to mix or split substances and may be either high-energy or low-energy

Brushes – devices consisting of bristles attached to a handle; brushes are used for sampling, cleaning, and microbrushing in pharmacy, microbiology, and other fields

Capsule-filling equipment – manual or automated machinery that can fill medicine capsules; used to put medications and other ingredients into capsule shells and then seal the capsule halves together so that they can be administered

Carts – heavy, two-wheeled, stainless steel vehicles, usually without springs; used to transport and/or store medications using 6-inch swivel wheels and brakes

Class A prescription balances – one- or two-pan torsion scales or balances that may be digital (electronic weight sensing) or spring-based in design; used for weighing medicinal (and other) substances required for prescriptions, or for other pharmaceutical compounding

Clean room – a work area that features highly regulated air quality, temperature, and humidity; used for compounding of medications and other products that require extremely contaminant-free states

Cocoa butter – a solid, oil-based product that melts at 34°C (93.2°F); commonly used as a base for suppositories

Counter balances – double-pan balances; used to weigh large quantities of bulk products, and are not indicated for prescription compounding

Crimpers – devices resembling pliers that can seal various containers; used to seal capped containers such as vials

Decappers – also known as "decrimpers," they resemble pliers; used to remove seals from capped containers such as vials

Droppers – plastic tubes attached to rubber bulbs that provide suction or propulsion when squeezed; used to deliver small doses of liquid medication

Dry baths – incubators that are used for a variety of applications in the laboratory, including denaturing **deoxyribonucleic acid**, melting various substances, and other uses; various types of dry baths may either heat or chill substances

Drying ovens – ovens containing several racks that are housed in steel panels; used for general laboratory drying, sterilization, stress testing, moisture analysis, and curing

Drying racks – racks with stainless steel pegboards and/or glassware drying racks, drip troughs, and catch drains; used to air-dry various types of equipment

Electronic single-pan balances – easier to use and more accurate than traditional double-pan torsion balances; used for weighing various laboratory-related substances

Ethyl alcohol (ethanol) – a clear, colorless, flammable type of alcohol that boils at 78°F, and has a characteristic odor; used as a solvent vehicle for the preparation of pharmaceutical dosage forms for internal or external use; an effective antiseptic-disinfectant, being germicidal in concentrations above 60%; its usual concentration as an antiseptic-disinfectant is 70%

Extemporaneous compounding – preparing, mixing, assembling, packaging, and labeling of drug products based on prescription orders from licensed practitioners for individual patients

Filters – usually devices made of paper or similar substances; used to trap undesired particles from solutions, drugs, and other substances

Forceps – devices that resemble tweezers; used to pick up prescription weights and other equipment in the laboratory

Funnel – tube with a wide mouth and a narrow bottom; used when pouring liquids from one container to another, usually with filter papers to remove particles

Glassine paper – a weighing paper with a smooth, shiny surface that does not absorb materials; used to easily transfer drugs and chemicals onto and off weighing pans

Gloves – protective gloves that may be made of latex, nylon, polyurethane, cotton, vinyl, or other substances; used to protect the hands from contaminants, electrostatic discharge, contact with allergens, temperatures, hazardous materials, and other substances

Glycerin – a sweet, colorless, oily fluid that is a pharmaceutical grade of glycerol; used as a moistening agent for chapped skin, as an ingredient of suppositories for constipation, and as a sweetening agent and vehicle for drug preparations; also spelled *glycerine*; glycerin suppositories are occasionally used vaginally, though they are not for rectal use

Glycols – alcohols that contain two hydroxyl groups; ethylene glycol is used in organic synthesis, fractionation, purification, and crystallization procedures

Graduates – conical graduates have wide tops and thinner bases, while cylindrical graduates are designed with a narrow diameter that is the same from top to base; used to measure liquids in the laboratory, and feature calibrated measurements

Hazardous waste – a solid waste that may threaten humans and/or the environment when improperly handled, due to its concentration, quantity, or characteristics

Heat guns – devices that resemble hair dryers; commonly used in the laboratory to heat temperature-sensitive materials, cure resins, and melt certain substances

Heat sealers – devices that consist of a heating surface and a movable "arm" that presses the object to be sealed between; primarily used to seal plastic containers such as bags to form a strong seal that keeps contents free from contact with the environment

High-efficiency particulate air filters – high-efficiency air filters that can remove more than 99 percent of airborne particles 0.3 micrometers or larger in diameter; used in laminar-airflow hoods to filter rapidly moving air

Homogenizers – bench-mounted or handheld devices that resemble mixers; used to blend, mix, and process various substances

Hot plates – small electric heating surfaces used to warm substances or keep them at a constant temperature; in the laboratory, substances are placed into glassware that is then put onto a hot plate – many lab hot plates use magnetic stirrers as part of their design

Intravenous bags – *polyvinyl chloride* bags used to hold fluids for intravenous administration

Intravenous tubing – plastic tubing used to transfer intravenous fluids from an IV bag or bottle to either a patient or another container

Isopropyl alcohol – a transparent, colorless, flammable liquid with a characteristic odor that is an effective disinfectant in concentrations equal or above 70 percent, and somewhat superior to ethyl alcohol as an antiseptic; used externally on body surfaces, and may also be used as a solvent-vehicle for drugs being formulated into topical products

Laminar airflow hoods – work stations that emit fast-flowing, HEPA-filtered air either horizontally or vertically (HEPA stands for "high-efficiency particulate air"); used for all types of sterile procedures

Locker facilities – an area where personnel involved in compounding sterile preparations can change their clothing before entering a clean room

Masks – cloths that cover the face and facial hair; used to prevent contamination of patients and work areas from the nose and mouth during procedures

Mortars – bowl-like vessels in which substances are crushed or ground with a cylindrical device known as a "pestle"

Ointment slabs – ground glass or porcelain plates that provide a hard, non-absorbable surface for mixing substances

Personal protective equipment – clothing, head coverings, goggles, and other equipment designed to protect from injury or infection in the work environment

Pestles – heavy, cylindrical, stick-like devices usually with an enlarged end; designed to crush or grind substances within a mortar

Pipettes – laboratory instruments that range from single-piece glass to complex instruments featuring pumps or electronic designs; used to transport measured amounts of liquids

Port adapters – also known as *male adapters*, these devices are external additive ports attached to an IV bag's additive post; used to inject different additives into an IV bag

Preservatives – substances used to preserve the quality and usability of medications or other substances; the most commonly used preservative is *benzyl alcohol*

Professional mixers – devices used to thoroughly mix substances, by rotation of blades, magnetic waves, or other methods

Purified water – a clear, colorless, odorless liquid; used as a solvent-vehicle for the preparation of pharmaceutical dosage forms for internal or external use

Quality assurance – activities ensuring that the procedures used in preparing compounded products result in products that will meet specific standards

Quality control – a set of testing activities used to determine the quality of compounded products

Refrigerators and freezers – specially designed units that maintain constant temperatures to cool or freeze substances at predetermined levels; many drugs and compounded sterile preparations require refrigeration to maintain stability, and some sterile preparations must be kept frozen to extend their stability and shelf life

Ringer's solution – a solution of recently boiled distilled water, sodium chloride, potassium chloride, and calcium chloride; commonly used to sustain tissue health and function

Safety glasses – also known as *safety goggles*, these are devices worn to protect the eyes from particulates, chemicals, and other substances

Sharps containers – red plastic containers used to deposit used medical needles, IV catheters, and other sharp medical instruments

Spatulas – utensils with long handles and flattened edges used for lifting substances during mixing or spreading

Spray bottles – devices that enable liquids to be sprayed through a pumping assembly; commonly used to spray cleaning fluids onto surfaces

Spring-based balances – devices used for weighing that operate by using spring tension

Sterile compounding – compounding using aseptic technique and a clean room environment to ensure that products are completely free of pathogens

Sterile products – pathogen-free drugs and drug products; these include medications for injection, aqueous and oil vehicles for injection, ophthalmic solutions, intravenous admixtures, inhalation solutions, irrigation solutions, and injected vitamins or minerals

Sterile purified water – a clear, colorless, odorless liquid; used as a solvent-vehicle for the preparation of pharmaceutical dosage forms, either for internal or external use

Sterile water for injection – a sterile, non-pyrogenic preparation of water for injection; used after addition of drugs that require dilution or that must be dissolved in an aqueous vehicle prior to injection

Stirring rods – rods made of glass, rubber, polypropylene, or bendable Teflon; used to stir a variety of solutions or mixtures in the laboratory

Tablet molds – metal devices used to form tablets; a tablet mold consists of a cavity plate, in which the tablet medication mixture is placed, and a peg plate, which pushes the formed tablets out of the mold

Tongs – commonly, tongs are steel devices used for picking up hot items, or those that cannot be safely lifted using the hands; types of tongs include crucible, laboratory, and beaker tongs

Ultrasonic cleaners – devices that use the process of *cavitation* to remove debris from various types of equipment; this process involves introducing high-intensity, high-frequency sound waves into a cleaning solution that envelops the objects to be cleaned

Vented spike adapters – devices used to vent glass bottles that are attached to intravenous tubing; vented tubing is used commonly to transfer the contents of one container to another

Weighing papers and boats – placed onto balance pans to contain drugs or chemicals to be weighed; used to protect balance pans from harmful or corrosive chemicals, or for preventing cross-contamination of drugs and chemicals

Weights – stainless steel weights used to accurately verify the mass of a substance; though available in different measurement systems, metric weights are the most common

GENERAL TERMINOLOGY RELATED TO COMPOUNDING

The following are common terms that relate to pharmacy compounding.

Term	Pronunciation	Definition
admixture	ad-MIKS-chur	a mixture of several ingredients
anteroom	AN-tee-room	a room located immediately outside of a clean room
aseptic	ah-SEP-tik	free of pathogenic microorganisms
autoclaved	AW-toh-klayvd	heated in an autoclave (a pressured device that boils substances to achieve sterilization)
beaker	BEE-ker	a cylindrical glass vessel with a "pouring lip" used for mixing and holding chemical substances
biohazard	BY-oh-hah-zard	a biological agent or condition that may harm humans or the environment
bolus	BOH-lus	an initial dose
calibration	kah-lih-BRAY-shun	the set of gradients that show position or value
compatibility	kom-pah-tih-BIH-lih-tee	capable of forming a stable chemical or biochemical system

compounding	kom-POWN-ding	to mix by combining two or more parts
cytotoxic	sy-toh-TOK-sik	toxic to cells
decontamination	dee-kon-tah-mih-NAY-shun	cleaning or deactivating by using alcohol or sodium hypochlorite (bleach)
deoxyribonucleic acid	dee-ok-see-ry-boh-noo-KLAY-ik AS-sid	a large, double-stranded helical molecule that is the carrier of genetic information
dextrose	DEKS-trohs	glucose; the sugar that is the chief source of energy in the human body
disinfectant	dih-sin-FEK-tant	an agent or chemical that is able to destroy, neutralize, or inhibit the growth of microorganisms
disposable product	dih-SPOH-suh-bul PRAW-dukt	designed to be disposed of after use
disposal	dih-SPOH-sul	the process of getting rid of a substance or object
distilled water	dih-STILD WAW-ter	water that has been purified by the process of distillation (the evaporation and subsequent collection of a liquid by condensation)
emulsion	ee-MUHL-shun	a suspension of small globules of one liquid inside another with which it will not mix
extemporaneous	ex-tem-poh-RAY-nee-us	a type of compounding wherein drug products are compounded based on prescription orders from licensed practitioners for individual patients
garment	GAR-ment	a fabric device used in health care practice; garments include gowns, lab coats, mats, linens, and scrubs
germicidal	jer-mih-SY-dul	killing pathogenic microorganisms; or, an agent that kills pathogenic microorganisms
gowning	GOW-ning	the donning of protective garments to guard against contamination, prevent the spread of infection, or act as protective barriers during medical procedures
graduate	GRAH-dyoo-ut	a graduated container, usually cylindrical in shape
homogenizer	hoh-MAW-jeh-ny-zer	a piece of electronic equipment, similar to a mixer or blender, that reduces particle size
infusion	in-FYOO-zhun	the passive introduction of a substance into a vein or between tissues
intravenous push	in-trah-VEE-nus PUSH	a method of intravenous injection wherein a syringe is connected to an IV access device and the medication is injected directly
irrigation	ih-rih-GAY-shun	a solution used for washing or cleaning out
large-volume parenteral	LARJ-VOL-yoom pah-REN-teh-rul	single-unit doses for injection that are greater than 100 mL in volume
levigate	LEH-vih-gayt	to make into a smooth, fine powder or paste, as by grinding when moist

(continues)

Term	Pronunciation	Definition
lozenge	LAW-zenj	a small, medicated candy to be dissolved slowly in the mouth for localized effects upon the mouth or throat; a *troche*
magma	MAG-muh	a suspension of particles in a liquid, an example of which is Milk of Magnesia
micelle	my-SELL	a large water drop surrounded by oil formation
miscible	MIH-sih-bul	susceptible to being mixed
ointment	OYNT-ment	a highly viscous or semisolid substance used on the skin as a *salve*
ophthalmic	off-THAL-mik	of or relating to the eye
piggyback	PIH-gee-bak	a supplementary ("added on") type of intravenous infusion
reconstitute	ree-KON-stih-toot	to mix a powdered agent with a diluent to form a liquid medication
reusable product	ree-YOO-zih-bul PRAW-dukt	does not need to be disposed of after a single use
sepsis	SEP-sis	the presence of microorganisms in the blood
shelf life	SHELF LYF	the length of time that a product may be used before it is considered unsuitable for use
small-volume parenteral	SMALL-VOL-yoom pah-REN-teh-rul	single-unit doses for injection that are less than 100 mL in volume
solubility	SAWL-yoo-bih-lih-tee	the degree of being able to dissolve into a substance
solvent	SAWL-vent	a substance that is capable of dissolving another substance
stability	stah-BIH-lih-tee	a state wherein a substance is not reactive in the environment or during normal use, retaining its useful properties
sterile	STEH-ril	aseptic; free from all living bacteria or other microorganisms and their spores
suspension	sus-PEN-shun	a mixture wherein one of the ingredients does not mix completely with the other(s); most suspensions should be shaken well before use
total parenteral nutrition	TOH-tul pah-REN-teh-rul noo-TRIH-shun	the practice of intravenous feeding, via a formula that contains glucose, amino acids, lipids, salts, vitamins, and other substances
trituration	try-tyoo-RAY-shun	the process of reducing the particle size of a substance by grinding it
troche	TROH-kee	a lozenge intended to be dissolved slowly in the mouth for localized effects
viscosity	vis-CAW-sih-tee	a physical property of fluids that determines the internal resistance to shear forces
volatile	VAW-lah-til	a substance that may give off vapors or fumes at room temperature, and may be otherwise unstable

ABBREVIATIONS

The following are common abbreviations that relate to pharmacy compounding.

Abbreviation	Meaning
comp	compound
DNA	deoxyribonucleic acid
DW	distilled water
D_5LR	dextrose 5% in lactated Ringer's
D_5NS	dextrose 5% in normal saline (0.9% sodium chloride)
D_5W	dextrose 5% in water
$D_{10}W$	dextrose 10% in water
HEPA	high-efficiency particulate air
IV bag	intravenous bag
LAFH	laminar-airflow hood
PVC	polyvinyl chloride
QA	quality assurance
QC	quality control
TPN	total parenteral nutrition
USP <797>	United States Pharmacopoeia Chapter 797 (sterile compounding)

REVIEW EXERCISES

Multiple Choice

Select the best answer and write the letter of your choice to the left of each number.

1. Which of the following devices resembles tweezers?

    A. pestle
    B. crimper
    C. drying rack
    D. forceps

2. A ground glass object that provides a hard, non-absorbable surface for mixing substances is referred to as a(n):

    A. stirring rod
    B. spatula
    C. tablet mold
    D. ointment slab

3. Which of the following devices are worn to protect the eyes from chemicals?

    A. safety gloves
    B. safety goggles
    C. safety masks
    D. laboratory coats

4. Which of the following devices is used to crush or grind substances?

    A. mortar
    B. homogenizer
    C. graduate
    D. funnel

5. Which of the following products is a solid, oil-based substance that melts at 93.2°F and commonly is used as a base for suppositories?

    A. glassine paper
    B. glycerin
    C. glycol
    D. cocoa butter

6. A sweet, colorless, oil fluid that is a pharmaceutical grade of glycerol is called:

    A. ethanol
    B. cocoa butter
    C. glycerin
    D. glycogen

7. Utensils with long handles and flattened edges used for lifting substances during mixing or spreading are referred to as:

   A. forceps
   B. spatulas
   C. tongs
   D. brushes

8. An initial dose of medication is called a:

   A. magma
   B. miscible
   C. lozenge
   D. bolus

9. The process of reducing the particle size of a substance by grinding it is known as:

   A. trituration
   B. fermentation
   C. habituation
   D. hyperhydration

10. Devices used in the laboratory that resemble ice tongs are called:

    A. blenders
    B. crimpers
    C. brushes
    D. beaker tongs

11. A physical property of fluids that determines the internal resistance of shear forces is referred to as:

    A. infusion
    B. germicidal
    C. viscosity
    D. solubility

12. Which of the following is not a factor related to increased pharmaceutical compounding?

    A. a shortage of drug products and combinations
    B. increasing special patient populations
    C. increasing number of pregnant women
    D. a limited number of dosage forms

13. Which of the following devices is used to remove seals on capped containers such as vials?

    A. crimpers
    B. droppers
    C. decappers
    D. filters

14. Heat sealers are primarily used to seal containers made of:

    A. plastic
    B. glass
    C. steel
    D. copper

15. Isopropyl alcohol is an effective disinfectant in concentrations equal to or above:

    A. 10%
    B. 25%
    C. 60%
    D. 70%

Fill in the Blank

Use your knowledge of medical terminology to insert the correct term from the list below.

spatula	pipette	funnel
port adapter	forceps	cocoa butter
mask	counter balance	blender
slab	beaker	mortar
graduate	hot plate	pestle

1. A device used to mix or split substances with low or high energy is called a(n) _____.

2. A container primarily used to mix and melt substances is referred to as a(n) _____.

3. A utensil with a long handle and a flattened edge used for lifting substances during mixing or spreading is known as a(n) _____.

4. Heavy, cylindrical, stick-like devices, usually with enlarged ends are called _____.

5. A solid, oil-based product is referred to as

   _____.

6. A ground glass or porcelain plate that provides a hard, non-absorbable surface for mixing substances is called a(n)

   _____.

7. A male adapter is also called a(n) _____.

8. A laboratory instrument used to transport measured amounts of liquids is known as a(n) _____.

9. A bowl-like vessel used for crushing or grinding substances is called a(n) _____.

10. A device used to weigh large quantities of bulk products is referred to as a(n) _____.

True / False

Identify each of the following statements as true or false by placing a "T" or "F" on the line beside each number.

_____ 1. Glycerin is a sweet, colorless fluid that is a pharmaceutical grade of benzyl alcohol.

_____ 2. The most commonly used preservative is cocoa butter.

_____ 3. Counter balances are used to weigh large quantities of bulk products.

_____ 4. A clean room is a work area that features highly regulated air quality, temperature, and humidity.

_____ 5. Class A prescription balances are made of only two-pan torsion scales that may be digital or spring-based in design.

_____ 6. A plastic tube attached to a rubber bulb that provides suction when squeezed and is used to deliver small doses of liquid medication is referred to as a *decapper*.

_____ 7. Ethanol is an effective antiseptic disinfectant.

_____ 8. A weighing paper with a smooth, shiny surface that does not absorb materials is called *glassine paper*.

_____ 9. A hazardous waste is a solid waste that may threaten humans or the environment when improperly handled.

_____ 10. A high-efficiency air filter can remove more than 50 percent of airborne particles 0.3 micrometers or smaller in diameter.

Definitions

Define each of the following words in one sentence.

1. sterile products: _____

2. tongs: _____

3. quality control: _____

    4. professional mixer: _____

    5. HEPA filter: _____

    6. glycol: _____

    7. dry bath: _____

    8. glassine paper: _____

    9. forceps: _____

    10. crimper: _____

Abbreviations

Write the full meaning of each abbreviation.

Abbreviation	Meaning
1. QA	_____
2. USP <797>	_____
3. HEPA	_____
4. DW	_____
5. comp	_____
6. PVC	_____
7. LAFH	_____
8. DNA	_____
9. D_5LR	_____
10. TPN	_____

Matching

Match each term with its correct definition by placing the corresponding letter on the line to its left.

_____ **1.** troche

_____ **2.** magma

_____ **3.** trituration

_____ **4.** piggyback

_____ **5.** garment

_____ **6.** bolus

_____ **7.** admixture

A. the presence of microorganisms in the blood

B. a fabric device used in health-care practice (such as lab coats and scrubs)

C. the passive introduction of a substance into a vein or between tissues

_____ **8.** infusion

_____ **9.** micelle

_____ **10.** sepsis

D. susceptible to being mixed

E. a suspension of particles in a liquid

F. an initial dose

G. the process of reducing the particle size of a substance by grinding it

H. a mixture of several ingredients

I. a supplementary type of intravenous infusion

J. a lozenge intended to be dissolved slowly in the mouth for localized effects

Spelling

Circle the correct spelling from each pairing of words.

1.	dicontamination	decontamination
2.	emolsion	emulsion
3.	extemporaneous	extemperaneous
4.	pigyback	piggyback
5.	lozenge	losenge
6.	homogeniser	homogenizer
7.	levigate	levygate
8.	troche	truche
9.	riconstitute	reconstitute
10.	gowning	guwning

Pharmacy Law

OBJECTIVES

Upon completion of this chapter, the reader should be able to:

1. Describe the purpose of the Pure Food and Drug Act.
2. Explain why knowledge of the law is important to pharmacy technicians.
3. Identify the sources of law.
4. Describe state law as it relates to pharmacy operation.
5. Explain the Controlled Substances Act.
6. Describe the Kefauver-Harris Amendment.
7. Interpret the meanings of the abbreviations presented in this chapter.
8. Identify the reason that Congress adopted the Harrison Narcotics Tax Act.

OVERVIEW

Pharmacy law has developed from many different sources. Important federal laws that pertain to pharmacy include the Food, Drug, and Cosmetic Act; the Controlled Substances Act; and the Poison Prevention Packaging Act. At the state level, pharmacy practice acts and codes regulate pharmacy operation. Several regulatory agencies have the authority to control pharmacy practice using regulations that have the force of law.

Laws that come from previous court decisions and interpret statutory and regulatory laws, or make new laws, are called "common" or "judge-made" laws, and were derived from the English court system. Civil law governs the relationships between individuals within society. Two subdivisions of civil law that affect pharmacists, pharmacy technicians, and pharmacy practice are contract law and tort law. Criminal law governs the relationship between an individual and society.

FEDERAL LAWS

The federal government enacts and interprets laws concerning the general public. Over the past 100 years, many federal laws and amendments have been enacted, shaping the current laws of today. These federal laws are as follows:

- **Pure Food and Drug Act of 1906**   This act prohibited interstate distribution or sale of **adulterated** (adding other ingredients) or **misbranded** (branded or labeled fraudulently) food and drugs. *Adulteration* is more completely defined as "tampering with or contaminating a product or substance." The Pure Food and Drug Act also prevented the manufacture, sale, or transportation of **impure**, misbranded, poisonous, or harmful drugs, foods, liquors, and medicines. This act also controlled the trafficking of these substances.

- **Harrison Narcotics Tax Act of 1914**   This act was implemented to regulate and tax the distribution, importation, and production of **opiates**. These substances include opium and products such as cocaine that are derived from coca plants.

- **Food, Drug, and Cosmetic Act of 1938**   The 1937 sulfanilamide tragedy influenced the passage of this act, under which pharmaceutical manufacturers were required to file a **New Drug Application** (NDA) with the Food and Drug Administration (FDA) for each new drug. Manufacturers had to ensure the packaging, purity, safety, and strength of their drugs, and foods and cosmetics were also regulated.

- **Durham-Humphrey Amendment of 1951**   This act created an exemption for drugs that could not be safely labeled for use. Drugs could not be dispensed without prescriptions, but specific drugs were not indicated by this amendment. It required that drugs intended for use by humans that were not safe to use without medical supervision be dispensed only via prescription, and bear the legend "℞". Drugs marketed as "by prescription only" were to be considered "misbranded" if dispensed without a prescription.

- **Kefauver-Harris Amendment of 1963**   This amendment to the Food, Drug, and Cosmetic Act of 1938 required that drug products (both prescription and non-prescription) must be effective, pure, and safe. Prescription drug advertising was required to be supervised by the FDA, and the qualifications of drug investigators became subject to review.

- **Comprehensive Drug Abuse Prevention and Control Act of 1970**   This act required the pharmaceutical industry to maintain physical security and strict record keeping for many drugs, and divided controlled substances into five schedules. Substances in Schedule I have the highest abuse potential, and Schedule V substances have the least. Any person involved in handling controlled substances is required to obtain a DEA registration, with the DEA limiting the amount of Schedule I and II substances that can be manufactured in the United States in a 1-year period. Anyone dispensing, distributing, or manufacturing controlled substances unlawfully is liable for prosecution under the Controlled Substances Act.

- **Poison Prevention Packaging Act of 1970**   This act created standards for child-resistant packaging, requiring nearly all **legend drugs**, and some OTC drugs, to be packaged in a manner so that they cannot be opened by most children younger than 5 years of age, but can be easily opened by most adults. This act was established due to prior poisonings, with aspirin being the first substance that had to be packaged with child-resistant lids.

- **Occupational Safety and Health Act of 1970**   This act was designed to prevent workplace diseases and injuries, and to ensure employee safety and health. It also established the Occupational Safety and Health Administration (which is also known as OSHA). The act requires employers to provide safe and healthy working conditions and environments.

- **Drug Listing Act of 1972**   This act assigned each drug a unique, permanent, 11-digit **National Drug Code** (NDC) number identifying the manufacturer or distributor, drug formulation, and size and type of packaging used. The FDA uses these numbers to maintain a drug database, and NDC numbers cannot be used for a product if any changes concerning the product's characteristics occur; a new number must be obtained for the modified product.

- **Medical Device Amendment of 1976**   This amendment classified medical devices and set up various "risk levels" depending upon their function. Life-sustaining and life-supporting devices were required to have pre-market approval by the FDA prior to becoming available for use. This amendment was chiefly influenced by problems with pacemakers and intrauterine devices (IUDs).

- **Resource Conservation and Recovery Act of 1976**   This act (also known as the Solid Waste Disposal Act) regulates the handling and disposal of solid wastes. It also authorizes environmental agencies to handle contaminated site cleanups and regulates solid-waste landfills. It was established due to disposal of hazardous wastes in ways that could harm the environment as well as potentially poison humans and animals.

- **Orphan Drug Act of 1983** This act offers financial incentives to developers of drugs that treat diseases and conditions affecting fewer than 200,000 people in the United States. These **orphan drugs** include those used to treat AIDS, blepharospasm, cystic fibrosis, snakebites, and other conditions. The act also offers tax breaks and a 7-year monopoly on drug sales in order to encourage orphan drug research, development, and marketing.

- **Drug Price Competition and Patent Term Restoration Act of 1984** This act gave generic drug marketers the ability to file "abbreviated new drug applications" for FDA approval, giving them more incentives to offset the time and money required to bring their new drugs to market. It extended most drug patents by 5 years. Generic versions of innovator drugs previously approved by the FDA could be approved without the manufacturer's having to submit a full NDA.

- **Prescription Drug Marketing Act of 1987** This act ensured that prescription drug products must be safe, effective, untainted, not counterfeited, and not misbranded. It protects the ability of manufacturers to maintain different pricing of drugs for different market segments, and allows for effective control of drug sources. It also regulates methods of selling certain drugs and controls the actions of participating companies and individuals.

- **Omnibus Budget Reconciliation Act of 1990 (OBRA-90)** This act affected Medicare and Medicaid costs by reducing inappropriate use of drugs for program participants. It also created a tax limit cap on taxable income of approximately $102,000. It requires Medicaid pharmacy providers to obtain, record, and maintain basic patient information, as well as expands rules about drug products to ensure safe, effective drug therapy. It also requires pharmacists to offer patient counseling and drug therapy review.

- **FDA Safe Medical Devices Act of 1990** This act gives the FDA greater regulatory capacity concerning medical devices and diagnostic products, requiring medical device reports to be filed on a timely basis. It established pre-market approval procedures concerning these devices and increased civil penalties for those violating the medical device policies of the Food, Drug, and Cosmetic Act.

- **Anabolic Steroids Control Act of 1990**   This act allowed the Controlled Substances Act to regulate anabolic steroids, the hormonal substances that promote muscle growth and are often used illegally by athletes. These "performance-enhancing drugs" have been shown to have serious health consequences when overused, and this act offered harsher penalties for abuse and misuse of anabolic steroids as a result.

- **Americans with Disabilities Act of 1990**   This act prohibits discrimination against the disabled, focusing on employment, public services and accommodations, transportation, commercial facilities, and telecommunications, among other areas. The ADA ensures that the disabled receive assistance in order to lead relatively normal lives, and also protects them against treatment that would not be given to completely normal individuals, including pre-employment examinations.

- **Dietary Supplement Health and Education Act of 1994 (DSHEA)**   This act amended the Food, Drug, and Cosmetic Act by changing the way in which dietary supplements can be labeled and regulated. The DSHEA holds supplement manufacturers responsible for the safety of their products, including amino acids, botanicals such as herbs, some hormones, minerals, vitamins, and others. It also affects the displaying, stocking, and recommendation of supplements.

- **Health Insurance Portability and Accountability Act (HIPAA) of 1996**   This act improved continuity and portability of health insurance, and was designed to focus on reduction of **fraudulent** activities, establish medical savings accounts, improve long-term health care access, and simplify health care administration. It is divided into three parts: "privacy regulations," "security regulations," and "transaction standards." Prior to HIPAA, many employees who changed or lost their jobs could not continue to have health insurance coverage.

- **FDA Modernization Act of 1997**   This act reformed the regulation of cosmetics, food, and medical products by focusing mostly on safe pharmacy compounding, food safety, regulation of medical devices, and user fees. It increased patient access to medical devices and experimental drugs, and gave manufacturers 6-month extensions on new pediatric drugs that had drug trial testing data on file. It also mandated risk assessment reviews of mercury-containing foods and drugs, and required legend drug manufacturers to label their packaging with the "℞" symbol.

- **Medicare Prescription Drug, Improvement, and Modernization Act of 2003**   Also known as the Medicare Modernization Act (MMA), this act greatly overhauled the Medicare program, introducing tax breaks and prescription drug subsidies. It presented new Medicare "Advantage" plans offering better choices to patients about care, providers, other coverage, and federal reimbursements. It partially privatized the Medicare system.

- **Combat Methamphetamine Epidemic Act of 2005**   This act focused on parts of the Patriot Act, intending to stop illegal use of the drug methamphetamine, as well as other drugs such as crack cocaine, and harshly penalize anyone found in violation. It came about because of the involvement of these drugs in financing terrorist activities. It limits the sale of precursors of methamphetamine, including ephedrine and pseudoephedrine, to only 9 grams per month per person (who must provide identification and sign sales logs recording the transactions). Everyone involved in selling these products must be registered with the U.S. Attorney General's office.

STATE LAWS

The practice of pharmacy is primarily regulated by state laws, not federal laws. State laws may be relatively independent of those of the federal government as long as they do not conflict with and are not inconsistent with federal laws. Most state pharmacy-related laws are similar regarding their fundamental principles, purposes, and the aims and objectives of pharmacy practice.

According to state law, no one may practice pharmacy without a license, with few exceptions. Most states, but not all, have a Board of Pharmacy as the regulatory agency that develops pharmacy regulations. In this book, the administrative agency in each state that governs the practice of pharmacy will therefore be referred to as a state's Board of Pharmacy. In some states, the Board of Pharmacy is a sub-agency of a larger state agency, often the Department of Health or Department of Licensing.

Every state has a pharmacy practice act regulating the profession, but these acts differ from state to state. Many state statutes are now out-of-date, and **amendments** are added in a rather haphazard manner. Many earlier acts regulated the profession at a time when it was more product-oriented and more solely focused on the preparation and delivery of drugs.

REGULATORY AGENCIES

There are many regulatory agencies that have specific functions related to how the public uses specific substances, and how the government controls these uses. The following agencies are listed alphabetically.

- **Board of Pharmacy (BOP)**   Each state's Board of Pharmacy is designed to regulate and control the practice of pharmacy. Laws are adopted by these boards that affect pharmacy practice, with each board's focus being the health of the general public.

- **Bureau of Alcohol, Tobacco, and Firearms (ATF)**   The ATF regulates alcohol, tobacco, firearms, and explosives, and investigates acts of arson. It is focused on the prevention of terrorism, reducing violent crime, and protecting the United States.

- **Centers for Medicare and Medicaid Service (CMS)**   The CMS promotes effective, up-to-date health care coverage as well as promoting quality health care for beneficiaries. It focuses on modernizing the U.S. health care system.

- **Department of Transportation (DOT)**   Focusing on protecting the public and environment from harm, the DOT regulates the safe transportation of hazardous and non-hazardous materials. Regulations became more consistent throughout all 50 states as a result of the Hazardous Materials Transportation Uniform Safety Act of 1990.

- **Drug Enforcement Agency (DEA)**   The DEA investigates and prosecutes those who violate controlled substance laws, focusing on gangs and individuals who use violence as part of their illegal activities. It strives to enforce controlled substances legislation while promoting the reduction of illicit substances, cooperating with local, regional, national, and international agencies. The DEA seizes assets of violators and also manages a national drug intelligence program.

- **Environmental Protection Agency (EPA)**   The EPA works to protect the environment and the health of the public by developing and enforcing environmental legislation. It offers grants to state environmental programs and publishes educational information.

- **Food and Drug Administration (FDA)**   The FDA works to promote public health, and was created from the Food, Drug, and Insecticide Administration in 1930. It controls the safety and effectiveness of foods, drugs, biological products, cosmetics, medical devices, and radioactive substances. Using a system called "MedWatch," the FDA encourages the reporting of adverse reactions, quality control issues, and product-use errors.

- **Institutional Review Boards (IRB)**   As regulated by the Office for Human Research Protections (OHRP), institutional review boards oversee biomedical and behavioral research. These boards can approve, reject, or require modifications in the research of new products.

- **Joint Commission on Accreditation of Healthcare Organizations**   The Joint Commission is an independent, non-governmental organization that accredits and certifies health care organizations with the intent of improving the safety and quality of health care. It is a not-for-profit commission with nationwide recognition of its efforts.

- **National Association of the Boards of Pharmacy (NABP)** This non-governmental agency assists state Boards of Pharmacy in protecting public health by developing uniform standards. The NABP's efforts are designed to reduce potential public harm that can be caused by the growing complexities of medications and delivery systems.

GENERAL TERMINOLOGY RELATED TO PHARMACY LAW

The following are common terms that relate to pharmacy law.

Term	Pronunciation	Definition
administrative law	ad-MIH-nih-stray-tiv LAW	the body of law governing the administrative agencies created by Congress or by state legislatures
adulteration	ah-dul-teh-RAY-shun	tampering with or contaminating a product or substance
amendments	ah-MEND-ments	revisions or intended improvements to an existing bill or other document
appeal	ah-PEEL	a legal process in which a case is brought to a higher court to review the decision of a lower court
autonomy	aw-TAW-no-mee	the ability or tendency to function independently
case law	KAYS LAW	a system of law based on judges' decisions and legal precedents rather than on statutes; in this system, judges may interpret statutory law, or apply common law

(continues)

Term	Pronunciation	Definition
code of ethics	KOHD OF EH-thiks	standards developed to affect quality and ensure the highest ethical and professional behavior
common law	KAH-mun LAW	a system of law derived from decisions of judges rather than from constitutions or statues
contract law	KON-trakt LAW	a system of law that pertains to agreements between two or more parties
criminal law	KRIH-mih-nul LAW	the body of law that defines criminal offenses against the public
disclosure	dis-KLOH-zher	transferring, releasing, providing access to, or divulging information in any manner
electronic data interchange	eh-lek-TRAW-nik DAY-tuh IN-ter-chaynj	a set of standards for structuring electronic information intended to be exchanged between different entities
electronic medical records	eh-lek-TRAW-nik MEH-dih-kul REH-kordz	the preferred method of record storage (over the use of paper records)
encryption	en-KRIP-shun	transforming information via an algorithm to make it unreadable to anyone who does not possess the code enabling them to "unlock" it
ethics	EH-thiks	the study of value, morals, and morality; includes concepts such as right, wrong, good, evil, and responsibility
extranet	EK-strah-net	a private network that uses Internet protocols, network connections, and sometimes telecommunication devices to share information with outside entities
facsimile	fak-SIH-mih-lee	a copy of an official document (such as a prescription or medication order) that is commonly transmitted via fax machine
felony	FEH-loh-nee	an offense punishable by imprisonment in a state or federal prison for more than 1 year, or punishable by death
fraud	FRAWD	the intentional use of deceit in order to deprive another person of his or her money, property, or rights
fraudulent	FRAW-dyoo-lent	deceitful; intending to deceive
infringements	in-FRINJ-ments	violations of laws, regulations, or agreements
investigational drugs	in-ves-tih-GAY-shuh-nul DRUGS	drugs used to provide detailed inquiry or systematic examination of their effects
jurisdiction	joo-ris-DIK-shun	the power and authority given to a court to hear a case and make a judgment
law	LAW	a rule of conduct or procedure established by custom, agreement, or authority

legal precedent	LEE-gul PREH-seh-dent	a legal principle created by a court decision that provides an example for judges deciding similar issues at a later date
legend drug	LEH-jend DRUG	a prescription drug
legislative law	LEH-jis-lay-tiv LAW	a law prescribed by legislature enactments; also known as "statutory law"
licensure	LY-sen-shur	the practice of granting a professional license to practice a profession
loyalty	LOY-ul-tee	a faithfulness or allegiance to a cause, ideal, custom, institution, or product
magistrates	MAH-jih-strayts	civil officers with the power to enforce laws
malfeasance	mal-FEE-zens	the execution of an unlawful or improper act
malpractice	mal-PRAK-tis	professional misconduct or demonstration of an unreasonable lack of skill with the result of injury, loss, or damage to the patient
medical code sets	MEH-dih-kul KOHD SETS	sets of alphanumeric codes used for encoding medical conditions, diseases, procedures, and other information
misbranding	mis-BRAN-ding	fraudulent or misleading labeling or marking
misdemeanor	MIS-deh-mee-nor	crimes punishable by fine or imprisonment in a facility other than a prison for less than 1 year
misfeasance	mis-FEE-zens	the improper performance of an act
morals	MOH-ruls	motivations based on ideas of right and wrong
National Drug Code	NAH-shuh-nul DRUG KOHD	the federal code that identifies a drug's manufacture, its formulation, and the size and type of its packaging
National Formulary	NAH-shun-nul FOR-myoo-leh-ree	a list of officially recognized drug names
negligence	NEH-glih-jens	a type of unintentional tort alleged when one may have performed, or failed to perform, an act that a reasonable person would or would not have done in similar circumstances
nonfeasance	non-FEE-zens	the failure to act when there is a duty to act, as a reasonably prudent person would, in similar circumstances
Notice of Privacy Practices	NO-tis OF PRY-vah-see PRAK-tih-ses	a document that explains to patients how their protected health information may be used and disclosed
opiates	OH-pee-ats	central nervous system depressants commonly prescribed to treat pain; common opiates include hydromorphone, morphine, and oxycodone
orphan drug	OR-fen DRUG	a drug used to treat a disease that affects fewer than 200,000 people in the United States
over-the-counter	OH-ver THE KOWN-ter	a non-prescription drug

(continues)

Term	Pronunciation	Definition
phocomelia	foh-koh-MEE-lee-uh	a severe birth defect, also known as "seal limbs," involving the malformation or non-formation of the arms and/or legs; it was shown to be caused by the drug known as "thalidomide"
professional ethics	pro-FEH-shuh-nul EH-thiks	moral standards and principles of conduct guiding professionals in performing their functions
prosecution	praw-seh-KYOO-shun	a legal proceeding against an individual
revocation	reh-voh-KAY-shun	recall of authority or power to act
revoked	ree-VOHKD	voided, annulled, recalled, withdrawn, or reversed
Schedules	SKEH-dyools	the five classifications of controlled substances, with the drugs having the highest abuse potential (and no medical use) listed as Schedule I and those with progressively less abuse potential (and accepted medical use) listed as Schedules II, III, IV, and V
statute of limitations	STAH-choot OF lih-mih-TAY-shuns	that period of time established by state law during which a lawsuit or criminal proceeding may be filed
statutory law	STAH-choo-toh-ree LAW	a law that is prescribed by legislative enactments; also known as "legislative law"
teratogenic	teh-rah-toh-JEH-nik	causing genetic defects
tort	TORT	a private wrong or injury, other than a breach of contract, for which the court will provide a remedy
United States Pharmacopoeia	yoo-NY-ted STAYTS far-mah-KOH-pee-uh	the officially recognized authority and standard on the prescribing of drugs, chemicals, and medicinal preparation in the United States
values	VAL-yoos	desirable standards or qualities
workers' compensation	WER-kers kom-pen-SAY-shun	laws that establish procedures for compensating workers who are injured on the job, with the employer paying the cost of the insurance premium for the employee

ABBREVIATIONS

The following are common abbreviations that relate to pharmacy law.

Abbreviation	Meaning
ADA	Americans with Disabilities Act
ATF	Bureau of Alcohol, Tobacco, and Firearms
BOP	Board of Pharmacy
CMS	Centers for Medicare and Medicaid Service
COBRA	Consolidated Omnibus Budget Reconciliation Act
CSA	Controlled Substances Act

DEA	Drug Enforcement Agency
DOT	Department of Transportation
DRS	designated records set
DSHEA	Dietary Supplement Health and Education Act
DUE	drug use evaluation
EDI	electronic data interchange
EMR	electronic medical records
EPA	Environmental Protection Agency
FDA	Food and Drug Administration
HHS	Health and Human Services
HIPAA	Health Insurance Portability and Accountability Act
IND	Investigational New Drug
IRB	Institutional Review Boards
IRS	Internal Revenue Service
JCAHO	Joint Commission on Accreditation of Healthcare Organizations
MA	Medicare Advantage
MMA	Medicare Modernization Act
NABP	National Association of the Boards of Pharmacy
NDA	New Drug Application
NDC	National Drug Code
NF	National Formulary
NOPP	Notice of Privacy Practices
OBRA-90	Omnibus Budget Reconciliation Act of 1990
OHRP	Office for Human Research
OIG	Office of the Inspector General
OSHA	Occupational Safety and Health Act
OTC	over-the-counter
PDP	prescription drug plan
PHI	protected health information
SMDA	Safe Medical Devices Act
TCS	transaction and code sets
USP	United States Pharmacopoeia

REVIEW EXERCISES

Multiple Choice

Select the best answer and write the letter of your choice to the left of each number.

1. Civil wrongs are often called:

   A. torts
   B. frauds
   C. malpractice
   D. misdemeanors

2. Drugs used to provide detailed inquiry are known as:

   A. national drug codes
   B. medical code sets
   C. teratogenic drugs
   D. investigational drugs

3. Which of the following terms describes "desirable standards or qualities"?

   A. laws
   B. ethics
   C. values
   D. morals

4. Crimes punishable by fine or by imprisonment in a facility other than a prison for less than 1 year are referred to as:

   A. misbranding
   B. misdemeanors
   C. malpractice
   D. malfeasance

5. Which of the following laws was passed as the result of the sulfanilamide tragedy?

   A. Kefauver-Harris Amendment
   B. Durham-Humphrey Amendment
   C. Pure Food and Drug Act
   D. Food, Drug, and Cosmetic Act

6. A violation of laws, regulations, or agreements is called:

   A. infringement
   B. fraud
   C. misfeasance
   D. facsimile

7. Any person who intends to handle controlled substances must obtain a(n):

   A. certification
   B. extranet
   C. autonomy
   D. Drug Enforcement Agency registration

8. Which of the following laws requires that drug products, both legend and non-prescription, be pure, effective, and safe?

   A. Pure Food and Drug Act
   B. Comprehensive Drug Abuse and Prevention Act
   C. Durham-Humphrey Amendment
   D. Kefauver-Harris Amendment

9. Which of the following laws includes regulations for physical workplaces and job-related materials?

   A. HIPAA
   B. OSHA
   C. OBRA
   D. MMA

10. Transforming information via an algorithm to make it unreadable to anyone who does not possess the key to unlock it is referred to as:

   A. encryption
   B. extranet
   C. magistrate
   D. misfeasance

11. The authority given to a court to hear a case, and to make a judgment, is called:

   A. legal precedent
   B. legal practice
   C. power of attorney
   D. jurisdiction

12. The Omnibus Budget Reconciliation Act of 1990 contained important amendments that affected:

   A. Medicaid
   B. drug recalls
   C. Medicare
   D. both A and C

13. Which of the following laws prohibits discrimination against disabled persons?

    A. OSHA
    B. HIPAA
    C. ADA
    D. ADHD

14. The study of values, morals, and morality is called:

    A. laws
    B. ethics
    C. legality
    D. loyalty

15. Tampering with a product or a substance is referred to as:

    A. malpractice
    B. adulteration
    C. fraudulence
    D. misdemeanor

Fill in the Blank

Use your knowledge of medical terminology to insert the correct term from the list below.

disclosure	appeal	encryption
fraud	licensure	felony
magistrate	misbranding	orphan drug
tort	phocomelia	misdemeanor
misfeasance	negligence	nonfeasance

1. A type of unintentional tort alleged when one may not have performed as required is referred to as _____.

2. The failure to act when there is a duty to act is called _____.

3. A civil officer with the power to enforce laws is known as a(n) _____.

4. A legal process in which a case is brought to a higher court to review the decision of a lower court is referred to as a(n) _____.

5. The term _____ means "transforming information via an algorithm to make it unreadable to anyone who does not possess the code enabling them to 'unlock' it."

6. A severe birth defect, which is known as "seal limbs," is referred to as _____.

7. The improper performance of an act is called _____.

8. Releasing information in any manner is referred to as _____.

9. Misleading labeling or marking is called _____.

10. A crime punishable by fine or imprisonment in a facility other than a prison for less than one year is known as a(n) _____.

True / False

Identify each of the following statements as true or false by placing a "T" or "F" on the line beside each number.

_____ 1. The sulfanilamide tragedy influenced the passage of the Kefauver-Harris Amendment.

_____ 2. The Durham-Humphrey Amendment required the pharmaceutical industry to maintain physical security and divided controlled substances into three schedules.

_____ 3. HIPAA was designed to prevent workplace diseases and injuries, and ensure employee safety and health.

_____ 4. The Drug Listing Act assigned each drug a unique, permanent 11-digit NDC.

_____ 5. The Medical Device Amendment offers tax breaks.

_____ 6. The Resource Conservation and Recovery Act regulates the handling and disposal of solid wastes.

_____ 7. Ephedrine is a precursor of methamphetamine; the law limits its sale to only 9 grams per month per person.

_____ 8. A rule of conduct or procedure established by custom, agreement, or authority is called a law.

_____ 9. A faithfulness or allegiance to a cause is referred to as "professional ethics."

_____ 10. The Harrison Narcotics Tax Act was the first federal law, passed in 1906.

Definitions

Define each of the following words in one sentence.

1. morals: _____

2. statutory law: _____

3. tort: _____

4. felony: _____

5. revocation: _____

6. malpractice: _____

7. teratogenic: _____

8. values: _____

9. amendment: _____

10. facsimile: _____

Abbreviations

Write the full meaning of each abbreviation.

Abbreviation	Meaning
1. NDC	_____
2. HHS	_____
3. EPA	_____
4. DEA	_____
5. BOP	_____
6. PHI	_____
7. OIG	_____
8. NDA	_____
9. NOPP	_____
10. DOT	_____

Matching

Match each term with its correct definition by placing the corresponding letter on the line to its left.

_____ **1.** 1938

_____ **2.** 1951

_____ **3.** 1963

_____ **4.** 1970

_____ **5.** 1972

_____ **6.** 1976

_____ **7.** 1986

A. Prescription Drug Marketing Act

B. Combat Methamphetamine Epidemic Act

C. Drug Price Competition and Patent Term Restoration Act

D. Food, Drug, and Cosmetic Act

_____ **8.** 1984

_____ **9.** 1987

_____**10.** 2005

E. Medical Device Amendment

F. Comprehensive Drug Abuse Prevention and Control Act

G. Drug Listing Act

H. Orphan Drug Act

I. Durham-Humphrey Amendment

J. Kefauver-Harris Amendment

Spelling

Circle the correct spelling from each pairing of words.

1. juridiction	jurisdiction
2. encryption	encription
3. misfeazance	misfeasance
4. misdimeanor	misdemeanor
5. magistrate	magestrate
6. revokation	revocation
7. phocomelia	phecomelia
8. malfeazance	malfeasance
9. apeal	appeal
10. adulteration	adulterration

Management of Pharmacy Operations

OBJECTIVES

Upon completion of this chapter, the reader should be able to:

1. Define *cost analysis* and *cost control*.

2. Explain why inventory control is vitally important.

3. Describe purchasing procedures.

4. Identify three basic types of budgets.

5. Define, pronounce, and spell the medical terms related to management of pharmacy operations.

6. Interpret the meanings of the abbreviations presented in this chapter.

7. Define *repackaging*.

8. Define the *ABC inventory method* and *inventory record card system*.

OVERVIEW

The management of a pharmacy starts with the people who work there: pharmacists, pharmacy technicians, clerks, and secretaries. A strong pharmacy setting benefits from strong leadership and management of all personnel. Pharmacy management includes overseeing many different areas of operations, including drug use control, costs, inventory control, repackaging, financial planning, and purchasing. The pharmacy manager must have enough knowledge and skills to be able to implement a good drug use control plan. The most effective way that pharmacists can achieve drug use control is by combining effective **management** of medication purchasing, prescribing, administration, and monitoring.

In an organized health care setting, drug use can be effectively managed by having appropriate policies, procedures, and programs in place that relate to both **pharmaceutical** services and therapeutics. These areas must be able to respond to needs that arise from customers, and also look forward to anticipate future needs. The role of the pharmacy technician in pharmacy operations and management includes assisting the pharmacy manager by providing good inventory control, record keeping, and **repackaging** of drugs for both cost analyses and purchasing procedures.

COST ANALYSIS

The most important concerns of pharmaceutical organizations are productivity, price, quality, and service. The pharmacist manager is responsible for the pharmacy's finances. The process of controlling these finances includes gathering information and data, and continually adjusting operations of the pharmacy to meet the standards that are developed. **Cost analysis** involves information about financial disbursements of an activity, agency, department, or program.

PURCHASING PROCEDURES

A pharmacy that offers more complex services will be more frequently involved with its **purchasing** department. Pharmacy services differ between types of pharmacies, and are also dependent on the size of the pharmacy. One of the most common and simplest methods of inventory control is the **want book**. The want book is a list of items that the pharmacist or pharmacy technician needs to order. In today's pharmacy, it is more likely to be entered into a handheld electronic device instead of an actual book. These devices allow easy entry of item numbers and quantities (Figure 26-1).

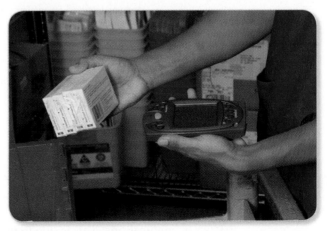

Figure 26-1 Inventory device.

RECORD KEEPING

Record keeping is an important part of a pharmacy technician's job, involving the accurate maintenance of patient records on the pharmacy information system. Patient records should include the patient's height, weight, diagnosis, treatment, diet plan, therapy, and blood and laboratory test results, and the name of his or her primary physician. Up-to-date records allow the pharmacist to provide better care and patient counseling.

Accurate and complete controlled substance records must be kept, including detailed receiving and dispensing information. Controlled substance records must be kept on hand for 2 years, with some states requiring them to be kept for 5 years.

INVENTORY CONTROL

Inventory control is vitally important because inventory is usually a pharmacy's largest **asset**. Control of a pharmacy's **inventory** directly affects the pharmacy's return on investment. Inventory control is also called *inventory management*. Computer systems allow accurate control of sales and inventory information. They can calculate and record very detailed areas of inventory information, identify low **turnover** items (in order to signify which items may be dropped from inventory), and can generate **wholesaler** or manufacturer orders.

In selecting a system for inventory management, the pharmacist may choose from any of the following:

- ABC inventory method
- computerized inventory system
- economic order quantity system
- economic order value system
- inventory record card system
- minimum/maximum level system
- order book system

REPACKAGING

The role of the pharmacist has changed from primarily a formulator and packager to a repackager of commercially prepared medications. This is due to pharmaceutical manufacturers' factory operations involving the preparation, packaging, and distribution of commonly prescribed medications. As a result, the pharmacist and pharmacy technician commonly repackage **bulk** containers of medication into patient-specific containers of medication (also known as **unit-of-use packaging**). Unit-of-use packaging or *repackaging* is used for both inpatients and outpatients.

FINANCIAL PLANNING

One of the most important financial management functions is budgeting. A budget is an annual plan, expressed in financial terms, that is an estimate of future revenues and expenses. A budget does not represent actual money that is available to be spent by the pharmacy, but is used to measure the pharmacy's financial performance. There are three basic types of budgets:

- the fixed budget
- the flexible budget
- the zero-based budget

GENERAL TERMINOLOGY RELATED TO MANAGEMENT OF PHARMACY OPERATIONS

The following are common terms that relate to pharmacy compounding.

Term	Pronunciation	Definition
annual report	AN-yoo-ul ree-PORT	a report focusing on a company's activities during the past year
assets	AH-sets	everything of value owned by a company
bar coding	BAR KOH-ding	placing a code on packaging to help standardize and regulate inventory control
batch repackaging	BATCH ree-PAH-kuh-jing	the reassembling of a specific dosage and dosage form of medication at a given time
budget	BUH-jet	a carefully compiled list of all planned expenses and revenues over a specified period
budget monitoring	BUH-jet MAW-nih-toh-ring	monitoring and controlling a budget's revenues and expenses
bulk	BULK	a larger amount of a substance or material to be broken down and repackaged into smaller amounts

(continues)

Term	Pronunciation	Definition
calendar year	KAH-len-dar YEER	January 1 to December 31
capital budget	KAH-pih-tul BUH-jet	a plan used to determine if a company's long-term investments are worth pursuing
cost analysis	KOST ah-NAH-lih-sis	all information regarding the disbursements of an activity, agency, department, or program
cost-benefit analysis	KOST-BEH-neh-fit ah-NAH-lih-sis	the procedure of evaluating costs and benefits of only those programs whose benefits are found to supersede costs
cost control	KOST kun-TROL	the implementation of managerial efforts to achieve cost objectives
expense budget	ek-SPENS BUH-jet	a limit to an amount anticipated as a future expense
expenses	ek-SPEN-ses	expenditures of money; costs
financial plan	fy-NAN-shul PLAN	a budgetary plan for spending and saving future income
fiscal year	FIH-skul YEER	a plan for financial activities of a company over a 12-month period
fixed budget	FIKSD BUH-jet	a budget that does not take into account possible variations in business activity
fixed expenses	FIKSD ek-SPEN-ses	fixed costs; those that do not change based upon production or sales
flexible budget	FLEK-sih-bul BUH-jet	revenue and expense projections that are able to change as production and sales levels change
group purchasing	GROOP PER-cha-sing	many hospital pharmacies working together to negotiate with pharmaceutical manufacturers to get better prices and benefits based upon the ability to promise high committed volumes
independent purchasing	in-dee-PEN-dent PER-cha-sing	contacting and negotiating pricing with pharmaceutical manufacturers
inventory	IN-ven-toh-ree	the stock of medications immediately on hand in a pharmacy
inventory control	IN-ven-toh-ree kun-TROL	controlling the amount of product on hand to maximize the return on investment
invoice	IN-voys	a form describing a purchase and the amount due
just-in-time system	JUST-in-time SIS-tem	an inventory control system in which stock arrives just before it is needed
management	MAH-nej-ment	the practice of handling, supervising, and controlling

material management	mah-TEE-ree-ul MAH-nej-ment	controlling tangible supplies
perpetual inventory system	per-PEH-choo-ul IN-ven-toh-ree SIS-tem	an inventory control system that allows review of drug use on a monthly basis
personnel expenses	per-soh-NEL ek-SPEN-ses	wages, salaries, stock options, pensions, and other expenses related to employees and staff
pharmaceutical	far-mah-SOO-tih-kul	a substance used in the treatment of disease
point-of-sale master	POYNT-OF-SAYL MAS-ter	an inventory control system that allows inventory to be tracked as it is used
prime supplier	PRYM suh-PLY-er	establishment of a relationship with a single supplier to obtain lower prices
procurement	pro-KYOOR-ment	acquisition of goods or services at the best possible cost in the most correct situation
purchase order	PER-chas OR-der	a document issued by a buyer to a seller that indicates the types, quantities, and prices of products or services
purchasing	PER-cha-sing	the acquiring of goods or services
recall	REE-kal	a request to return some or all of a manufactured drug product to the manufacturer, usually due to safety issues, mislabeling, incorrect packaging, or adulteration
record keeping	REH-kord KEE-ping	maintaining, usually via computer, the operating activities history of an organization
repackaging	re-PAH-kah-jing	to package again; in pharmacy, this means to package drug products from bulk containers into patient specific containers
revenue budget	REH-veh-noo BUH-jet	a type of budget that monitors actual financial performance against approved financial targets or goals
salary	SAH-luh-ree	a type of fixed, regular payment from an employer to an employee which is not based on "piece" work or pay per hour or per job
tangible	TAN-jih-bul	anything real, factual, or touchable; something that has monetary value
time purchase	TYM PER-chus	the actual time that a purchase order is made
turnover	TER-noh-ver	the amount of business done, shown by the rate at which goods are sold and replaced
turnover rate	TER-noh-ver RAYT	the rate of drug inventory calculated by dividing total dollars spent to purchase a drug over 1 year by the actual pharmacy inventory dollars

(continues)

Term	Pronunciation	Definition
unit-of-use packaging	YOO-nit-of-yoos PAH-kuh-jing	packaging from bulk containers into patient-specific containers
variance analysis	VAH-ree-ans ah-NAH-lih-sis	analysis by a pharmacy manager of significant variances from the monthly budget
want book	WANT BOOK	a list of drugs and devices that routinely need to be reordered
wholesaler	HOLE-say-ler	the sale of goods in large amounts, especially to retail stores that resell them to actual users
zero-based budget	ZE-roh-baysd BUH-jet	a budgeting system wherein all expenditures must be individually reviewed and approved

ABBREVIATIONS

The following are common abbreviations that relate to management of pharmacy operations.

Abbreviation	Meaning
CY	calendar year
EOQ	economic order quantity
EOV	economic order value
FY	fiscal year
GPOs	group purchasing organizations
JIT	just-in-time
POS	point of sale

REVIEW EXERCISES

Multiple Choice

Select the best answer and write the letter of your choice to the left of each number.

1. Packaging of drug products from bulk containers into patient-specific containers is referred to as:

   A. repackaging
   B. record keeping
   C. replacement therapy
   D. unit-of-use packaging

2. The stock of medications that a pharmacy keeps so that it is immediately available, on hand, is called:

   A. inventory control
   B. inventory
   C. assets
   D. acquisition

3. A calendar year is defined as:

   A. January 1 to June 1
   B. January 1 to July 1
   C. July 1 to December 31
   D. January 1 to December 31

4. Expenditures of money are referred to as:

   A. expenses
   B. expense budgets
   C. budget monitors
   D. fixed budgets

5. The actual time that a purchase order is made is called a:

   A. turnover
   B. point-of-sale master
   C. time purchase
   D. just-in-time system

6. Purchasing goods or services at the best possible cost, in the most correct situation, is referred to as:

   A. group purchasing
   B. turnover
   C. prime supplier
   D. procurement

7. Contacting and negotiating pricing with pharmaceutical manufacturers is called:

   A. group purchasing
   B. independent purchasing
   C. financial planning
   D. cost analysis

8. A revenue budget is a type of budget that monitors actual financial performance against:

   A. purchase orders
   B. approved financial targets
   C. approved personnel expenses
   D. the fiscal year

9. A special form describing a purchase and the amount due is referred to as a(n):

   A. want book
   B. purchase order
   C. invoice
   D. material management form

10. Which of the following is/are important concern(s) of pharmaceutical organizations?

    A. productivity
    B. price
    C. quality
    D. all of the above

11. Which of the following is the simplest and most common method of inventory control?

    A. handheld electronic device
    B. want book
    C. iPod
    D. recording voice

12. Most states require pharmacies to keep controlled substance records for:

    A. 1 year
    B. 2 years
    C. 3 years
    D. 4 years

13. Control of a pharmacy's inventory directly affects the pharmacy's return on:

    A. investment
    B. invoices

C. purchase orders
D. turnover rate

14. A budgeting system wherein all expenditures must be individually reviewed and approved is referred to as a(n):

    A. revenue budget
    B. fixed budget
    C. zero-based budget
    D. flexible budget

15. Inventory control is also called:

    A. independent purchasing
    B. perpetual inventory
    C. revenue budget
    D. inventory management

Fill in the Blank

Use your knowledge of pharmacy terminology to insert the correct term from the list below.

wholesaler	variance analysis	recall
invoice	flexible budget	inventory
fixed budget	cost analysis	procurement
budget	batch repackaging	bar coding
bulk	fixed expenses	capital budget

1. An amount of a substance to be broken down into smaller amounts is referred to as a(n) _____ amount.

2. Fixed costs are also known as _____ .

3. A budget that does not take into account possible variations in business activity is referred to as a(n) _____ .

4. Analysis by a pharmacy manager of significant changes from the monthly budget is called _____ .

5. Acquisition of goods or services at the best possible cost in the most correct situation is referred to as _____ .

6. A plan used to determine if a company's long-term investments are worth pursuing is called a(n) _____ .

7. Revenue and expense projections that are able to change as production and sales levels change are known as a(n) _____ .

8. The reassembling of a specific dosage and dosage form of medication at a given time is called _____ .

9. The stock of medications immediately on hand in a pharmacy is called _____.

10. A form explaining a purchase and the amount due is referred to as a(n) _____.

True / False

Identify each of the following statements as true or false by placing a "T" or "F" on the line beside each number.

_____ 1. The most effective way that pharmacists can achieve drug use control is by combining effective management of medication purchasing, administration, and monitoring.

_____ 2. The role of the pharmacy technician in pharmacy operations and management is overseeing drug use control, costs, and financial planning.

_____ 3. The most important concerns of pharmaceutical organizations are quality, price, and service.

_____ 4. The want book is a list of staff personnel including pharmacists, technicians, clerks, and secretaries.

_____ 5. Turnover is the operating activity history of an organization.

_____ 6. Material management is controlling tangible supplies.

_____ 7. A plan for financial activities of a company over a 12-month period is referred to as a *financial plan*.

_____ 8. A type of fixed, regular payment from an employer to an employee is called a *revenue budget*.

_____ 9. The sale of goods in large amounts is called *inventory*.

_____ 10. A prime supplier relationship involves the ordering of supplies from a single supplier in order to obtain lower prices.

Definitions

Define each of the following words in one sentence.

1. time purchase: _____

2. point-of-sale master: _____

3. purchasing: _____

4. just-in-time system: _____

5. expenses: _____

6. budget: _____

7. assets: _____

8. expense budget: _____

9. invoice: _____

10. pharmaceutical: _____

Abbreviations

Write the full meaning of each abbreviation.

Abbreviation	Meaning
1. EOQ	_____
2. POS	_____
3. JIT	_____
4. FY	_____
5. CY	_____
6. EOV	_____

Spelling

Circle the correct spelling from each pairing of words.

1. reveneu   revenue

2. perpetual   perpitual

3. asetts   assets

4. pharmoceutical   pharmaceutical

5. purchasing   perchasing

6. bolk   bulk

7. fiscal   fisical

8. repackaging   repackeging

9. tanjible   tangible

10. variance   varience

Health Insurance Billing

OBJECTIVES

Upon completion of this chapter, the reader should be able to:

1. Discuss the purpose of health insurance.
2. Differentiate between various types of insurance policies.
3. Explain how insurance benefits are determined.
4. List and discuss major private insurance policies.
5. Define the various types of Medicare.
6. Interpret the meanings of the abbreviations presented in this chapter.
7. Discuss the different types of fee schedules.
8. Define, spell, and pronounce the terms listed in the general vocabulary of this chapter.

OVERVIEW

Health insurance is designed to help individuals and families to offset the costs of their medical care. It is defined as "protection against financial losses due to illness or injury." Monetary benefits are paid for covered sicknesses or injuries depending on the type of insurance policy purchased. Various types of health insurance include accident insurance, **disability income insurance**, hospitalization, medical expense insurance (including prescription medications), and accidental death and dismemberment insurance.

Health insurance commonly covers medically necessary procedures and services. Most insurance policies do not cover procedures that are considered "elective," which include certain cosmetic surgeries not considered to be medically necessary.

Types of Health Insurance

The various types of available health insurance include group insurance, individual insurance, government-sponsored insurance, self-insured plans, and medical savings accounts.

Group Insurance

A group policy covers a number of people under one master contract that is issued to their employer, or to an association with which they are affiliated. Group insurance usually provides greater benefits at lower premiums. This is because of the large number of people from whom the premiums are collected.

Individual Policies

Individuals who cannot qualify for group insurance or government-sponsored plans may apply to insurance companies who offer individual policies. These policies are also often called *personal insurance policies.*

Governmental Plans

Governmental insurance plans cover eligible individuals. The federal government provides coverage under plans known as Medicare, Medicaid, TRICARE (formerly the Civilian Health and Medical Program of the Uniformed Services, or CHAMPUS), and the Civilian Health and Medical Program of the Veterans' Administration (CHAMPVA). These plans cover large groups of people, and are also known as *entitlement programs.*

Medicare (A, B, C, D)

Medicare is a federal health insurance program that was established in 1965 to provide health care coverage for individuals age 65 and older. It also covers certain disabled persons under age 65, such as the permanently disabled, blind, or people receiving dialysis for permanent kidney failure. Medicare was developed by the Health Care Financing Administration (now called the Centers for Medicare and Medicaid Services), as part of Title XVIII of the Social Security Act. Medicare is administered by the Centers for Medicare and Medicaid Services (CMS), which was previously known as the Health Care Financing Administration (HCFA). CMS is a division of the Department of Health and Human Services. Medicare is regulated by laws that were enacted by Congress, with two parts that cover health care services: Part A and Part B.

Medicare Part A is hospital insurance. Retired people 65 years of age and older, and people who receive monthly Social Security checks or checks from previous employment on railroads, are automatically enrolled for hospital insurance benefits. They do not have to pay any premiums for this insurance.

Medicare Part B is medical insurance. Persons eligible for Part A are also eligible for Part B. However, they must apply for Part B coverage and pay a monthly premium. A patient with Medicare Part B is required to meet an annual deductible before benefits become available. After this occurs, Medicare pays 80 percent of the covered (allowed) benefits.

Those with Medicare may also carry supplemental private insurance. This pays the deductible as well as the 20 percent co-payment not covered by Medicare. A supplemental policy that covers these items is referred to as a *Medigap policy*.

A new program called *Medicare & Choice* was added in 1997. It is commonly called "Medicare Part C," and offers expanded benefits for a fee by contracting with private health insurance programs such as HMOs and PPOs. As a result of congressional reforms, Medicare & Choice was renamed *Medicare Advantage* in 2004.

Drug and prescription benefits were added to Medicare in 2006. This new part of the program became known as "Medicare Part D." Under this program, people can choose, with reduced costs, a prescription drug plan that offers them the ability to obtain their prescriptions by paying only a small co-payment, with the plan covering the remainder of the cost. All Medicare patients can get this coverage, which may help lower prescription drug costs and help protect against future higher costs.

Medicaid

Medicaid provided for medically indigent patients via Title XIX of Public Law 89-97, under the Social Security Amendments of 1965. The federal government enacted Medicare in agreement with state jurisdictions for federal assistance concerning medical care for people who met certain eligibility criteria.

TRICARE (Formerly CHAMPUS)

Formerly called CHAMPUS when created in 1956, TRICARE was established by the federal government, authorizing dependents of military personnel to receive treatment from civilian physicians at government expense.

CHAMPVA

This program, which is similar to TRICARE, was established in 1973 for spouses and dependent children of veterans suffering from total, permanent, service-connected disabilities, and for surviving spouses and dependent children of veterans who died as a result of service-related disabilities.

Workers' Compensation

Every state legislature has passed workers' compensation laws to protect workers against loss of wages and costs of medical care due to occupational accidents or diseases. State laws differ as to the types of employees included, and the benefits which they are allowed.

Self-Insured Plans

Many large companies and organizations with many employees choose to fund their own insurance programs. These are called **self-insured plans**, but are technically not insurance plans because the employer pays employee health care costs out of the firm's own funds. These plans are usually similar in benefits and premium costs to group plans. Often, a **third-party administrator** or fiscal **intermediary** handles paperwork and claims for self-insured groups.

Medical Savings Account

In 1996, Congress made tax-free **medical savings accounts**, a type of self-insurance, available to 750,000 American workers and their families. These accounts combine personal savings accounts with high-deductible health insurance policies. Individuals must first purchase a health insurance policy before deposits can be made, up to a predetermined limit, into the savings account. Annual deductibles vary. Qualified medical expenses are not subject to taxation, and money remaining in the account at the end of each tax year rolls over into the next year's account with no penalty.

TYPES OF INSURANCE BENEFITS

Insurance packages are tailored to the needs of each individual or group policy. The combination of benefits are unlimited. A policy may contain one or any combination of the following:

- *Hospitalization* – Hospital coverage pays all or part of an insured person's hospital room and board costs, as well as those of specific hospital services, including surgery within a hospital.

- *Surgical* – Surgical coverage pays all or part of a surgeon's fee. **Surgery** may be done in a hospital, a physician's office, or elsewhere.

- *Basic medical* – This coverage pays all or part of a physician's fee for non-surgical services. These may include hospital, office, or home visits. A **deductible** amount is usually payable by the patient, as well as a **co-payment** or **co-insurance** payment, each time service is received.

- *Major medical* – Major medical insurance (formerly known as *catastrophic coverage*) provides protection against very large medical bills that may result from a catastrophe or a prolonged illness. This type of insurance may supplement basic medical coverage.

- *Disability protection* – This coverage offers weekly or monthly cash benefits to employed policyholders who become unable to work because of an accident or illness.

- *Dental care* – This coverage is included in many **fringe-benefit** packages. Policies may be based on a co-payment and **incentive** program, wherein preventive dental care (including x-rays) is 100 percent covered, while most other coverage is paid at 50 percent.

- *Vision care* – This type of insurance may reimburse all or part of the costs for **refraction**, lenses, and frames.

- *Medicare supplement* – Many Medicare beneficiaries purchase supplemental health insurance to help **defray** medical costs that are not covered, or only partially covered by Medicare.

- *Liability insurance* – There are many different types of **liability** insurance, including automobile, business, and homeowners' policies.

- *Long-term care insurance* – This newer type of insurance covers long-term, broad-range maintenance and health services to chronically ill, disabled, or mentally retarded persons.

HEALTH INSURANCE PROVIDERS

Health insurance providers include managed care plans, Blue Cross/Blue Shield, **commercial insurance** companies, and federal or state government programs such as Medicare, Medicaid, TRICARE, workers' compensation, and disability insurance.

Managed Care

Managed care is a term that stands for all health care plans that provide coverage in return for pre-set, scheduled payments as well as coordinated care through a defined network of physicians and hospitals. Managed care plans coordinate health care through a network of **primary care providers**, hospitals, and other providers.

A **health maintenance organization** is one that provides comprehensive health care to an enrolled group of people for a fixed, periodic payment. Some of these plans are paid for by **capitation**, regardless of the number of provided services. Under this system, providers collect only the contracted rate even if expenses cost much more than that rate for the specified coverage period.

Blue Cross/Blue Shield (BC/BS)

Blue Cross/Blue Shield is the oldest and largest system of independent health insurers in the U.S. It offers incentive contracts to health care providers. A provider who chooses to sign a member contract becomes a **participating provider**, and then agrees to accept BC/BS reimbursement as payment in full for the covered services. BC/BS reimburses providers directly, and in a shorter time.

BC/BS identification (ID) cards carry the subscriber's name, ID number, and a three-character alphabetic prefix. These prefixes must be included on each claim form because they are important in verifying the ID number and subscriber.

Models of Managed Care

The two basic models of managed care are the *health maintenance organization* and the **preferred provider organization**. The health maintenance organization can be structured as an independent practice association, staff, or group model—or as an exclusive provider organization. The preferred provider organization consists of doctors, hospitals, and other health care providers working with insurers or third-party administrators to offer reduced health care coverage to the insurers' or administrators' clients.

TERMINOLOGY RELATED TO HEALTH INSURANCE BILLING

The following are common terms that relate to health insurance billing.

Term	Pronunciation	Definition
allowed charge	ah-LOUD CHARJ	the maximum amount that most third-party payers allow for a specific procedure or service
authorization	aw-thoh-rih-ZAY-shun	a term used in managed care for an approved referral
beneficiary	beh-nih-FIH-shee-eh-ree	an individual entitled to receive benefits from an insurance policy, program, or governmental entitlement program; also known as a *subscriber, member*, etc.
benefits	BEH-nih-fits	amounts payable from an insurance company to cover an individual's monetary loss

(continues)

Term	Pronunciation	Definition
capitation	cah-pih-TAY-shun	a method of payment used by managed care organizations involving a fixed amount reimbursed to a provider for enrolled patients within a certain time period, no matter what services were provided or how many visits occurred
co-insurance	KOH-in-shoo-rens	an insurance provision wherein the policyholder and insurer share costs of covered losses in specified ratios (commonly 80 percent by the insurer and 20 percent by the policyholder)
co-payment	KOH-pay-ment	a sum paid at the time of medical service; a type of co-insurance
deductibles	dee-DUK-tih-buls	amounts that a policyholder must pay out of pocket before the insurer begins paying, usually ranging from $100 to $500 per year or per incident
dependents	dee-PEN-dents	spouses, children, domestic partners, or others designated by a policyholder who are covered under his or her plan
effective date	ee-FEK-tiv DAYT	the date that a policy or plan takes effect and benefits become payable
eligibility	eh-lih-jih-BIH-lih-tee	a term describing effective insurance coverage of a policyholder and his or her ability to receive benefits
exclusions	ek-SKLOO-zhuns	limitations on policies for which benefits will not be paid
explanation of benefits (EOB)	ek-spluh-NAY-shun OF BEH-nih-fits	insurer paperwork describing benefits paid, denied, or reduced in payment, as well as deductible amounts, co-insurance, and allowed amounts
explanation of Medicare benefits (EOMB)	ek-spluh-NAY-shun OF MEH-dih-kayr BEH-nih-fits	an explanation of benefits from Medicare, similar to EOB above
fee for service	FEE FOR SER-vis	established fee schedule for provider services and payments to a patient
fiscal intermediary	FIH-skal in-ter-MEE-dee-eh-ree	an organization working with the government to handle insurance claims from medical facilities, home health care, and those who provide medical services or supplies
government plans	GUH-vern-ment PLANS	entitlement programs or plans sponsored or subsidized by federal or state government; these include Medicaid and Medicare
group policy	GROOP PAW-lih-see	an insurance policy covering a number of people under a single master contract issued to the employer or to an employer-affiliated association
guarantor	GAH-ran-tor	a person responsible for paying a medical bill

indemnity plan	in-DEM-nih-tee PLAN	traditional plans that pay for covered services regardless of which provider is used; policyholders and their dependents may choose when and where to obtain care
individual policy	in-dih-VIH-dyoo-al PAW-lih-see	a policy designed for one person and his or her dependents, usually involving higher premiums than group policies; also called *personal insurance*
insured	in-SHOORD	a covered person or organization, with premiums usually paid by the person or organization; also called a *subscriber*
Medicaid	MEH-dih-kayd	a federal- and state-sponsored health insurance program for those who cannot afford medical care
Medicare	MEH-dih-kayr	a federally sponsored health insurance program for people over 65, or disabled people under 65
Medigap	MEH-dih-gap	a term used for private insurance coverage that supplements Medicare benefits
participating provider	par-TIH-sih-pay-ting pro-VY-der	a provider who contracts with an insurer, agreeing to follow certain rules and regulations set forth by the insurer
policyholder	PAW-lih-see-hol-der	a person who pays premiums to an insurer, and in whose name the policy is written
preauthorization	pree-aw-thoh-rih-ZAY-shun	a process that some insurers require wherein the provider obtains permission to perform certain services, or to refer the patient to a specialist
premium	PREE-mee-um	periodic payments to an insurer for which the insurer provides certain benefits
primary care provider (PCP)	PRY-meh-ree KAYR pro-VY-der	a non-specialist medical provider responsible for patients under certain HMOs; also called a *gatekeeper*
remittance advice (RA)	ree-MIH-tens ad-VYS	a Medicaid-oriented explanation of benefits
rider	RY-der	provisions that may be added to a policy to affect the benefits that are normally payable; a rider amends an original contract
self-insured plan	SELF-in-SHOORD PLAN	a plan funded by a large organization that chooses to fund its own employee insurance program
third-party payors	THIRD-PAR-tee PAY-ors	payors that cover obligations or debts without being party to the contract that created the obligations or debts
TRICARE	TRY-KAYR	a government program that offers medical care to authorized dependents of military personnel; originally called CHAMPUS

ABBREVIATIONS

The following abbreviations are related to terms and procedures concerning health insurance billing.

Abbreviation	Meaning
BC/BS	Blue Cross/Blue Shield
BIC	benefits ID card
CHAMPUS	CHAMPVA
CMS	the Center for Medicare and Medicaid Services
EOB	explanation of benefits
EOMB	explanation of Medicare benefits
EPO	exclusive provider organization
HCFA	Health Care Financing Administration
HHS	Health and Human Services
HICN	health insurance claim number
HMO	health maintenance organization
MSA	medical savings accounts
PAR	participating provider
PCP	primary care provider
PIN	provider identification number
PPO	preferred provider organization
RA	remittance advice
TPA	third-party administrator
UCR fee	Usual, Customary, and Reasonable fee
VA	Department of Veterans Affairs

REVIEW EXERCISES

Multiple Choice

Select the best answer and write the letter of your choice to the left of each number.

1. Which of the following types of medical insurance is designed to offset medical expenses resulting from prolonged injury or illness?

    A. hospital coverage
    B. major medical
    C. disability protection
    D. liability insurance

2. Which of the following is a third-party health plan that is funded by the federal government?

    A. Blue Cross and Blue Shield
    B. medical savings account
    C. self-insured plan
    D. TRICARE

3. Which of the following individuals would not normally be eligible for Medicare?

    A. a 66-year-old retired man
    B. a person on dialysis
    C. a 25-year-old recipient of AFDC
    D. a blind teenager

4. Medicare Part B covers:

    A. hospital care
    B. outpatient services
    C. hospice care
    D. nursing facility care

5. Which of the following is a federation of nonprofit organizations offering private insurance plans?

    A. CHAMPVA
    B. TRICARE
    C. Medicare
    D. Blue Cross and Blue Shield Association

6. Which of the following plans covers spouses of veterans with permanent, service-related disabilities?

   A. Medigap
   B. Medicare
   C. Medicaid
   D. CHAMPVA

7. An independent practice association (IPA) is a type of:

   A. Blue Cross and Blue Shield provider
   B. Medicare
   C. Medicaid
   D. HMO

8. TRICARE was formerly known as:

   A. BCBS
   B. Medicaid
   C. Medicare
   D. CHAMPUS

9. A patient whose 65th birthday was yesterday arrives at the hospital. Under the guidelines of the Social Security Act, she is now entitled to receive benefits under:

   A. workers' compensation
   B. CHAMPUS
   C. Medicaid
   D. Medicare Part A

10. An addition to an insurance policy is called a(n):

   A. rider
   B. premium
   C. expansion
   D. exclusion

11. All of the following insurance programs are sponsored by the federal government, except:

   A. TRICARE
   B. CHAMPVA
   C. Medicaid
   D. workers' compensation

12. Health insurance designed for military dependents and retired military personnel is known as:

   A. Medicare
   B. Medicaid
   C. TRICARE
   D. CHAMPVA

13. Organizations that fund their own insurance programs offer employees:

    A. group coverage
    B. individual coverage
    C. government plans
    D. self-insured plans

14. A pharmacist who enters into a contract with an insurance company and agrees to certain rules and regulations is called a(n):

    A. participating provider
    B. paying provider
    C. pharmacist provider
    D. inclusion provider

15. Which part of Medicare covers prescription drug services?

    A. Part A
    B. Part B
    C. Part C
    D. Part D

Fill in the Blank

Use your knowledge of medical terminology to insert the correct term into the list below.

payors	co-payment	policyholder
compensation	authorization	fee for service
Medigap	deductible	insured
exclusions	eligibility	dependents
capitation	beneficiary	co-insurance

1. A term sometimes applied to private insurance products that supplement Medicare insurance benefits is

    _____ .

2. A payment method used by many managed care organizations wherein a fixed amount of money is reimbursed to the provider for patients is referred to as

    _____ .

3. A term which describes whether a patient's insurance coverage is in effect is _____ .

4. A specific amount of money that a patient must pay out of pocket before the insurance carrier begins paying is called a(n) _____ .

5. A policy provision frequently found in medical insurance whereby the policyholder and the insurance company share the cost of covered losses in a specific ratio is called _____.

6. An individual covered by an insurance policy according to the policy's terms is referred to as the _____.

7. A person who pays a premium to an insurance company, and in whose name the policy is written in exchange for the insurance protection provided, is called the _____.

8. A sum of money that is paid at the time of medical service is called a(n) _____.

9. Limitations on an insurance contract for which benefits are not payable are referred to as _____.

10. An established schedule of fees set for services performed is known as _____.

True / False

Identify each of the following statements as true or false by placing a "T" or "F" on the line beside each number.

_____ 1. The person responsible for paying the medical bill is always the patient.

_____ 2. Medicare was established in 1995.

_____ 3. The world's largest insurance program is Medicaid.

_____ 4. Plans that provide benefits in the form of certain surgical and medical services rendered, rather than cash, are called *service benefit plans*.

_____ 5. Liability insurance never covers medical expenses.

_____ 6. A person who is blind may be covered by Medicare.

_____ 7. A co-payment is a sum of money paid at the time of the medical services.

_____ 8. An established schedule of fees set for services performed by providers and paid by the patient is called an indemnity plan.

_____ 9. An organization that contracts with the government to handle and mediate insurance claims from medical facilities or providers is called a *fiscal intermediary*.

_____ 10. A medical savings account can be established only if the individual does not have any other health insurance.

Definitions

Define each of the following words in one sentence.

1. premium: _____

2. benefits: _____

3. authorization: _____

4. dependent: _____

5. preauthorization: _____

6. referral: _____

7. guarantor: _____

8. rider: _____

9. exclusions: _____

10. indemnity: _____

Abbreviations

Write the full meaning of each abbreviation.

Abbreviation	Meaning
1. BIC	_____
2. EOB	_____
3. HMO	_____
4. TPA	_____
5. RA	_____
6. MSA	_____
7. PCP	_____
8. HCFA	_____
9. VA	_____
10. HICN	_____

Matching

Match each term with its correct definition by placing the corresponding letter on the line to its left.

_____ 1. deductible

_____ 2. Medicaid

_____ 3. CHAMPVA

A. covered by Medicare Part D

B. a federation of non-profit organizations offering private insurance plans

_____ **4.** TRICARE

_____ **5.** workers' compensation

_____ **6.** self-insured plans

_____ **7.** Blue Cross/ Blue Shield

_____ **8.** prescription only

_____ **9.** hospital care

_____ **10.** outpatient services

C. covered by Medicare Part B

D. protects workers from loss of wages after an industrial accident that happened on the job

E. covered by Medicare Part A

F. the amount of money that the policyholder pays per claim before the insurer will pay on the claim

G. formerly known as CHAMPUS

H. a plan that covers the spouses of military personnel who have permanent, service-related disabilities

I. those that are created by large companies to insure their own employees using their own funding

J. the federal- and state-sponsored health insurance program for the medically indigent

Spelling

Circle the correct spelling from each pairing of words.

1. priauthorization   preauthorization

2. remittance   remitance

3. guarrantor   guarantor

4. exclutions   exclusions

5. indemnity   indemnety

6. Medigape   Medigap

7. referal   referral

8. catastrofic coverage   catastrophic coverage

9. hospitalization   hospitalisation

10. compensation   compencation

Computer Applications in the Pharmacy

OUTLINE

OBJECTIVES

Upon completion of this chapter, the reader should be able to:

1. Describe computer components.
2. List the software and hardware components used in pharmacy computers.
3. Identify the advantages of computers in the pharmacy setting.
4. Discuss the various types of input and output devices.
5. Interpret the meaning of the abbreviations presented in this chapter.
6. Define, pronounce, and spell the terms used in this chapter.
7. Differentiate computers in the hospital pharmacy versus computers in the community pharmacy.
8. Describe how personal digital assistants may be used for working with outpatients and their information.

OVERVIEW

The pharmacy setting has been revolutionized by the use of computers. In both hospital and community pharmacies, computer applications are used in conjunction with drug administration, ambulatory care, clinical practice, and drug distribution. Computers have become the main component of pharmacy practice. It is essential for pharmacists and pharmacy technicians to become computer literate, and comfortable using the common software programs made for pharmacies. Computers can help in reducing errors and potential patient harm by keeping information up-to-date, accessible, accurate, standardized, concise, and correct.

COMPUTER COMPONENTS

A **computer** can be used in the pharmacy for many different activities, including billing, finance, inventory control, shipping, and receiving. Computers are programmable and able to process, store, and retrieve massive amounts of data, which can be analyzed and used to improve the efficiency of the pharmacy. Computer systems consist of four areas:

- *Data* – the raw facts manipulated by a computer, including images, letters, numbers, and sounds

- *Hardware* – the physical components of a computer, including its monitor, motherboard, central processing unit, memory, input/output devices, and storage devices

  - Most hardware designed for pharmacy use allows computers to be connected through *local area networks* to the **World Wide Web**. As a pharmacy grows, additional workstations, printers, servers, and other hardware may be easily added (Figure 28-1).

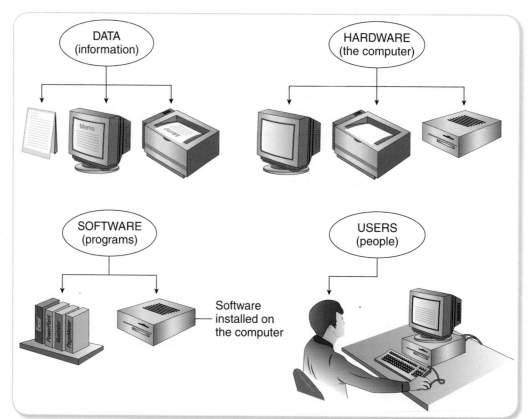

Figure 28-1 Components of a computer.

- *Software* – electronic **programs**, which contain complex sets of instructions allowing the computer hardware to perform desired functions

  - Computer software programs include *operating systems*, which actually run computer activities, and *applications*, which allow users to achieve specific computing tasks.

  - Specialized pharmacy software allows the user to easily perform data entry, track patient information, and store patient records. Forms, reports, labels, and many other printed materials are easily generated using pharmacy software programs.

  - Other forms of pharmacy software allow security measures to be set up, including video surveillance technology, to ensure the pharmacy's record keeping controls and avoid theft of inventory. Drug information can be easily cross-referenced between pharmacies across the country, and, if required, the world.

  - A unique type of software integrates with the pharmacy's phone system and allows customers to use an **automated touch-tone response system** to phone in prescription refill orders.

- *Users* – pharmacy personnel who work with the pharmacy computer system

Prescription orders are entered into the pharmacy computers, which check them for potential adverse interactions with other medications that the patient is currently taking. Pharmacists can easily review this information to quickly verify accuracy. Pharmacy staff can also use computers to integrate with insurance providers, control inventory, and keep pricing up-to-date.

Computer data is processed in the **central processing unit**, or *processor*, of which there may be one or several. **Memory** is the term used to describe the main storage component of a computer, and is commonly divided into two types: *random access memory* and *read-only memory*. A computer **file** consists of data sets or program instructions that have been "saved" with an identifying name or title.

Storage devices are those that consist of anything other than the main computer memory, including removable disks, hard drives, and optical media. Backup drives are also considered to be storage devices. Electronic medical records are easily stored and retrieved using the storage devices that are commonly used in pharmacy today—an immense improvement over early storage of paper records. Also, electronic storage takes up less space than paper-based storage.

Input devices such as the keyboard, touch screen, scanner, modem, and *mouse* are used to bring information into a computer. *Keyboards* resemble typewriters and contain alphabetic characters, numbers, symbols, and punctuation marks. Certain specific keys may be included that trigger specific actions within the pharmacy computer. *Touch screens* are types of monitors that have touch-sensitive surfaces, allowing the user to select a function by touching the screen instead of making the selection via a keyboard or mouse.

Scanners are devices that can "see" printed information and convert it into data that can be interpreted by the computer. *Modems* are used to transfer information from one computer to another using telephone lines and servers. A *mouse* is a device that allows users to move a pointer (known as a *cursor*) across the monitor screen in order to make selections or move information.

In the pharmacy, computers are often connected to robotic machinery that can count, dispense, package, and label medications. Once information is input, these machines can carry out many of the tasks that would otherwise require a pharmacist or pharmacy technician to complete. **Output devices** carry information out of a computer; examples of output devices include monitors and printers. *Monitors* resemble television screens, and are also known as "displays," enabling a user to view information that is being worked on. *Printers* produce paper copies of information, though specialized printers can be used to print a variety of other items, including prescription labels.

COMPUTERS IN THE HOSPITAL PHARMACY

In the hospital pharmacy, computer systems offer automatic screening for drug interactions, allergies, food interactions, therapeutic duplication, and single-screen order entry. Also, unit-dose distribution for hospitalized patients is easily coordinated via computer, supporting medication cart exchanges, automated distribution, a counting machine, **automation** and **robotics**, physician order entry interfaces, and many other areas of operation. Labels are easily printed, pick/fill lists prepared, on-screen patient profiles viewed, customized forms prepared, bedside charting updated, and automatic stop orders given—all using common hospital pharmacy computer systems. Hospital formularies are easily managed via these systems.

Many physicians use a **personal digital assistant** to manage patient information. These devices resemble handheld video games and allow easy input of data that can later be integrated into the hospital computer system. Physicians regularly use these devices to enter notes into patient charts and get information on prescription drugs instantaneously. Software used by these devices offer risk assessments, emergency dose calculation, mathematical conversions, dosing equivalencies, diabetic drug databases, etc.

There are several different types of drug information software. These include Micromedex® and Lexicomp®, both of which allow the accessing of many different types of clinical information, including detailed drug information, emergency data, acute care data, and disease data. Electronic Medication Administration Records are now used more widely than ever before to electronically store and track unlimited numbers of medication administration records. Automated distribution systems in the hospital pharmacy may include "automated drug cabinets" such as Pyxis® and Omnicell®. Similar automated "picking" systems are used to retrieve medications. These include robotic machinery as well as carousel-based systems such as Tay1st®. Many hospital pharmacies utilize centralized delivery devices to receive prescriptions from different departments and to send medications to these departments when they are ready. These devices include pneumatic tubes and robotic delivery systems such as TUG®. Some advanced hospitals utilize automated sterile compounding systems such as RIVA®. They also utilize "smart" IV pumps.

COMPUTERS IN THE COMMUNITY PHARMACY

Community pharmacies use many of the same computer applications that hospital pharmacies use. Some areas of the community pharmacy that may differ, however, include the stocking and pricing of commercial drug products that would not be found in a hospital pharmacy. Community pharmacy computer systems offer instant credit card authorizations, allowing pharmacy staff to quickly process payments for prescriptions and other items sold. **Bar code scanners** may also be used to quickly scan in a product's bar code, determining its pricing and other important product information.

Most community pharmacies have between one and six individual computer workstations. In the community pharmacy, technicians commonly use computers to create and maintain patient profiles, manage the inventory, and handle insurance billing. Also, the computer system can easily verify DEA numbers for accuracy, patient contact information, dosage information, and refill information, and ultimately serve to help reduce medication errors.

When a patient brings his or her prescription into a community pharmacy, it should first be reviewed and properly translated, then entered into the computer system, with medication labels being printed. The entering of a prescription requires the pharmacy technician to search for the patient in the computer database, bring up the prescription entry screen, search for the prescriber, verify the DEA number, enter the date of the prescription, select the prescribed drug or drugs, enter the quantity, enter the prescriber's directions for administration, and enter the number of refills and other pertinent information. Product dispensing information is then verified, inventory is updated, and insurance information is processed. The pharmacy technician must alert the pharmacist about any *drug use review* messages that appear, and then the pharmacist must review the prescription for accuracy.

GENERAL TERMINOLOGY RELATED TO COMPUTER APPLICATIONS IN THE PHARMACY

The following are general terms related to the use of computers and their applications within the pharmacy.

Term	Pronunciation	Definition
application	ah-plih-KAY-shun	a computer program with a user interface
automated touch-tone response system	AW-toh-MAY-ted TUCH-TOAN ree-SPONS SYS-tem	a system that allows customers to phone in prescription refill orders by using the keypad on the telephone to integrate with a pharmacy computer system
automation	aw-toh-MAY-shun	the use of computers to control machinery
backup	BAH-kup	the action of copying important data to a second location to protect against data loss through equipment failure or unforeseen events
banner	BAN-ner	an advertisement that extends across the width of a Web page
bar-coding	BAR-koh-ding	placing a machine-readable representation of information (in the form of, usually, black and white lines) onto an item so that it can be "read" by a bar code scanner
bar code scanner	BAR KOHD SKAH-ner	an electronic device that reads printed bar codes via a light source, a lens, and a light sensor
bit	BIT	binary digit; the smallest unit of information on a computer
booting	BOO-ting	the act of starting up a computer and loading the system software into memory

browsers	BROUW-sers	user interfaces on computers that allow navigation of objects, access to the World Wide Web, or management of files and related objects
bubble jet	BUH-bul JET	a type of inkjet printer that uses ink-containing nozzles that form an image when the ink is heated and expanded, forcing it out onto a sheet of paper
byte	BYT	binary term; a unit of storage capable of holding a single character
cache	KASH	a special type of high-speed storage that may be a part of a computer's main memory or a separate storage device
central processing unit	SEN-trul PRAW-seh-sing YOO-nit	a computer processor; the part of the computer that controls all computations
cipher text	SY-fer TEKST	encrypted text
clock speed	KLAWK SPEED	the rate at which a computer performs its most basic functions; also known as *clock rate*
computer	kum-PYOO-ter	a piece of programmable equipment that processes, retrieves, and stores data
cookies	KUH-kees	groups of information that are sent to a computer via its browser each time a specific server is accessed
crash	KRASH	a sudden and unexpected system failure
cursor	KER-ser	a symbol used to point to objects on a computer monitor
cyberspace	SY-ber-spays	the Internet, or the online "digital world" in general
data	DAH-tuh (or DAY-tuh)	the raw facts that a computer can manipulate
databases	DAH-tuh-bay-ses (or DAY-tuh-bay-ses)	collections of information organized for rapid search and retrieval by a computer
dialog box	DY-uh-log BOKS	a movable "window" displayed on a computer monitor in response to the user's selecting a menu option
dot matrix	DAWT MAY-triks	a pattern of dots that forms character and graphic images on printers
driver	DRY-ver	a piece of software that tells the computer how to operate an external or added device, such as a printer or hard disk drive
ecommerce (or e-commerce)	EE-kaw-mers	commerce conducted over the Internet, and most often, over the World Wide Web
electronic mail	eh-lek-TRAW-nik MAYL	messages and data exchanged between computers; also known as *e-mail*
encrypted data	en-KRIP-ted DAH-tuh (or DAY-tuh)	data that is converted into a difficult-to-interpret format (cipher text) to protect the information it contains

(continues)

Term	Pronunciation	Definition
Ethernet	EE-ther-net	a common method of networking computers used in local area network systems
file	FYL	a set of data or program instructions that has been given a name or title
firewalls	FYR-wahls	computer security systems that control the flow of data from one computer or network to another
floppy disk	FLAW-pee DISK	flexible plastic storage mediums for use in computers; they contain a magnetic material that actually holds the data
formatting	FOR-mat-ting	arranging data for correct recording and recovery
hardware	HARD-wair	the part of a computer that can be touched, including the processor, memory, storage, and input/output devices
hard drive		a nonremovable magnetic medium inside a computer where information is stored
icon	EYE-kon	a small pictorial on-screen representation of hardware, software, or data
inkjet printer	INK-jet PRIN-ter	a printer that propels droplets of ink in order to form characters or images
input devices	IN-put dee-VY-ses	those devices that bring information into a computer; they include the keyboard, mouse, touch screen, scanner, and modem
instruction set	in-STRUK-shun SET	machine language instructions that a computer can follow
keyboard	KEE-bord	a set of input keys used with a computer
laser printer	LAY-zer PRIN-ter	a common type of printer that rapidly produces high-quality text and graphics on plain paper
megabyte	MEH-gah-byt	a unit of storage equivalent to approximately 1 million bytes
memory	MEH-moh-ree	the main storage component of a computer; it includes random access and read-only memory
modem	MOH-dem	a device used to transmit and receive digital data
monitor	MAW-nih-ter	a display screen used to present output
mouse	MOUWS	hand-controlled device for interacting with a computer
multimedia	muhl-ty-MEE-dee-uh	software and applications that combine text, sound, graphics, animation, photos, and video
output devices	OUT-put dee-VY-ses	those that bring information out of a computer; they include monitors and printers

peripheral device	peh-RIH-feh-rul dee-VYS	any input, output, or storage device connected to a computer's CPU; examples include keyboards, monitors, printers, etc.
personal digital assistant	PER-soh-nul DIH-jih-tul ah-SIS-tant	a small, portable device that can store and transfer information into computer systems and other devices (such as digital cameras, scanners, and cellular phones); used commonly by physicians for their hospitalized patients
purging	PER-jing	the process of removing outdated data from computer disks or drives
printer	PRIN-ter	computer output device that reproduces data on paper or other media
programs	PRO-grams	software with specific purposes
robotics	roh-BOT-iks	the science and technology of robots, combining electronics, mechanics, and software
scanner	SKAH-ner	an optical device that can "read" text or illustrations printed on paper and translate the information into a form that the computer can use
software	SOFT-wair	sets of electronic instructions that tell computer hardware how to operate
telepharmacy	teh-leh-FAR-mah-see	a combination of pharmacy computer software, remote control dispensing, and telecommunications technology that allows pharmaceutical services to be provided from a distance
terabyte	TEH-rah-byt	a unit of storage equivalent to approximately 1 trillion bytes
upload	UP-lohd	to send a file to another computer
users	YOO-sers	people who use computers
virus detector	VY-rus dee-TEK-ter	a program that can detect software that is intended to damage a computer's programs
voicemail	VOYS-mayl	electronic system for recording oral messages sent by telephone
workstation	WERK-stay-shun	any computer that is attached to a network
zip drive	ZIP DRYV	a disk drive that uses hard disks to store information externally to the computer; zip drives are commonly used to back up computers

ABBREVIATIONS

The following are common abbreviations related to computer applications in the pharmacy.

Abbreviation	Meaning
CAN	campus area network
CD-R	compact disk recordable
CD-ROM	compact disk read-only memory
CD-RW	compact disk rewritable
CPU	central processing unit
DEA	Drug Enforcement Agency
DOS	disk operating system
DSL	digital subscriber line
DUR	drug use review
DVD	digital video disk
eMAR	electronic medication administration record
HAN	home area network
HIS	hospital information system
HTML	hypertext markup language
HTTP	hypertext transfer protocol
LAN	local area network
PDA	personal digital assistant
RAM	random access memory
RIVA	robotic intravenous automation
ROM	read-only memory
URL	uniform resource locator
WAN	wide area network
WWW	World Wide Web

REVIEW EXERCISES

Multiple Choice

Select the best answer and write the letter of your choice to the left of each number.

1. Microcomputers perform which of the following functions?

   A. input
   B. output
   C. storage
   D. both A and C

2. An application program is software that is designed to:

   A. interpret program instructions
   B. provide the computer with a set of basic instructions for executing other programs
   C. perform word processing, database functions, and patient billing
   D. back up the computer system

3. Which of the following is the most commonly used input device that allows the computer operator to select commands by interfacing with the monitor screen?

   A. scanner
   B. mouse
   C. printer
   D. cursor

4. What type of printer would be the most beneficial for printing multi-part insurance claim forms?

   A. laser
   B. inkjet
   C. dot matrix
   D. bubble jet

5. Which of the following electronic systems or devices is able to record oral messages sent by telephone?

   A. e-mail
   B. firewalls
   C. voicemail
   D. printer

6. Which of the following is not a peripheral device?

   A. digital camera
   B. zip drive
   C. light pen
   D. keyboard

7. Which of the following devices is used to transmit and receive digital data?

   A. memory
   B. mouse
   C. keyboard
   D. modem

8. A special type of high-speed storage that is a separate storage device is called a:

   A. zip drive
   B. device driver
   C. byte
   D. cache

9. Which of the following is an example of computer software?

   A. Word 2003
   B. e-mail
   C. internal memory
   D. floppy disk

10. The Internet, or the online "digital world" in general, is referred to as:

    A. cyberspace
    B. cache
    C. browser
    D. banner

11. Which of the following prevent access to private networks?

    A. virus detectors
    B. scanners
    C. blogs
    D. firewalls

12. A mouse is a(n):

    A. output device
    B. input device
    C. storage device
    D. processor

13. Which of the following is not one of the items that will differentiate microprocessors?

    A. memory
    B. clock speed
    C. bandwidth
    D. instruction set

14. The most common use of disks or diskettes today is for:

    A. giving instructions to the computer while it is being used
    B. substituting for a zip drive
    C. storing information
    D. formatting the computer

15. A series of computers that are linked together allowing them to share information is a(n):

    A. database
    B. clearinghouse
    C. network
    D. Internet

Fill in the Blank

Use your knowledge of medical terminology to insert the correct terms from the list below.

cache	icon	e-commerce
disk drives	data	icon
bar-coding	firewalls	megabyte
crash	zip drive	scanner
dialog box	cursor	booting

1. A picture, often on the desktop of a computer, that represents a program or an object is called a(n) _____.

2. The word used to describe selling and buying goods over the Internet is _____.

3. Devices that load a program or data stored on a disk into a computer are called _____.

4. A disk drive that uses hard disks to store large amounts of information externally to the computer is called a(n) _____.

5. Placing a machine-readable representation of information onto an item is called _____.

6. The act of starting up a computer is called _____.

7. The raw facts that a computer can manipulate are collectively known as _____.

8. A sudden and unexpected system failure is referred to as a(n) _____.

9. A special type of high-speed storage that may be a part of a computer's main memory is called _____.

10. The pointer, or flat bar, appearing on the monitor that shows where the next character will appear is called the _____.

True / False

Identify each of the following statements as true or false by placing a "T" or "F" on the line beside each number.

_____ 1. A scanner is used to burn a new CD from information on a computer.

_____ 2. Advertisements found on a Web page that can be animated to attract the user's attention are called *banners.*

_____ 3. Computers may help in reducing medication errors and potential harm by keeping information up-to-date.

_____ 4. Computer data is processed in the computer memory.

_____ 5. The term *software* refers to electronic programs.

_____ 6. A unique type of software integrates with the pharmacy's phone system and allows customers to use an automated touch-tone response system to phone in prescription refill orders.

_____ 7. Input devices are used to carry information out of a computer.

_____ 8. A modem is a device that allows users to move a pointer across the monitor screen in order to make selections or move information.

_____ 9. Community pharmacy computer systems offer instant credit card authorizations.

_____ 10. Most community pharmacies have one or two individual computer workstations.

Definitions

Define each of the following words in one sentence.

1. keyboard: _____

2. firewalls: _____

3. laser printer: _____

4. zip drive: _____

5. cookies: _____

6. cyberspace: _____

7. dot matrix: _____

8. crash: _____

9. booting: _____

10. peripheral device: _____

Abbreviations

Write the full meaning of each abbreviation.

Abbreviation	Meaning
1. LAN	_____
2. PDA	_____
3. CPU	_____
4. RAM	_____
5. WWW	_____
6. DOS	_____
7. HIS	_____
8. CD-ROM	_____
9. URL	_____
10. CAN	_____

Matching

Match each term with its correct definition by placing the corresponding letter on the line to its left.

_____ 1. virus detector

_____ 2. firewalls

_____ 3. inkjet printer

_____ 4. Ethernet

A. placing a machine-readable representation of information onto an item so that it can be "read" with a special scanner

_____ **5.** bar-coding

_____ **6.** monitor

_____ **7.** laser printer

_____ **8.** zip drive

_____ **9.** cipher text

_____ **10.** databases

B. collections of information organized for rapid search and retrieval by a computer

C. rapidly produces high-quality text and graphics on plain paper

D. a display screen used to present output

E. control the flow of data from one computer or network to another

F. a type that is encrypted

G. uses hard disks that store large amounts of information externally to the computer

H. a method of networking computers in local area network systems

I. detects software that is intended to damage a computer's programs

J. propels droplets of ink in order to form characters or images

Spelling

Circle the correct spelling from each pairing of words.

1. formating   formatting

2. scanner   scaner

3. modum   modem

4. encrypted   encripted

5. floppie disk   floppy disk

6. corsor   cursor

7. booting   bouting

8. buble jet   bubble jet

9. cache   cashe

10. cipher text   cypher text

MATHEMATICS REVIEW

Basic Mathematics

OBJECTIVES

Upon completion of this chapter, the reader should be able to:

1. Define *percents*, *decimals*, and *ratios*.
2. Describe the Roman numeral system.
3. Define the *Arabic system*.
4. Explain fractions and the various types of fractions.
5. Recognize the symbols used to represent numbers in the Roman numeral system.
6. Distinguish between the various types of fractions.
7. Describe the concept of proportions.
8. Interpret the meaning of symbols presented in this chapter.

OVERVIEW

   Basic math skills are essential for students studying to become pharmacists and pharmacy technicians. Fractions and decimals are the building blocks of accurate dosage calculations. To prepare yourself mathematically, you must be able to understand the terminology and abbreviations used in basic mathematics. You should keep in mind that a minor mistake may result in a major error affecting a patient's medication.

ROMAN NUMERALS

Pharmacy students and pharmacy technicians must be familiar with Roman numerals. Most medication dosages are prescribed using the metric system, also using Arabic numbers such as 1, 2, 3, 4, 5, 6, 7, 8, 9, and 10. Occasionally, orders involve apothecary system weights and measures, using Roman numeral **symbols** such as I, V, and X. The following are basic Roman numerals:

Roman Numerals	Arabic Numbers
I	1
II	2
III	3
IV	4
V	5
VI	6
VII	7
VIII	8
IX	9
X	10
L	50
C	100
D	500
M	1,000

GENERAL TERMINOLOGY RELATED TO BASIC MATHEMATICS

The following are common terms that are related to basic mathematics.

Arabic number – a mathematical object used in counting and measuring

Common fractions – fractions represented as equal parts of a whole

Complex fractions – fractions in which the numerator, denominator, or both may either be whole numbers, proper fractions, or mixed numbers

Decimals – fractions with denominators of 10, 100, 1,000, or any multiple or power of 10; also known as *decimal fractions*

Denominator – a number that the whole is divided into; for example, in the fraction ¾, the denominator is 4

Dimensional analysis – a conceptual tool used to understand physical situations involving mixes of different kinds of physical quantities

Dividend – the number being divided

Divisor – the number performing the division

Equation – a mathematical statement used to express equivalency between two variables

Extremes – the two outside terms in a ratio

Fractions – expressions of division with a number that is the portion or part of a whole

Improper fractions – fractions with numerators larger or equal to the denominators

Means – the two inside terms in a ratio

Mixed numbers – whole numbers combined with proper fractions

Multiplicand – a number to be multiplied by another number

Multiplier – a number by which another is multiplied

Numerator – the portion of the whole being considered; for example, in the fraction ¾, the numerator is 3

Percents – fractions whose numerators are expressed and whose denominators are understood to be 100

Prime number – a number that can only be divided by itself and 1

Proper fractions – fractions with numerators that are smaller than the denominators

Proportion – the relationship between two equal ratios

Quantity – an amount

Quotient – the answer to a division problem

Ratio – a mathematical expression comparing two numbers by division

Roman numeral – a symbol devised in ancient Rome that depicts Arabic number equivalencies by using letters such as I, V, and X

MATHEMATICAL SYMBOLS

The following symbols are commonly used in basic mathematics.

Symbol	Meaning
+	plus
−	minus
×	multiplied by
÷	divided by
=	equal to
<	less than
>	greater than
.	decimal
#	number
%	percent
:	signifies a ratio
::	signifies a proportion

REVIEW EXERCISES

Multiple Choice

Select the best answer and write the letter of your choice to the left of each number.

1. Which of the following Roman numeral symbols is equivalent to the Arabic number 100?

   A. M
   B. VIII
   C. L
   D. C

2. Fractions represented as equal parts of a whole are called:

   A. complex fractions
   B. common fractions
   C. improper fractions
   D. proper fractions

3. Whole numbers combined with proper fractions are called:

   A. numerators
   B. prime numbers
   C. mixed numbers
   D. extremes

4. Fractions whose numerators are expressed and whose denominators are understood to be 100 are referred to as:

   A. percents
   B. fractions
   C. decimals
   D. proportions

5. The answer to a division problem is called a(n):

   A. quantity
   B. prime number
   C. divisor
   D. quotient

6. A number to be multiplied by another number is referred to as a:

   A. mixed number
   B. multiplicand
   C. multiplier
   D. numerator

7. A conceptual tool used to understand physical situations involving mixes of different kinds of physical quantities is called (a):

   A. ratio
   B. proportion
   C. dimensional analysis
   D. complex fraction

8. The portion of the whole being considered is referred to as the:

   A. numerator
   B. denominator
   C. mixed number
   D. proportion

9. The two inside terms in a ratio are called the:

   A. extremes
   B. mixed numbers
   C. means
   D. equations

10. The number performing the division is referred to as the:

    A. prime number
    B. denominator
    C. dividend
    D. divisor

11. Fractions in which the numerator, denominator, or both may either be whole numbers, proper fractions, or mixed numbers are called:

    A. improper fractions
    B. complex fractions
    C. proper fractions
    D. common fractions

12. The symbol "M" in the Roman numeral system is equivalent to the Arabic number:

    A. 5
    B. 10
    C. 100
    D. 1,000

13. The number being divided is referred to as the:

    A. dimensional analysis
    B. dividend
    C. divisor
    D. extreme

14. A number that can only be divided by itself and 1 is called the:

   A. multiplier
   B. multiplicand
   C. equation
   D. prime number

15. The relationship between two equal ratios is known as a:

   A. proportion
   B. ratio
   C. percent
   D. fraction

Fill in the Blank

Use your knowledge of mathematics terminology to insert the correct term from the list below.

equation	quantity	quotient
numerator	proportion	ratio
extremes	denominator	dividend
percents	means	multiplier
multiplicand	decimals	complex fractions

1. A number by which another is multiplied is referred to as a(n) _____.

2. A number that a whole number is divided into is called a(n) _____.

3. A mathematical statement used to express equivalency between two variables is called a(n) _____.

4. The portion of the whole being considered is known as the _____.

5. The two inside terms in a ratio are referred to as the _____.

6. A mathematical expression comparing two numbers by division is called a(n) _____.

7. The answer to a division problem is the _____.

8. The relationship between two equal ratios is a(n) _____.

9. The two outside terms in a ratio are called the _____.

10. The number being divided is known as the _____.

True / False

Identify each of the following statements as true or false by placing a "T" or "F" on the line beside each number.

_____ **1.** A number that can only be divided by itself and 1 is a mixed number.

_____ **2.** Expressions of division with a number that is the portion or part of a whole are called *percents*.

_____ **3.** A quotient is the total of two numbers when they are added.

_____ **4.** A mathematical expression comparing two numbers by division is called a *ratio*.

_____ **5.** Expressions of division with a number that is the portion or part of a whole are known as *fractions*.

_____ **6.** The number being divided is called the *divisor*.

_____ **7.** The portion of the whole being considered is the denominator.

_____ **8.** Fractions whose numerators are expressed and whose denominators are understood to be 100 are called *percents*.

_____ **9.** The two outside terms in a ratio are called the *means*.

_____**10.** Whole numbers combined with proper fractions are called *mixed numbers*.

Definitions

Define each of the following words in one sentence.

1. improper fractions: _____

2. mixed numbers: _____

3. multiplier: _____

4. quantity: _____

5. proportion: _____

6. ratio: _____

7. dividend: _____

8. equation: _____

9. means: _____

10. divisor: _____

Symbols

Write the full meaning of each symbol.

	Symbol	**Meaning**
1.	#	_____
2.	<	_____
3.	×	_____
4.	: :	_____
5.	=	_____
6.	−	_____
7.	>	_____
8.	÷	_____
9.	%	_____
10.	:	_____

Measurement Systems

OBJECTIVES

1. Define the term "measurement system."
2. Describe the system of measurement accepted worldwide, and the household system.
3. List the basic units of weight, volume, and length of the metric system.
4. Define the term "International Unit."
5. Interpret the meaning of the abbreviations presented in this chapter.
6. Recognize the symbols used for the terms *ounce, grain,* and *drop*.
7. Describe the apothecary system.
8. Define *milliequivalents* and *units*.

OVERVIEW

In order to calculate drug dosage and convert units, it is essential to understand measurement systems. The major and most common system of weights and measures used in medicine is the metric system. The metric system is one of the two systems of measurement used in medication dispensation and administration, the other being the apothecary system. Today, the metric system is preferred in all countries for prescribing medications.

The use of the apothecary system in the prescribing of medications has greatly diminished, and the household system is not accurate. While the household system is perfectly safe to use for cooking, it should be avoided when administering medications. However, it is also important that you be familiar with this system. Dosage calculations are mostly concerned with the measurement of weight and volume. It is important to be familiar with all three of the systems of measurement in this chapter as well as their common terminology.

THE METRIC SYSTEM

The **metric system** was developed in France in the eighteenth century for use in scientific study and calculations. It is sometimes referred to as the *International System of Units* (derived from the French "**systeme International**"). In the United States, most people use the English system instead of the metric system. The English system use *inches, feet, miles, pounds,* and *tons* to describe length and weight. The basic units making up the metric system are the **gram** (for weight), **liter** (for volume), and the **meter** (for length).

THE HOUSEHOLD SYSTEM

The **household system** was designed so that dosages could be measured in the home. It uses ordinary containers found in the kitchen, including the teaspoon, tablespoon, and cup. The household system is sometimes called the "English system."

THE APOTHECARY SYSTEM

The **apothecary** system is the oldest system still in use, but is used rarely today. It is very difficult to use in comparison to the others. Because of this, its use has led to many medication errors. The Joint Commission and others have suggested that the apothecary system be discontinued in the United States and elsewhere. Apothecary system measurements are no longer used in package inserts and other references for recommended medication dosages. However, you should still become familiar with the terminology and units used in the apothecary system.

MILLIEQUIVALENTS AND UNITS

Other measurements used for quantities of medication include **units, milliunits, International Units,** and **milliequivalents.** The quantity is shown in Arabic numbers followed by its symbol.

GENERAL TERMINOLOGY RELATED TO MEASUREMENT SYSTEMS

The following are common terms relating to measurement systems.

Term	Pronunciation	Definition
apothecary system	ah-PAW-theh-kah-ree SIS-tem	a system of measurement that was used in pharmacies until the early twentieth century; it has been replaced by the metric system
avoirdupois system	ah-vwahr-doo-PWAH SIS-tem	a French system of measurement used in the United States for the measurement of weight only
centimeter	SEN-tih-mee-ter	a metric measurement of length equivalent to one one-hundredth of a meter
cubic centimeter	KYOO-bik SEN-tih-mee-ter	a metric unit of volume equal to one one-thousandth of a liter
deciliter	DEH-sih-lee-ter	a metric unit of volume equal to one tenth of a liter
dram	DRAM	a unit of mass equivalent to an apothecary's measure of 60 grains or 1/8 ounce
fluid dram	FLOO-id DRAM	a unit of liquid measure equivalent to 3.696 milliliters
fluid ounce	FLOO-id OUWNS	an apothecary system measure of liquid volume, equivalent to 8 fluid drams or 29 mL
foot	FOOT	a household (English) measure of length equivalent to 12 inches or 0.3048 meters
gallon	GAH-lon	a quantity of fluid in the household (English) system of weights and measures; a gallon is equivalent to 4 quarts or 3.785 liters
gram	GRAM	the basic unit of weight in the metric system, equal to one one-thousandth of a kilogram
inch	INCH	a household (English) measure of length equivalent to 1/12 of a foot or 2.54 centimeters
International Unit	in-ter-NAH-shuh-nul YOO-nit	a measurement used to describe potency of vitamins and chemicals
kilogram	KIH-loh-gram	a metric unit of mass that equals 1,000 grams; a kilogram is equivalent to 2.2 pounds
liter	LEE-ter	a metric unit of volume of 1 kilogram of water at 25° Celsius; a liter consists of 1,000 milliliters and is the basic unit of measure in the metric system for volume

(continues)

Term	Pronunciation	Definition
meter	MEE-ter	the basic unit of measure in the metric system for length
metric system	MEH-trik SIS-tem	the most commonly used system of measurement
microgram	MY-kro-gram	a metric measurement comprised of one one-millionth of a gram
milliequivalent	mih-lee-KWIH-vah-lent	one one-thousandth of an equivalent measurement
milligram	MIH-lih-gram	a metric measurement comprised of one one-thousandth of a gram
millimeter	MIH-lih-mee-ter	a metric unit of length comprised of one one-thousandth of a meter
milliunit	MIH-lee-yoo-nit	one one-thousandth of a unit
minim	MIH-nim	an apothecary unit of volume originally equivalent to one drop (of water); one minim equals 0.06 mL
nanogram	NAH-noh-gram	a metric measurement equal to one one-billionth of a gram
ounce	OUWNS	a household (English) measurement of weight that equals 1/16 of a pound, or 28 grams
pint	PYNT	a household (English) measurement of fluid weight that equals 16 fluid ounces or 473 milliliters
pound	POWND	a household (English) measurement of weight that equals 16 ounces or 454 grams
quart	KWART	a household (English) measurement of fluid volume equivalent to ¼ gallon, 2 pints, 32 ounces, or 946.24 mL
unit	YOO-nit	a standard of measurement based on the biological activity of a drug rather than its weight

ABBREVIATIONS

The following are common abbreviations that relate to measurement systems.

Abbreviation	Meaning
cc	cubic centimeter
cm	centimeter
dL	deciliter
dm	decimeter
dr	dram

fl. oz	fluid ounce
ft	foot
g	gram
gal	gallon
gr	grain
gtt	drop
in	inch
IU	International Unit
kg	kilogram
L	liter
lb	pound
m	meter
mcg	microgram
mEq	milliequivalent
mg	milligram
min	minim
mL, ml	milliliter
mm	millimeter
mU	milliunits
ng	nanogram
oz	ounce
pt	pint
qt	quart
T, tbsp	tablespoon
t, tsp	teaspoon
U	unit

REVIEW EXERCISES

Multiple Choice

Select the best answer and write the letter of your choice to the left of each number.

1. Which of the following is the oldest system of measurement?

   A. household system
   B. apothecary system
   C. international system
   D. metric system

2. A unit of mass equivalent to an apothecary's measure of 60 grains is called a:

   A. pint
   B. microgram
   C. minim
   D. dram

3. A unit of volume fluid measure equivalent to ¼ gallon is known as a(n):

   A. minim
   B. ounce
   C. quart
   D. pint

4. A weight of the English system that equals 1/16 of a pound is referred to as a(n):

   A. ounce
   B. pint
   C. liter
   D. quart

5. A unit of mass that equals 1,000 grams is called a:

   A. microgram
   B. milligram
   C. kilogram
   D. minim

6. Two pints, or 32 ounces, are equal to a:

   A. minim
   B. quart
   C. fluid ounce
   D. milliunit

7. A measurement used to describe the potency of a vitamin is called a(n):

   A. household measurement
   B. apothecary measurement
   C. avoirdupois measurement
   D. International Unit

8. A measure of liquid volume in the apothecary system which is equal to 8 fluid drams or 29 milliliters is known as a:

   A. fluid ounce
   B. pint
   C. quart
   D. minim

9. The volume of 1 kilogram of water at 25° Celsius is called a(n):

   A. ounce
   B. pint
   C. liter
   D. pound

10. A weight in the English system that equals 16 ounces is called a(n):

    A. gram
    B. kilogram
    C. pound
    D. ounce

Fill in the Blank

Use your knowledge of measurement terminology to insert the correct term from the list below.

gram	meter	pint
liter	dram	pound
gallon	minim	microgram
ounce	quart	millimeter
kilogram	milliunit	unit

1. A weight in the English system that equals 454 grams is a(n) _____.

2. A weight in the English system that equals 28 grams is a(n) _____.

3. A unit of mass that equals 1,000 grams is called a(n) _____.

4. A unit of mass equivalent to an apothecary measure of 60 grains is known as a(n) _____.

5. The basic unit of weight in the metric system is the _____.

6. The basic unit of volume in the metric system is the _____.

7. The basic unit of length in the metric system is the _____.

8. A standard of measurement based on the biological activity of a drug rather than its weight is a(n) _____.

9. A unit of fluid volume that is equivalent to 946.24 milliliters is a(n) _____.

10. A fluid measure in the English system equivalent to 473 milliliters is a(n) _____.

True / False

Identify each of the following statements as true or false by placing a "T" or "F" on the line beside each number.

_____ 1. A measurement in the metric system that is comprised of one-thousandth of a gram is a kilogram.

_____ 2. The basic metric system unit of length is the liter.

_____ 3. One kilogram is approximately equivalent to 2.2 pounds.

_____ 4. A liter consists of 1,000 milliliters.

_____ 5. A measurement of volume in the apothecary system that originally was equivalent to one drop of water is the quart.

_____ 6. The apothecary system is commonly used in the pharmacy today.

_____ 7. The household system was designed so that dosages could be measured at home-care facilities.

_____ 8. A gram is used to measure weight, and a meter is used to measure length.

_____ 9. Inches, feet, and pounds are used in the English system.

_____ 10. The metric system is sometimes referred to as the *avoirdupois system*.

Definitions

Define each of the following words in one sentence.

1. nanogram: _____
2. minim: _____
3. dram: _____
4. foot: _____
5. gram: _____
6. quart: _____
7. unit: _____
8. meter: _____
9. pint: _____
10. inch: _____

Abbreviations

Write the full meaning of each abbreviation.

Abbreviation	Meaning
1. dr	_____
2. ft	_____
3. g	_____
4. IU	_____
5. mcg	_____
6. T	_____
7. mm	_____
8. gtt	_____
9. gr	_____
10. ng	_____

Answer Keys

Chapter 1

Multiple Choice

1. A	2. C	3. B	4. D	5. C
6. C	7. B	8. D	9. B	10. B
11. A	12. B	13. A	14. C	15. C

Fill in the Blank

1. word root
2. prefix
3. combining vowel
4. suffix
5. combining form
6. *primi*
7. *an*
8. *hemi*
9. *bi*
10. *poly*

True / False

1. F	2. T	3. T	4. F	5. T
6. T	7. F	8. T	9. F	10. T

Definitions

1. male
2. skin
3. water
4. vessel
5. walk
6. blood
7. cell
8. joint
9. white
10. milk

Chapter 2

Multiple Choice

1. A	2. C	3. D	4. D	5. B
6. D	7. A	8. C	9. D	10. D
11. B	12. C	13. A	14. D	15. B

Fill in the Blank

1. neuron
2. chromosome
3. coronal
4. cephalic
5. cilia
6. ventral
7. endoplasmic reticulum
8. cytoplasm

9. flagellum

10. gene

Labeling – The Abdominal Regions

A. right inguinal region

B. left hypochondriac region

C. left lumbar region

D. umbilical region

E. hypogastric region

F. epigastric region

True / False

1. T	2. F	3. F	4. T	5. F
6. T	7. F	8. F	9. T	10. T

Definitions

1. the midline of the sagittal plane

2. the study of body structures

3. situated below

4. a condition of internal stability and constancy

5. the study of the tissues

6. the depressed area of the abdominal wall near the thigh

7. the smallest unit of life

8. the study of the functions of the structures of the body

9. a group of cells that act together for a specific purpose

10. the basic structural element of the nervous system

Abbreviations

1. endoplasmic reticulum

2. deoxyribonucleic acid

3. anteroposterior

4. left lower quadrant

5. lateral

6. ventral

7. posterior

8. ribonucleic acid

9. right upper quadrant

10. umbilical

Matching – Terms and Definitions

1. H	2. J	3. G	4. F	5. I
6. B	7. C	8. A	9. D	10. E

Spelling

1. homeostasis

2. lysosome

3. sagittal

4. hypochondriac

5. flagellum

6. visceral

7. umbilical

8. mitochondria

9. nucleus

10. chromosome

Chapter 3

Multiple Choice

1. C	2. D	3. B	4. D	5. C
6. D	7. A	8. C	9. B	10. D
11. B	12. A	13. C	14. A	15. D

Fill in the Blank

1. mast cells

2. diaphoresis

3. abscess

4. gangrene

5. ulcer

6. sebum

7. keratin

8. melanocyte

9. furuncle

10. erythema

Labeling

A. epidermis

B. sebaceous gland

C. dermis

D. subcutaneous fatty tissue

E. sweat gland

True / False

1. F	2. F	3. T	4. F	5. F
6. T	7. T	8. T	9. F	10. T

Definitions

1. itching
2. a sweat gland
3. a hard-fibrous protein that is found in the epidermis, hair, and nails
4. redness of the skin due to capillary dilation
5. peeling or sloughing off of tissue cells
6. a bruise or a black-and-blue mark
7. a diffuse, acute infection of the skin and subcutaneous tissue

Abbreviations

1. discoid lupus erythematosus
2. biopsy
3. xeroderma pigmentosum
4. ultraviolet A
5. sun protection factor
6. lupus erythematosus
7. purified protein derivative
8. incision and drainage
9. frozen section
10. body surface area

Matching – Terms and Definitions

1. J	2. G	3. I	4. A	5. H
6. B	7. C	8. D	9. F	10. E

Spelling

1. xeroderma
2. verruca
3. tinea
4. psoriasis
5. pemphigus
6. nevus
7. pruritus
8. impetigo
9. ecchymosis
10. melanocyte

Chapter 4

Multiple Choice

1. B	2. D	3. B	4. C	5. B
6. C	7. C	8. B	9. A	10. D
11. C	12. D	13. C		

Fill in the Blank

1. osteoblast
2. tibia
3. femur
4. patella
5. ulna
6. humerus
7. coccyx
8. vomer
9. scapula
10. conchae

Labeling the Skull

A. vomer

B. mandible

C. orbit

D. maxillary bone

E. temporal bone

True/False

1. T   2. F   3. F   4. F   5. T
6. F   7. T   8. T   9. T   10. F

Labeling – The Anterior View of the Ribs, Shoulder, and Arm

A. xiphoid process
B. humerus
C. ulna
D. sternum
E. clavicle
F. ribs
G. radius
H. scapula

Definitions

1. grows mostly by elongation of the diaphysis
2. includes the skull, vertebral column, and thoracic cage
3. include the malleus, incus, and stapes
4. forms the side and roof of the cranium
5. an agent that reduces inflammation without the use of steroids
6. five lower ribs on either side of the ribcage that do not unite directly with the sternum
7. immature bone cells
8. a cavity, opening, or hollow space within a bone
9. a hunched deformity of the back
10. softening of the bones due to defective bone mineralization

Abbreviations

1. fracture
2. total hip replacement
3. temporomandibular joint
4. lumbar vertebra 1–5
5. thoracic vertebra 1–12
6. computerized tomography
7. estrogen replacement therapy
8. osteoarthritis
9. rheumatoid arthritis
10. cervical vertebra 1–7

Matching – Terms and Definitions

1. I   2. J   3. G   4. F   5. D
6. E   7. C   8. H   9. B   10. A

Spelling

1. osteoporosis
2. arthritis
3. osteomalacia
4. scoliosis
5. analgesic
6. zygomatic bone
7. sesamoid bone
8. hyoid bone
9. vertebrae
10. fissure

Chapter 5

Multiple Choice

1. C   2. D   3. C   4. D   5. B
6. C   7. B   8. D   9. D   10. A
11. C   12. D   13. A   14. D   15. C

Fill in the Blank

1. fascia
2. ataxia
3. arthralgia
4. dorsiflexion
5. pronation
6. supination
7. insertion
8. strains
9. adduction
10. origin

Labeling – Superficial Muscles of the Body (Anterior View)

A. orbicularis oculi
B. vastus lateralis
C. rectus femoris
D. flexor carpi
E. pectoralis major
F. serratus anterior
G. sartorius
H. gastrocnemius

True / False

1. F	2. T	3. T	4. F	5. F
6. T	7. F	8. F	9. T	10. T

Labeling – Superficial Muscles of the Body (Posterior View)

A. hamstring
B. teres minor
C. latissimus dorsi
D. extensors of the hand and fingers
E. Achilles tendon
F. deltoid
G. trapezius
H. gluteus maximus

Definitions

1. a movement of a joint that decreases the angle between the bones of (usually) a limb
2. shortening of a muscle or tendon in response to stress
3. joint pain, generally when there is no joint inflammation
4. the main part of the body, from the neck to the genitals, including the thorax and abdomen
5. rotation of a body part that turns it upward or forward
6. movement of a body part in a circular motion
7. contractile tissue that is labeled individually based on its location and function
8. a fibrous, collagenous tissue that connects bones to other bones
9. general discomfort or a feeling of uneasiness often indicating disease
10. skeletal or cardiac muscle that appears striped, with separate, parallel fibers

Abbreviations

1. systemic lupus erythematosus
2. rheumatoid arthritis
3. muscular dystrophy
4. electromyography
5. rheumatoid factor
6. deep tendon reflexes
7. metatarsophalangeal
8. left upper extremity
9. metacarpophalangeal (joint)
10. right lower extremity

Matching – Terms and Definitions

1. F	2. I	3. E	4. D	5. H
6. G	7. C	8. J	9. B	10. A

Spelling

1. tremor
2. dystrophy
3. ganglion
4. leiomyoma
5. ataxia
6. sciatica
7. asthenia
8. supination
9. fascia
10. myalgia

Chapter 6

Multiple Choice

1. A	2. C	3. D	4. B	5. A
6. C	7. D	8. B	9. D	10. A
11. D	12. B	13. C	14. A	15. B

Fill in the Blank

1. stye
2. entropion
3. cochlear
4. nystagmus
5. pupil
6. vitreous humor
7. cornea
8. exotropia
9. diplopia
10. astigmatism

Labeling – The Structures of the Eye

A. lens
B. choroid
C. fovea centralis
D. suspensory ligament
E. iris
F. pupil
G. optic nerve
H. ciliary body

True / False

1. T	2. F	3. F	4. T	5. F
6. T	7. T	8. F	9. F	10. T

Labeling – The Structures of the Ear

A. malleus
B. semicircular canals
C. cochlea
D. pinna
E. tympanic membrane
F. incus
G. vestibule
H. stapes

Definitions

1. located along the edges of the eyelids
2. the vascular middle layer of the eye
3. relating to the cornea of the eye
4. the constriction of the iris muscle to decrease the size of the pupil
5. a clouding of the lens of the eye
6. an inflammation of a sebaceous gland of the eyelid
7. ear pain
8. containing pus as a result of infection
9. surgical repair of the eardrum
10. relating to hearing

Abbreviations

1. right ear
2. left eye
3. retinitis pigmentosa
4. tympanic membrane
5. external auditory canal
6. each eye
7. astigmatism
8. hertz
9. serous otitis media
10. bilateral otitis media

Matching – Terms and Definitions

1. I	2. J	3. A	4. F	5. G
6. H	7. E	8. D	9. B	10. C

Spelling

1. astigmatism
2. dacryocystitis
3. pupil

4. uvea
5. vitreous
6. miosis
7. nystagmus
8. emmetropia
9. cholesteatoma
10. otorrhea

Chapter 7

Multiple Choice

1. B	2. D	3. C	4. A	5. B
6. D	7. C	8. A	9. A	10. C
11. D	12. B	13. D	14. B	15. C

Fill in the Blank

1. agnosia
2. microglia
3. dyslexia
4. stupor
5. plexus
6. lethargy
7. pons
8. craniotomy
9. paraplegia
10. aneurysm

Labeling – The Neuron

A. myelin sheath
B. cell body
C. dendrites
D. axon
E. axon terminals
F. nucleus

True/False

1. F	2. T	3. F	4. F	5. F
6. T	7. T	8. F	9. F	10. T

Labeling – The Brain

A. pons
B. spinal cord
C. cerebrum
D. hypothalamus
E. cerebellum
F. thalamus
G. midbrain
H. medulla

Definitions

1. the absence of most of the brain, skull, and scalp
2. star-shaped glial cells of the brain
3. located between the cerebrum and midbrain; contains the thalamus, hypothalamus, and pineal gland
4. the lower part of the brain stem; it is continuous with the spinal cord
5. an electrical-insulating covering that protects the axon and speeds up impulse transmission
6. the functional unit of the nervous system
7. the small endocrine gland in the brain that produces melatonin
8. the spaces that exist between two nerves
9. the second-largest part of the brain
10. a mass of white matter composed of nerve fibers that connects the cerebral hemispheres of the cerebrum

Abbreviations

1. acetylcholine
2. amyotrophic lateral sclerosis
3. cerebrospinal fluid
4. Alzheimer's disease
5. cerebrovascular accident
6. lumbar puncture

7. magnetic resonance imaging

8. multiple sclerosis

9. position emission tomography

10. peripheral nervous system

Matching – Terms and Definitions

1. C	2. E	3. H	4. A	5. G
6. J	7. D	8. I	9. B	10. F

Spelling

1. ataxia

2. aneurysm

3. cerebellum

4. anesthesia

5. astrocyte

6. bradykinesia

7. dyslexia

8. dementia

9. corpus callosum

10. melatonin

Chapter 8

Multiple Choice

1. C	2. D	3. A	4. C	5. B
6. D	7. A	8. D	9. C	10. B
11. D	12. C	13. A	14. A	15. A

Fill in the Blank

1. aldosterone

2. thymus

3. anterior pituitary

4. epinephrine

5. cretinism

6. thyroid gland

7. pancreas

8. myxedema

9. posterior pituitary

10. adrenal cortex

Labeling – The Structures of the Endocrine System

A. pancreatic islets

B. thyroid gland

C. pineal gland

D. thymus gland

E. adrenal gland

F. ovaries

G. pituitary gland

H. hypothalamus

True / False

1. F	2. F	3. F	4. T	5. T
6. T	7. F	8. T	9. F	10. F

Definitions

1. higher-than-normal levels of sodium in the blood

2. regulates the growth of bone, muscle, and other body tissue

3. excessive secretion of gonadal hormones

4. a physician who specializes in disease and disorders of the endocrine system

5. a male steroid hormone

6. lower-than-normal levels of glucose in the blood

7. excessive or abnormal appetite

8. an enlargement of the thyroid gland due to low iodine in the blood

9. the hormone released from the alpha cells of the pancreas

10. the primary type of female sex hormone

Abbreviations

1. thyroid-stimulating hormone

2. melanocyte-stimulating hormone

3. protein-bound iodine

4. blood urea nitrogen

5. radioactive iodine

6. basal metabolic rate
7. glucose tolerance test
8. insulin resistance syndrome
9. antidiuretic hormone
10. diabetes insipidus

Matching – Terms and Definitions

| 1. C | 2. I | 3. H | 4. J | 5. G |
| 6. B | 7. E | 8. F | 9. D | 10. A |

Spelling

1. cretinism
2. aldosterone
3. hirsuitism
4. norepinephrine
5. gigantism
6. pheochromocytoma
7. virilism
8. cortex
9. glycosuria
10. oxytocin

Chapter 9

Multiple Choice

1. D	2. C	3. B	4. B	5. D
6. D	7. B	8. A	9. D	10. A
11. C	12. A	13. D	14. A	15. D

Fill in the Blank

1. rugae
2. chyme
3. gavage
4. villi
5. hepatomegaly
6. lavage
7. uvula
8. pyloric sphincter

9. jejunum
10. peristalsis

Labeling – The Major Structures and Accessory Organs

A. rectum and anus
B. pancreas
C. pharynx
D. liver
E. small intestine
F. stomach
G. gallbladder
H. appendix

True / False

| 1. T | 2. T | 3. F | 4. F | 5. T |
| 6. T | 7. F | 8. T | 9. F | 10. F |

Labeling – Structures of the Stomach

A. pylorus
B. fundus
C. rugae
D. pyloric sphincter
E. antrum
F. lower esophageal sphincter

Definitions

1. the breaking down of food into an absorbable form
2. the gums; the tissue that surrounds the teeth
3. a liver cell involved in many normal liver functions
4. the intestine from the pyloric opening of the stomach to the anus
5. the taking up of a substance by cells, tissues, or organs
6. chewing food with the teeth as it is mixed with saliva

7. the clear fluid secreted by the salivary and mucous glands in the mouth

8. the muscle at the juncture of the stomach and the duodenum

9. the double sheets of the peritoneum that hold some of the organs in their proper positions in the abdominal cavity

10. the outermost serous layer of a visceral structure that lies in a body cavity, such as the abdomen or thorax

Abbreviations

1. gastroesophageal reflux disease
2. irritable bowel syndrome
3. hepatitis C virus
4. stomach and duodenum
5. total parenteral nutrition
6. nausea and vomiting
7. bowel movement
8. nasogastric
9. inflammatory bowel disease
10. gastrointestinal

Matching – Terms and Definitions

1. H	2. G	3. I	4. J	5. A
6. C	7. F	8. D	9. E	10. B

Spelling

1. sphincter
2. jejunum
3. pylorus
4. gavage
5. chyme
6. cecum
7. glycogen
8. rugae
9. serosa
10. deglutition

Chapter 10

Multiple Choice

1. C	2. C	3. A	4. D	5. B
6. D	7. C	8. D	9. D	10. C
11. C	12. D	13. A	14. C	15. D

Fill in the Blank

1. murmur
2. hepatomegaly
3. arteriosclerosis
4. bruit
5. ischemia
6. myocarditis
7. endocarditis
8. malaise
9. systole
10. Tetralogy of Fallot

Labeling – The Anterior External View of the Heart

A. right ventricle
B. right pulmonary artery
C. vena cava
D. left ventricle
E. right atrium
F. left pulmonary artery
G. aorta
H. right pulmonary veins
I. apex
J. left pulmonary veins

True / False

1. F	2. T	3. T	4. F	5. T
6. F	7. F	8. T	9. F	10. T

Labeling – The Anterior Cross-section View of the Heart

A. inferior vena cava
B. tricuspid valve

C. left atrium
D. aorta
E. mitral valve
F. interventricular septum
G. left ventricle
H. pulmonary semilunar valve

Definitions

1. Irregularity in the rhythm of the heartbeat
2. Atrioventricular valve on the left side of the heart
3. The period when the heart relaxes after each contraction
4. The innermost layer of the heart tissue
5. An abnormal heart sound made by blood rushing past an obstructed blood vessel
6. The outer layer of the heart tissue
7. A sudden drop in the supply of blood to the blood vessels
8. The SA node, which generates electrical impulses in the heart
9. A small red or purple spot caused by a minor capillary hemorrhage
10. Localized blood insufficiency caused by an obstruction

Abbreviations

1. atrial fibrillation
2. coronary artery disease
3. blood pressure
4. cardiovascular disease
5. low-density lipoprotein
6. mitral stenosis
7. cardiopulmonary accident
8. lactate dehydrogenase
9. left ventricle
10. myocardial infarction or mitral insufficiency

Matching – Terms and Definitions

1. J	2. C	3. G	4. H	5. I
6. A	7. E	8. B	9. D	10. F

Spelling

1. dysrhythmia
2. aneurysm
3. malaise
4. thrombosis
5. ischemia
6. varicose
7. prophylactic
8. aorta
9. palpitation
10. fibrillation

Chapter 11

Multiple Choice

1. C	2. D	3. B	4. D	5. C
6. A	7. B	8. D	9. D	10. B
11. C	12. D	13. B	14. A	15. B

Fill in the Blank

1. leukemia
2. erythremia
3. hemolysis
4. granulocyte
5. thalassemia
6. hemostasis
7. myeloma
8. purpura
9. thrombocytopenia
10. erythropoiesis

True / False

1. F	2. F	3. T	4. T	5. F
6. F	7. T	8. T	9. T	10. F

Definitions

1. the termination of bleeding by the complex coagulation process of the body
2. the process of erythrocyte production in the bone marrow
3. a substance that stimulates formation of antibodies
4. anti-clotting agent
5. the breakdown of red blood cells and release of hemoglobin
6. cancer of the white blood cells
7. pinpointed red or purple skin hemorrhages
8. excessive iron deposits in the tissue of the body
9. a type of cell in bone marrow that generates all other blood cells
10. a tumor that develops in the blood cell forming tissue of the bone marrow

Abbreviations

1. B-lymphocyte
2. packed cell volume
3. prothrombin tissue activator
4. low-density lipoprotein
5. complete blood (cell) count
6. pernicious anemia
7. prostate-specific antigen
8. hemoglobin
9. antibody
10. cholesterol

Matching – Terms and Definitions

1. H	2. J	3. F	4. I	5. B
6. C	7. D	8. E	9. G	10. A

Spelling

1. oxyhemoglobin
2. fibrinogen
3. anaphylaxis
4. anisocytosis
5. bilirubin
6. agglutination
7. hemorrhage
8. lipoprotein
9. splenomegaly
10. hemophilia

Chapter 12

Multiple Choice

1. C	2. A	3. D	4. A	5. C
6. B	7. C	8. B	9. B	10. D
11. D	12. C	13. B	14. A	15. D

Fill in the Blank

1. antigen
2. cytotoxic cells
3. humoral immunity
4. T helper cells
5. lymphocyte
6. antigen
7. suppressor cell
8. macrophage
9. autoimmune
10. immunoglobulin

True / False

1. F	2. T	3. F	4. F	5. F
6. T	7. T	8. T	9. F	10. T

Definitions

1. a hormone secreted by the thymus gland
2. the engulfing of foreign material by white blood cells
3. a preparation of material derived from microorganisms administered to confer immunity to an infectious disease

4. the state or condition of being resistant to invading microorganisms

5. a substance that stimulates formation of antibodies

6. a natural glycoprotein formed by cells exposed to a virus

7. a substance developed within the immune system and designed to identify and destroy foreign substances

8. the protein of blood plasma that contains antibodies

9. any substance that can produce a hypersensitive allergic reaction in the body

10. a clear fluid of slightly yellowish color that is produced by many organs of the body and enters into the lymphatic vessels

Abbreviations

1. immunoglobulin M
2. systemic lupus erythematosus
3. Kaposi's sarcoma
4. acquired immunodeficiency syndrome
5. antigen
6. human immunodeficiency virus
7. Epstein-Barr virus
8. AIDS-related complex
9. antibody
10. severe combined immunodeficiency

Matching

1. I	2. H	3. J	4. F	5. G
6. C	7. B	8. E	9. D	10. A

Spelling

1. immunosuppressed
2. humoral immunity
3. phagocytosis
4. macrophage
5. surveillance

6. thymosin
7. immunoglobulin
8. interferon
9. anaphylaxis
10. globulin

Chapter 13

Multiple Choice

1. C	2. D	3. A	4. D	5. A
6. B	7. D	8. D	9. C	10. B
11. D	12. D	13. D	14. C	15. D

Fill in the Blank

1. hemothorax
2. oropharynx
3. aphonia
4. hilum
5. apex
6. snore
7. intubation
8. aspiration
9. anoxia
10. dyspnea

Labeling – The Structures of the Upper Respiratory Tract

A. esophagus
B. frontal sinus
C. epiglottis
D. nasopharynx
E. lingual tonsil
F. sphenoid sinus
G. trachea
H. oropharynx
I. pharyngeal tonsil
J. vocal cords

True / False

1. F   2. T   3. F   4. F   5. F
6. F   7. T   8. T   9. T   10. F

Labeling – The External View of the Lungs

A. superior lobe
B. primary bronchus
C. thyroid cartilage
D. trachea
E. middle lobe
F. bronchioles

Definitions

1. an inflammation of the pleura
2. an inflammation of the nose
3. the absence of breathing
4. a lung disease caused by long-term inhalation of coal dust
5. a deficient amount of oxygen in tissue
6. accumulation of blood in the pleural cavity
7. normal breathing
8. a hoarseness usually caused by laryngitis
9. a collapse of a lung or part of a lung
10. popping sounds heard in lung collapse

Abbreviations

1. anteroposterior
2. chronic obstructive lung disease
3. acute respiratory failure
4. dyspnea on exertion
5. respiratory distress syndrome
6. left upper lobe
7. infant respiratory distress syndrome
8. respiratory disease
9. tuberculosis
10. shortness of breath

Matching – Terms and Definitions

1. I   2. F   3. G   4. H   5. J
6. C   7. B   8. E   9. D   10. A

Spelling

1. alveoli
2. mediastinum
3. epiglottis
4. tonsils
5. epistaxis
6. trachea
7. pharynx
8. snore
9. wheezes
10. asphyxia

Chapter 14

Multiple Choice

1. C   2. D   3. D   4. D   5. A
6. C   7. B   8. A   9. D   10. C
11. A   12. D   13. B   14. A   15. C

Fill in the Blank

1. bladder
2. ureter
3. prostate
4. calyx
5. glomerulus
6. hilum
7. trigone
8. renal pelvis
9. meatus
10. cortex

Labeling – The Urinary System

A. prostate gland
B. renal cortex
C. adrenal glands

D. urethra
E. urethral orifices
F. urinary bladder
G. renal medulla
H. abdominal aorta

True / False

1. F	2. F	3. T	4. T	5. T
6. F	7. F	8. F	9. T	10. F

Labeling – The Internal Anatomy of the Kidney

A. ureter
B. renal pelvis
C. renal papilla
D. hilum
E. renal pyramid
F. cortex
G. renal vein

Definitions

1. stone formations occurring in the kidney
2. urinary bladder inflammation and infection
3. decreased production of urine associated with kidney failure
4. the presence of pus in the urine
5. enzyme production in the kidneys to regulate the filtration rate of blood
6. waste product of nitrogen metabolism excreted in normal adult urine
7. increased frequency of urination during the night
8. a malignant kidney tumor that occurs in adulthood
9. enlargement of the kidney due to constant pressure from backed-up urine in the ureter
10. excessive production of urine associated with diabetes mellitus and diabetes insipidus

Abbreviations

1. culture and sensitivity
2. antidiuretic hormone
3. chronic renal failure
4. erythropoietin
5. intravenous pyelogram
6. urinalysis
7. potassium
8. blood urea nitrogen
9. acute renal failure
10. hemodialysis

Matching – Terms and Definitions

1. J	2. E	3. G	4. H	5. I
6. D	7. A	8. C	9. F	10. B

Spelling

1. trigone
2. peritoneum
3. glomerulus
4. papillae
5. hilum
6. nocturia
7. calyx
8. filtration
9. nephrolithiasis
10. micturition

Chapter 15

Multiple Choice

1. C	2. B	3. A	4. D	5. B
6. C	7. A	8. C	9. B	10. A
11. D	12. C	13. B	14. D	15. C

Fill in the Blank

1. varicocele
2. testicular torsion
3. genital warts

4. perineum
5. orchidopexy
6. epispadias
7. chancre
8. priapism
9. circumcision
10. ductus deferens

Labeling – The Organs and Ducts of the Male Reproductive System

A. epididymis
B. pubis
C. vas deferens
D. seminal vesicle
E. ejaculatory duct
F. anus
G. urethra
H. scrotum
I. bulbourethral gland
J. prostate gland

True / False

1. F	2. T	3. F	4. F	5. T
6. T	7. F	8. F	9. F	10. T

Definitions

1. a male hormone secreted by the testes
2. the structure that carries sperm from the epididymis to the urethra
3. the sensitive area at the tip of the penis
4. a structure composed of a fibrous network in the center of each testis
5. the pouch of skin containing the testes and parts of the spermatic cords
6. the extension of the epididymis of the testis that ascends from the scrotum into the abdominal cavity
7. a congenital defect in which the urethra opens on the dorsum of the penis

8. a skin lesion of primary syphilis that is painless
9. the inability of an adult male to ejaculate after achieving an erection
10. a dilation of the pampiniform venous complex of the spermatic cord

Abbreviations

1. serological test for syphilis
2. genitourinary
3. prostate-specific antigen
4. human papillomavirus
5. penile erectile dysfunction
6. sexually transmitted disease
7. herpes simplex virus
8. testicular self-examination
9. venereal disease
10. digital rectal examination

Matching – Terms and Definitions

1. I	2. G	3. J	4. H	5. F
6. B	7. E	8. C	9. D	10. A

Spelling

1. scrotum
2. testicles
3. purulent
4. epididymis
5. chancre
6. perineum
7. prepuce
8. balanitis
9. epispadias
10. chlamydia

Chapter 16

Multiple Choice

1. C	2. D	3. C	4. C	5. D
6. B	7. A	8. A	9. D	10. B
11. C	12. A	13. D	14. C	15. B

Fill in the Blank

1. ovulation
2. parturition
3. coitus
4. zygote
5. fimbriae
6. areola
7. contraception
8. menopause
9. estrogen
10. menstruation

Labeling – The Structures of the Female Reproductive System

A. vaginal orifice
B. cervix
C. labia minora
D. uterus
E. ovary
F. urethra
G. vagina
H. Fallopian tube
I. clitoris
J. labia majora

True / False

1. F	2. F	3. T	4. F	5. T
6. T	7. T	8. F	9. F	10. T

Labeling – The Female Reproductive Organs

A. myometrium
B. ovary
C. fimbriae
D. fundus
E. infundibulum
F. perimetrium
G. mature ovum
H. Fallopian tube
I. interior of uterus
J. endometrium

Definitions

1. the normal discharge of blood and tissue from the uterus
2. the two tubes that lead from the ovaries to the uterus
3. sexual intercourse or copulation
4. the first menstrual period
5. two glands on either side of the vagina that secrete fluid into the vagina
6. the fold of skin at the top of the labia minora
7. the premature ending of a pregnancy
8. a polyurethane contraceptive device filled with spermicide
9. a fertilized egg
10. an immature ovum produced in the ovary

Abbreviations

1. dysfunctional uterine bleeding
2. previous menstrual period
3. dilation and curettage
4. intrauterine device
5. estrogen replacement therapy
6. oral contraceptive pill
7. toxic shock syndrome
8. pelvic inflammatory disease
9. endometrial biopsy
10. abortion

Matching – Terms and Definitions

1. J	2. H	3. G	4. I	5. F
6. D	7. B	8. E	9. A	10. C

Spelling

1. fertilization
2. menarche
3. fimbriae
4. diaphragm
5. coitus
6. isthmus
7. menorrhea
8. colostrum
9. leukorrhea
10. zygote

Chapter 17

Multiple Choice

1. D	2. C	3. A	4. B	5. D
6. B	7. D	8. B	9. C	10. C
11. B	12. D	13. A	14. D	15. C

Fill in the Blank

1. congenital
2. meningocele
3. head circumference
4. microcephalus
5. chickenpox
6. mumps
7. neonatology
8. German measles
9. kernicterus
10. impetigo

True / False

1. F	2. T	3. F	4. T	5. T
6. F	7. F	8. T	9. T	10. F

Definitions

1. the delivery of a fetus that died before or during the birthing process
2. existing at the time of birth
3. to expel an embryo or fetus before completion of pregnancy
4. pertaining to the mental activities associated with thinking, learning, and memory
5. an inflammation of the umbilical area
6. an excessive accumulation of cerebrospinal fluid in the cerebral ventricles
7. a congenital birth defect consisting of one or more clefts in the upper lip
8. a serous discharge from the umbilicus
9. a whistling, musical, or puffing sound made by air passing through the narrowed airway
10. a deformity of the foot and ankle

Abbreviations

1. attention deficit disorder
2. fetal alcohol syndrome
3. Down syndrome
4. respiratory distress syndrome
5. sudden infant death syndrome
6. newborn
7. patent ductus arteriosus
8. hyaline membrane disease
9. attention deficit hyperactivity disorder
10. phenylketonuria

Matching

1. G	2. J	3. F	4. H	5. C
6. I	7. D	8. B	9. E	10. A

Spelling

1. meningocele
2. kernicterus

3. omphalorrhea

4. atresia

5. paroxysmal cough

6. anencephaly

7. pertussis

8. talipes

9. impetigo

10. myelomeningocele

Chapter 18

Multiple Choice

1. D	2. B	3. D	4. C	5. B
6. D	7. A	8. D	9. B	10. D
11. D	12. A	13. C	14. B	15. C

Fill in the Blank

1. presbyopia

2. delusion

3. agitation

4. hallucination

5. malignant

6. thrombus

7. ketosis

8. insomnia

9. tremor

10. impotence

True / False

1. T	2. F	3. F	4. T	5. T
6. F	7. T	8. F	9. F	10. T

Definitions

1. unusual or irregular

2. the smallest blood vessel in the cardiovascular system

3. a hormone produced by the pancreas that lowers blood sugar

4. to invade other body cells

5. an abnormal growth of new tissue that forms into a tumor

6. extreme emotional disturbance

7. a type of white blood cell that performs a vital role in the immune system

8. loss of memory

9. loss of voluntary movement in a part of the body

10. the accumulation of ketone bodies in the blood

Abbreviations

1. myocardial infarction

2. prostatic-specific antigen

3. cerebrovascular accident

4. chronic lymphocytic leukemia

5. hip fracture

6. benign prostatic hypertrophy

7. Alzheimer's disease

8. decubitus ulcer

9. thyroid hormone

10. basal cell carcinoma

Matching

1. F	2. I	3. H	4. J	5. G
6. C	7. B	8. D	9. E	10. A

Spelling

1. rickettsiae

2. protozoa

3. thromboembolism

4. hallucination

5. benign

6. deterioration

7. metastasize

8. ketosis

9. tremor

10. menopause

Chapter 19

Multiple Choice

1. D	2. C	3. A	4. D	5. A
6. C	7. D	8. B	9. A	10. D
11. C	12. A	13. D	14. B	15. D

Fill in the Blank

1. oncogenes
2. ovarian cancer
3. oncology
4. mutation
5. osteosarcoma
6. prostatic cancer
7. dysplasia
8. hepatoma
9. carcinoma
10. retinoblastoma

True / False

1. F	2. F	3. T	4. F	5. F
6. T	7. T	8. F	9. F	10. F

Definitions

1. a malignant tumor arising in the epithelial tissue
2. its growth is relatively slow and remains localized
3. a highly malignant tumor of the connective tissue
4. a malignant neoplasm composed of lymphoreticular cells that causes destruction of the jaw
5. a malignant tumor that develops from bone marrow, usually in long bones and the pelvis
6. any of the largest group of primary tumors of the brain
7. a sarcoma that contains unstriated muscle cells
8. a malignant growth of primitive fat cells
9. a malignant cancer of the bones
10. a malignant cancer of the testes

Abbreviations

1. carcinoembryonic antigen
2. digital rectal exam
3. x-ray or radiation therapy
4. prostate-specific antigen
5. estrogen receptor
6. progesterone receptor
7. bone marrow transplantation
8. acute myelogenous leukemia
9. biopsy
10. ribonucleic acid

Matching

1. I	2. H	3. J	4. F	5. G
6. D	7. A	8. B	9. C	10. E

Spelling

1. osteosarcoma
2. medulloblastoma
3. leukoplakia
4. chondrosarcoma
5. carcinoid
6. glioma
7. astrocytoma
8. squamous cell
9. benign
10. rhabdomyosarcoma

Chapter 20

Multiple Choice

1. B	2. D	3. A	4. C	5. D
6. D	7. C	8. B	9. D	10. A
11. B	12. D	13. C	14. B	15. A

Fill in the Blank

1. half-life
2. potency
3. cumulation
4. bacteriostatic
5. efficacy
6. potentiation
7. peak effect
8. antagonist
9. tolerance
10. adverse

True / False

1. F	2. T	3. F	4. F	5. F
6. T	7. T	8. T	9. F	10. F

Definitions

1. a drug that produces a functional change in a cell
2. the intended effect of a drug
3. a change that takes place in the body as a result of drug action
4. the measure of a drug's effectiveness
5. a drug that may be obtained without a prescription
6. the study of the biochemical and physiological effects of drugs
7. the first dose of a medication
8. promotes easy bowel emptying
9. destroys or inhibits fungal growth
10. the study of the absorption, distribution, metabolism, and excretion of drugs

Abbreviations

1. adverse drug reaction
2. contraindicated
3. over-the-counter
4. therapeutic index
5. *United States Pharmacopoeia*

6. mechanism of action
7. nonsteroidal anti-inflammatory drug
8. birth control
9. half-life
10. tricyclic antidepressants

Matching

1. J	2. H	3. E	4. I	5. D
6. G	7. C	8. F	9. B	10. A

Spelling

1. anaphylactic
2. bactericidal
3. hepatotoxicity
4. idiosyncrasy
5. pharmacognosy
6. potentiation
7. bioavailability
8. pharmacokinetics
9. druggist
10. hemostatic

Chapter 21

Multiple Choice

1. D	2. C	3. B	4. D	5. A
6. C	7. C	8. B	9. D	10. A
11. D	12. A	13. B	14. D	15. C

Fill in the Blank

1. ointment
2. prefilled
3. topical
4. gavage
5. aerosol
6. gelcap
7. injector pen
8. buffered tablet
9. plaster
10. gauge

True / False

1. T 2. F 3. F 4. T 5. F
6. T 7. F 8. F 9. F 10. T

Definitions

1. through the skin
2. injection into the layer of fat and blood vessels beneath the skin
3. an alcoholic solution prepared from vegetable sources or chemical substances
4. pertaining to the inside of the cheek
5. a liquid preparation of filtered vegetable medications, containing alcohol
6. a soft, pliable drug such as a gel or suppository
7. injection between the layers of the skin
8. pertaining to the area under the tongue
9. a small glass or plastic bottle containing medication
10. an object inserted into the body for prosthetic, therapeutic, diagnostic, or experimental reasons

Abbreviations

1. intradermal
2. total parenteral nutrition
3. sublingual
4. suspension
5. intravenous push
6. dextrose 5% in water
7. fluid
8. intravenous piggyback
9. powder
10. suppository

Matching

1. J 2. G 3. E 4. I 5. B
6. H 7. D 8. C 9. F 10. A

Spelling

1. anesthetic
2. lozenge
3. emulsion
4. liniment
5. suppository
6. troche
7. parenteral
8. gavage
9. buffered tablet
10. spirits

Chapter 22

Multiple Choice

1. D 2. B 3. A 4. D 5. C
6. A 7. D 8. A 9. C 10. A
11. C 12. D 13. C 14. A 15. B

Fill in the Blank

1. oncology
2. dispensing
3. compounding
4. certification
5. quality control
6. authorization
7. licensure
8. externship
9. extemporaneous
10. infusion devices

True / False

1. T 2. T 3. F 4. F 5. T
6. F 7. T 8. F 9. F 10. T

Definitions

1. relating to the management of an organization
2. the following of qualified instructions

3. the giving of legal approval to conduct business in a specified manner

4. a doctor of pharmacy

5. relating to a job, occupation, or trade

6. supplying a certain amount of specified products and devices

7. a professional record of qualification

8. a system designed to ensure that products or services meet customer requirements

9. to prepare and distribute medications

10. being qualified to do a specific type of work

Abbreviations

1. United States Pharmacopoeia

2. Pharmacy Technician Certification Examination

3. Board of Pharmacy

4. American Association of Pharmaceutical Scientists

5. American Council on Pharmaceutical Education

6. American Association of Pharmacy Technicians

7. American Pharmacists Association

8. Pharmacy Technician Educators Council

9. American Association of Colleges of Pharmacy

10. American College of Clinical Pharmacy

Matching

1. J	2. F	3. G	4. H	5. I
6. A	7. B	8. D	9. C	10. E

Spelling

1. extemporaneous

2. competency

3. institutional

4. pharmacognosy

5. oncology

6. licensure

7. dispensing

8. radionuclide

9. vocational

10. compliance

Chapter 23

Multiple Choice

1. D	2. B	3. D	4. A	5. D
6. B	7. D	8. C	9. D	10. A

Fill in the Blank

1. fume hood

2. dose calibrator

3. chart review

4. radioactive

5. in-house pharmacy

6. outpatient pharmacy

7. e-prescribing

8. dosimeter

9. Internet pharmacy

10. adulterated drug

True / False

1. F	2. F	3. T	4. T	5. F
6. F	7. T	8. T	9. F	10. F

Definitions

1. a pharmacy that provides special care for an extended period of time

2. a pharmacy that dispenses medications to terminally ill patients who are at home or in institutions

3. a pharmacy that is specially licensed to work with radioactive materials

4. provides pharmaceutical care to patients at a distance via the use of telecommunication and information technology

5. a licensed pharmacy that dispenses maintenance medications to members via delivery through the mail or overnight carriers and parcel services

6. an institutional long-term care facility staffed by nurses

7. the presence of a foreign chemical in a radiopharmaceutical

8. a hollow tube that passes food into the stomach

9. a device that controls the infusion of intravenous solutions

10. the area in a nuclear pharmacy where empty or unused radiopharmaceutical containers are returned and dismantled to be re-used

Abbreviations

1. intravenous
2. gastrointestinal
3. drug regimen review
4. total parenteral nutrition
5. enteral nutrition

Matching

1. H	2. G	3. J	4. I	5. B
6. A	7. D	8. E	9. F	10. C

Spelling

1. hospice
2. telepharmacy
3. radiopharmacy
4. ambulatory
5. terminally
6. dosimeter
7. reimbursement
8. nuclear
9. radionuclide
10. adulterated

Chapter 24

Multiple Choice

1. D	2. D	3. B	4. A	5. D
6. C	7. B	8. D	9. A	10. D
11. C	12. C	13. C	14. A	15. D

Fill in the Blank

1. blender
2. beaker
3. spatula
4. pestles
5. cocoa butter
6. slab
7. port adapter
8. pipette
9. mortar
10. counter balance

True / False

1. F	2. F	3. T	4. T	5. F
6. F	7. T	8. T	9. T	10. F

Definitions

1. pathogen-free drug products

2. steel device used for picking up hot items

3. a set of testing activities used to determine the quality of compounded products

4. a device used to thoroughly mix substances

5. a high-efficiency air filter that can remove more than 99% of airborne particles 0.3 micrometers or larger

6. alcohol that contains two hydroxyl groups

7. an incubator that is used for a variety of applications in the laboratory

8. a weighing paper with a smooth, shiny surface that does not absorb materials

9. a device that resembles tweezers, used to pick up prescription weights and other equipment in the laboratory
10. a device that can seal various containers

Abbreviations

1. quality assurance
2. United States Pharmacopoeia Chapter 797
3. high-efficiency particulate air
4. distilled water
5. compound
6. polyvinyl chloride
7. laminar airflow hood
8. deoxyribonucleic acid
9. dextrose 5% in lactated Ringer's
10. total parenteral nutrition

Matching

1. J	2. E	3. G	4. I	5. B
6. F	7. H	8. C	9. D	10. A

Spelling

1. decontamination
2. emulsion
3. extemporaneous
4. piggyback
5. lozenge
6. homogenizer
7. levigate
8. troche
9. reconstitute
10. gowning

Chapter 25

Multiple Choice

1. A	2. D	3. C	4. B	5. D
6. A	7. D	8. D	9. B	10. A
11. D	12. D	13. C	14. B	15. B

Fill in the Blank

1. negligence
2. nonfeasance
3. magistrate
4. appeal
5. encryption
6. phocomelia
7. misfeasance
8. disclosure
9. misbranding
10. misdemeanor

True / False

1. F	2. F	3. F	4. T	5. F
6. T	7. T	8. T	9. F	10. F

Definitions

1. motivations based on ideas of right and wrong
2. a law that is prescribed by legislative enactments
3. a private wrong or injury, other than a breach of contract
4. an offense punishable by imprisonment in a state or federal prison for more than one year, or punishable by death
5. a private wrong or injury, other than a breach of contract
6. professional misconduct of an unreasonable lack of skill with the result of injury, loss, or damage to the patient
7. causing genetic defects
8. desirable standards or qualities
9. a revision or intended improvement to an existing bill or other document
10. a copy of an official document that is commonly transmitted via fax machine

Abbreviations

1. National Drug Code
2. Health and Human Services
3. Environmental Protection Agency
4. Drug Enforcement Agency
5. Board of Pharmacy
6. Protected Health Information
7. Office of Inspector General
8. New Drug Application
9. Notice of Privacy Practices
10. Department of Transportation

Matching

1. D	2. I	3. J	4. F	5. G
6. E	7. H	8. C	9. A	10. B

Spelling

1. jurisdiction
2. encryption
3. misfeasance
4. misdemeanor
5. magistrate
6. revocation
7. phocomelia
8. malfeasance
9. appeal
10. adulteration

Chapter 26

Multiple Choice

1. D	2. B	3. D	4. A	5. C
6. D	7. B	8. B	9. C	10. D
11. B	12. B	13. A	14. C	15. D

Fill in the Blank

1. bulk
2. fixed expenses
3. fixed budget
4. variance analysis
5. procurement
6. capital budget
7. flexible budget
8. batch repackaging
9. inventory
10. invoice

True / False

1. T	2. F	3. T	4. F	5. F
6. T	7. F	8. F	9. F	10. T

Definitions

1. the actual time that a purchase order is made
2. system that allows inventory to be tracked as it is used
3. the acquiring of goods or services
4. system in which stock arrives just before it is needed
5. expenditures of money, or costs
6. a list of planned expenses and revenues over a specified period
7. everything of value owned by a company
8. a limit to an amount anticipated as a future expense
9. a form describing a purchase and the amount due
10. a substance used in the treatment of disease

Abbreviations

1. economic order quantity
2. point of sale
3. just-in-time
4. fiscal year
5. calendar year
6. economic order value

Spelling

1. revenue
2. perpetual
3. assets
4. pharmaceutical
5. purchasing
6. bulk
7. fiscal
8. repackaging
9. tangible
10. variance

Chapter 27

Multiple Choice

1. C	2. D	3. C	4. B	5. D
6. D	7. D	8. D	9. D	10. A
11. D	12. C	13. D	14. A	15. D

Fill in the Blank

1. Medigap
2. capitation
3. eligibility
4. deductible
5. co-insurance
6. insured
7. policyholder
8. co-payment
9. exclusions
10. fee for service

True / False

1. F	2. F	3. F	4. T	5. F
6. T	7. T	8. F	9. T	10. F

Definitions

1. the periodic payment for insurance coverage
2. the amounts payable by an insurance company for a monetary loss to an individual insured by that company
3. a term used in managed care for an approved referral
4. a spouse, child, and sometimes domestic partner of an insured person
5. the process required by some insurance carriers by which the provider obtains permission to perform certain procedures or services
6. the insurance term used when a provider sends a patient to another provider for consultation
7. the individual responsible for the payment for medical services
8. a special provision or group of provisions attached to an insurance policy to expand or limit coverage
9. limitations on an insurance contract for which benefits are not payable
10. a traditional health insurance plan that pays for all, or a share of the cost of, covered services

Abbreviations

1. benefits identification care
2. explanation of benefits
3. health maintenance organization
4. third-party administrator
5. remittance advice
6. medical savings account
7. primary care provider
8. Health Care Financing Administration
9. Department of Veterans Affairs
10. health insurance claim number

Matching

1. F	2. J	3. H	4. G	5. D
6. I	7. B	8. A	9. E	10. C

Spelling

1. preauthorization
2. remittance

3. guarantor
4. exclusions
5. indemnity
6. Medigap
7. referral
8. catastrophic coverage
9. hospitalization
10. compensation

Chapter 28

Multiple Choice

1. D	2. C	3. B	4. C	5. C
6. D	7. D	8. D	9. A	10. A
11. D	12. B	13. A	14. C	15. C

Fill in the Blank

1. icon
2. e-commerce
3. disk drives
4. zip drive
5. bar-coding
6. boating
7. data
8. crash
9. cache
10. cursor

True / False

1. F	2. T	3. T	4. F	5. T
6. T	7. F	8. F	9. T	10. F

Definitions

1. a set of input keys used with a computer
2. computer security systems that control the flow of data from one computer or network to another
3. a common type of printer that rapidly produces high-quality text and graphics on plain paper
4. a disk drive that uses hard disks that store large amounts of information externally to the computer; commonly used to back up computers
5. groups of information that are sent to a computer via its browser each time a specific server is accessed
6. the Internet, or the online "digital world" in general
7. a pattern of dots that forms character and graphic images on printers
8. a sudden and unexpected system failure
9. the act of starting up a computer and loading the system software into memory
10. any input, output, or storage device connected to a computer's CPU; examples include keyboards, monitors, printers, etc.

Abbreviations

1. local area network
2. personal digital assistant
3. central processing unit
4. random access memory
5. World Wide Web
6. disk operating system
7. hospital information system
8. compact disk read-only memory
9. uniform resource locator
10. campus area network

Matching

1. I	2. E	3. J	4. H	5. A
6. D	7. C	8. G	9. F	10. B

Spelling

1. formatting
2. scanner
3. modem
4. encrypted
5. floppy disk

6. cursor

7. booting

8. bubble jet

9. cache

10. cipher text

Chapter 29

Multiple Choice

1. D	2. B	3. C	4. A	5. D
6. B	7. C	8. A	9. C	10. D
11. B	12. D	13. B	14. D	15. A

Fill in the Blank

1. multiplier

2. denominator

3. equation

4. numerator

5. means

6. ratio

7. quotient

8. proportion

9. extremes

10. dividend

True / False

1. F	2. F	3. F	4. T	5. T
6. F	7. F	8. T	9. F	10. T

Definitions

1. fractions with numerators larger or equal to their denominators

2. whole numbers combined with proper fractions

3. a number by which another is multiplied

4. an amount

5. the relationship between two equal ratios

6. a mathematical expression comparing two numbers by division

7. the number being divided

8. a mathematical statement used to express equivalency between two variables

9. the two insider terms in a ratio

10. the number performing the division

Symbols

1. number

2. less than

3. multiplied by

4. a proportion

5. equal to

6. minus

7. greater than

8. divided by

9. percent

10. a ratio

Chapter 30

Multiple Choice

1. B	2. D	3. C	4. A	5. C
6. B	7. D	8. A	9. C	10. C

Fill in the Blank

1. pound

2. ounce

3. liter

4. dram

5. gram

6. liter

7. meter

8. unit

9. quart

10. pint

True / False

1. F	2. F	3. T	4. T	5. F
6. F	7. F	8. T	9. T	10. F

Definitions

1. a metric measurement equal to one one-billionth of a gram
2. an apothecary unit of volume originally equivalent to one drop of water
3. a unit of mass equivalent to an apothecary's measure of 60 grains
4. a household (English) measure of length equivalent to 12 inches
5. the basic unit of weight in the metric system
6. a household measurement of fluid volume equivalent to 2 pints
7. a standard of measurement based on the biological activity of a drug rather than its weight
8. the basic unit of measure in the metric system for length
9. a household measurement of fluid weight that equals 16 fluid ounces
10. a household measure of length equivalent to 25 centimeters

Abbreviations

1. dram
2. foot
3. gram
4. International Unit
5. microgram
6. tablespoon
7. millimeter
8. drop
9. grain
10. nanogram

Index

Note: Page numbers followed by a *t* refer to tables. Page numbers followed by an *f* refer to figures.